Non-Parkinsonian Movement Disorders

NEUROLOGY IN PRACTICE:

SERIES EDITORS: ROBERT A. GROSS, DEPARTMENT OF NEUROLOGY,
UNIVERSITY OF ROCHESTER MEDICAL CENTER, ROCHESTER, NY, USA

JONATHAN W. MINK, DEPARTMENT OF NEUROLOGY,
UNIVERSITY OF ROCHESTER MEDICAL CENTER, ROCHESTER, NY, USA

Non-Parkinsonian Movement Disorders

EDITED BY

Deborah A. Hall, MD, PhD
Department of Neurological Sciences
Section of Movement Disorders
Rush University Medical Center, Chicago
Illinois, USA

Brandon R. Barton, MD, MS
Department of Neurological Sciences
Section of Movement Disorders
Rush University Medical Center, Chicago
Illinois, USA

Department of Neurological Sciences
Rush University Medical Center; Neurology Section
Jesse Brown VA Medical Center
Chicago, Illinois, USA

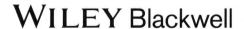

This edition first published 2017, © 2017 by John Wiley & Sons, Ltd.

Registered Office
John Wiley & Sons, Ltd, The Atrium, Southern Gate, Chichester, West Sussex, PO19 8SQ, UK

Editorial Offices
9600 Garsington Road, Oxford, OX4 2DQ, UK
The Atrium, Southern Gate, Chichester, West Sussex, PO19 8SQ, UK
111 River Street, Hoboken, NJ 07030-5774, USA

For details of our global editorial offices, for customer services and for information about how to apply for permission to reuse the copyright material in this book please see our website at www.wiley.com/wiley-blackwell

Library of Congress Cataloging-in-Publication Data

Names: Hall, Deborah A., editor. | Barton, Brandon R., editor.
Title: Non-Parkinsonian movement disorders / edited by Deborah A. Hall and Brandon R. Barton.
Description: Chichester, West Sussex ; Hoboken, NJ : John Wiley & Sons Inc., 2016. |
    Includes bibliographical references and index.
Identifiers: LCCN 2016023027 | ISBN 9781118473924 (Paperback) | ISBN 9781118474068 (Adobe PDF) |
    ISBN 9781118474051 (epub)
Subjects: | MESH: Movement Disorders–diagnosis | Diagnosis, Differential | Diagnostic Techniques, Neurological
Classification: LCC RC376.5 | NLM WL 390 | DDC 616.8/3–dc23
LC record available at https://lccn.loc.gov/2016023027

A catalogue record for this book is available from the British Library.

Wiley also publishes its books in a variety of electronic formats. Some content that appears in print may not be available in electronic books.

Background cover image: iStockphoto.com

Set in 8.75/11.75pt Utopia by SPi Global, Pondicherry, India
Printed and bound in Malaysia by Vivar Printing Sdn Bhd

10   9   8   7   6   5   4   3   2   1

Contents

List of Contributors

Pinky Agarwal MD
Movement Disorders Center
Evergreen Health Neuroscience Institute
Kirkland, WA

Brandon R. Barton MD, MS
Department of Neurological Sciences
Section of Movement Disorders
Rush University Medical Center
Jesse Brown VA Medical Center
Chicago, IL

Nina Browner MD
National Parkinson Foundation Center of Excellence
University of North Carolina
Chapel Hill, NC

Daniel Burdick MD
Movement Disorders Center
Evergreen Health Neuroscience Institute
Kirkland, WA

Florence C. F. Chang MBBS, FRACP
Neurology Department
Westmead Hospital
Wentworthville, NSW

Khashayar Dashtipour MD, PhD
Department of Neurology, Movement Disorders
Loma Linda University School of Medicine
Loma Linda, CA

Rohit Dhall MBBS, MSPH
Parkinson's Institute and Clinical Center
Sunnyvale, CA

Alberto J. Espay MD, MSc
Gardner Center for Parkinson's Disease and Movement Disorders
Department of Neurology
University of Cincinnati
Cincinnati, OH

Steven J. Frucht MD
Mount Sinai Medical Center
NY

Janice Fuentes MD
Department of Neurology, Movement Disorders
Loma Linda University School of Medicine
Loma Linda, CA

Deborah A. Hall MD, PhD
Department of Neurological Sciences
Section of Movement Disorders
Rush University Medical Center
Chicago, IL

Samantha Holden MD
University of Colorado School of Medicine,
Aurora, Colorado, USA

Un Jung Kang MD
Department of Neurology
Columbia University Medical Center
NY

Olga Klepitskaya MD
Department of Neurology
School of Medicine, University of Colorado
Aurora, CO

Jeff Kraakevik MD
Assistant Professor
Oregon Health and Science University
Portland, OR

Stephanie Lessig MD
Department of Neurosciences
University of California San Diego
La Jolla, CA

Shyamal H. Mehta MD, PhD
Department of Neurology
Movement Disorders Division
Mayo Clinic
Phoenix, AZ

Ifeoma Nwaneri MD
Reston Hospital Center
Springfield, VA

Gian Pal MD, MS
Department of Neurological Sciences
Section of Movement Disorders
Rush University Medical Center
Chicago, IL

Kathleen L. Poston MD, MS
Department of Neurology and Neurological
Sciences
Stanford University
Stanford, CA

Michael Rotstein MD
Tel Aviv Sourasky Medical Center
Tel Aviv, Israel

Bernadette Schoneburg MD
Northshore Medical Group
Glenview, IL

Lauren Schrock MD
University of Utah
Department of Neurology
Salt Lake City, UT

David Shprecher DO, MSc
Cleo Roberts Center, Banner Sun Health
Research Institute in Sun City, AZ

Christina L. Vaughan MD, MS
Hospice and Palliative Medicine Program
University of California San Diego/Scripps Health
La Jolla, CA

Aleksandar Videnovic MD
Department of Neurology
Massachusetts General Hospital
Harvard Medical School
Boston, MA

Padmaja Vittal MD, MS
Northwestern Medicine Regional Medical Group
Winfield, IL

Tao Xie MD, PhD
Department of Neurology
University of Chicago Medical Center
Chicago, IL

S. Elizabeth Zauber MD
Department of Neurology
Indiana University School of Medicine
Indianapolis, IN

Series Foreword

The genesis for this book series started with the proposition that, increasingly, physicians want direct, useful information to help them in clinical care. Textbooks, while comprehensive, are useful primarily as detailed reference works but pose challenges for uses at the point of care. By contrast, more outline-type references often leave out the "hows and whys"—pathophysiology, pharmacology—that form the basis of management decisions. Our goal for this series is to present books, covering most areas of neurology, that provide enough background information to allow the reader to feel comfortable, but not so much as to be overwhelming, and to associate that with practical advice from experts about care, combining the growing evidence base with best practices.

Our series will encompass various aspects of neurology, with topics and the specific content chosen to be accessible and useful.

Chapters cover critical information that will inform the reader of the disease processes and mechanisms as a prelude to treatment planning. Algorithms and guidelines are presented, when appropriate. "Tips and Tricks" boxes provide expert suggestions, while other boxes present cautions and warnings to avoid pitfalls. Finally, we provide "Science Revisited" sections that review the most important and relevant science background material, and references and further reading sections that guide the reader to additional material.

Our thanks, appreciation, and respect go out to our editors and their contributors, who conceived and refined the content for each volume, assuring a high-quality, practical approach to neurological conditions and their treatment.

Our thanks also go to our mentors and students (past, present, and future), who have challenged and delighted us; to our book editors and their contributors, who were willing to take on additional work for an educational goal; and to our original publisher, Martin Sugden, for his ideas and support, for wonderful discussions and commiseration over baseball and soccer teams that might not quite have lived up to expectations. And thanks, too, to Claire Bonnett, our current publisher, for her efforts to bring this volume forward.

This volume represents the end of our series. As readers will recognize, neurology encompasses far more than we have presented; still, we hope that the high points encompassed by these books will serve well.

We have dedicated the series to Marsha, Jake, and Dan, and to Janet, Laura, and David. And also to Steven R. Schwid, MD, our friend and colleague, whose ideas helped shape this project and whose humor brightened our lives; but he could not complete this goal with us. Our thanks to them are undiminished.

Robert A. Gross
Jonathan W. Mink
Rochester, NY, USA

Foreword

Non-Parkinsonian Movement Disorders, edited by my colleagues, Drs. Brandon Barton and Deborah Hall, is a new entry in the larger series, *Neurology in Practice* and an immediate compendium of the *Parkinsonian Movement Disorders*. The topics covered in this volume provide the practicing neurologist, psychiatrist, and primary care health professional with expert reviews that cover both hypokinetic and hyperkinetic disorders. Hypokinetic disorders discussed include stiff-person syndrome, catatonia, and catalepsy as well as a variety of stiff-muscle conditions. For the hyperkinetic disorders, the editors have assembled a group of expert authors to cover tremors, myoclonus, tics, chorea, dystonia, and involuntary movements due to toxins and drugs. Importantly, because neurological disorders can be both out-patient and in-patient consultations, a chapter on ICU movement disorders emergencies is included, and an important chapter on the knotty and complex problem of psychogenic movement disorders that focuses on a variety of functional movements, both consciously and unconsciously generated.

Each presentation is anchored in very practical descriptions of phenomenology, key clinical information from the history and neurological examination that guide the physician to the correct diagnosis and treatment options. The text is enriched with tables and figures and a number of unique learning tools not found in other books on this topic. These tools include special boxed "Tips and Tricks" and "Caution" warnings that can help prevent errors. Besides the focus on practical clinical medicine, the authors provide two special highlights in each chapter, "Science Revisited" to remind clinicians of the scientific anchors related to the disorders and "Evidence at a Glance" where clinical trial evidence-based review information is provided. All these special additions allow a reader to study the full text, but also to retrieve rapidly needed key points.

With a long career devoted to the treatment of movement disorders, research, and education, I laud the editors and their recruited authors in providing the medical community with an accessible and accurate book with a unique format. In a busy environment, this text serves as a very solid neurological work with the essentials delivered in a succinct and highly readable format.

Because a movement disorders diagnosis always starts with accurate visual identification, a very strong advantage of this text is the video material that accompanies each chapter. The elegant examples assembled are well synchronized with the text materials and allow the reader to study very good examples of the disorders under consideration. I suggest that readers start a chapter with a short examination of the video materials, so as to be clear on the type of movement under discussion, then read the text, finally returning to the videos for a focused re-examination of the details of the carefully prepared examples. With this emphasis on the key role of expert visual recognition in movement disorders, the words of the celebrated nineteenth-century neurologist, Jean-Martin Charcot, resonate, and I offer this citation as the reader embarks on the very pleasant road of reading this volume:

> Let someone say of a doctor that he really knows his physiology or anatomy, that he is dynamic—these are not real compliments; but if you say he is an observer, a man who knows how to see, this is perhaps the greatest compliment one can make (Charcot, 1888, *Leçons du mardi).*

Christopher G. Goetz, MD, Chicago, IL, USA,
2016

About the Companion Website

This book is accompanied by a companion website:

www.wiley.com/go/hall/non-parkinsonian_movement_disorders

The website includes:

Videos

Approach to Movement Disorders

Deborah A. Hall, MD, PhD[1] and Brandon R. Barton, MD, MS[1,2]

[1]Department of Neurological Sciences, Section of Movement Disorders, Rush University Medical Center, Chicago, Illinois, USA
[2]Department of Neurological Sciences, Rush University Medical Center; Neurology Section, Jesse Brown VA Medical Center, Chicago, Illinois, USA

Introduction

Patients with movement disorders typically present with a change in their overall pattern of movements: this may represent an increase of movement (hyperkinetic), decrease (hypo- or akinetic), uncoordinated movement (ataxia), or a combination of the aforementioned. The initial task is to properly categorize the appearance or "phenomenology" of the movement disorder, as this is the essential step to guide the clinician in developing a differential diagnosis and treatment plan. Given recent advances in neurology, the majority of movement disorder patients are candidates for treatment, such as medication, physical therapy, or surgical interventions.

The first part of this book provides a short chapter on non-parkinsonian hypokinetic movement disorders; parkinsonian disorders are covered in another volume in this series. The second part includes hyperkinetic disorders. Part three includes various syndromes that do not fit into the other categories or that overlap between categories. Broader chapters in part four, on genetics, neuroimaging, rating scales, and videotaping suggestions, are intended to serve as clinician resources.

This introductory chapter provides an approach that will facilitate the evaluation of a movement disorder patient. The phenomenological categorization of the most common movement disorders falls into seven major categories: parkinsonism, tremor, dystonia, myoclonus, chorea, ataxia, and

tics. Most of the commonly encountered disorders can be classified into one of these categories, but given the breadth of the diseases in the field, there are many unusual or rare types of movement that may not be easily categorized or may be consistent with more than one phenomenological category. A thorough history and examination are essential to defining the phenomenology. Home videotapes of the patient may also be useful if the movements are intermittent, variable, or not seen clearly in the office. Laboratory testing and imaging are necessary in some movement disorders, but are less helpful in many circumstances given that the disorders are diagnosed mainly on history and examination.

History

Start by asking *six questions* in the history.

1. Can you describe the movements?

Patients will usually be able to describe a decrease or increase (or both) in their overall movement from baseline, although often hyperkinetic aspects of abnormal movements can overshadow the hypokinetic movements from the patient's perspective. Hypokinetic movement disorders, also termed bradykinesia (slowed movement) or akinesia (loss of movement) are characterized by an overall decrease in the speed or amplitude of movement in any area of the body. Signs and symptoms could include decreased facial expression, slowed speech, reduced

Non-Parkinsonian Movement Disorders, First Edition. Edited by Deborah A. Hall and Brandon R. Barton.
© 2017 John Wiley & Sons, Ltd. Published 2017 by John Wiley & Sons, Ltd.
Companion website: www.wiley.com/go/hall/non-parkinsonian_movement_disorders

dexterity of the extremities, decreased arm swing, and slowed walking speed. Hyperkinetic movement disorders, also generally termed dyskinesia (abnormal movements), are characterized by an increase in baseline movements. Hyperkinetic movement disorders have highly variable manifestations, ranging from increased eye closure to arm flailing to jerking of the legs. Lastly, patients may complain of a change in the character of voluntary movements, such as becoming clumsy or unsteady with walking, which may be seen in ataxic disorders.

Certain features of abnormal movements are very important to elicit in the patient's description. Defining the conditions under which the movement occurs, such as with rest or with action, is necessary for accurate diagnosis and categorization of tremor. An ability to suppress the movement or an increase in the movement with suggestion are features common to tics. Specific triggers of the movements, especially with certain tasks, may be reported in dystonic disorders or paroxysmal movement disorders. Myoclonus can be triggered by startle. Asking about worsening of the disorder or improvement with certain foods or alcohol can narrow the differential diagnosis in forms of dystonia, myoclonus, or tremor disorders. A history of falls, especially the temporal course, is helpful in disorders that affect gait and balance, as falls are seen earlier or more frequently in some disorders as opposed to others.

2. When did the movements start and how have they changed over time?

Most movement disorders are subacute or chronic in nature. An acute onset is less common and may signify a secondary movement disorder related to an underlying inciting event, such as a stroke or medication change. Acute onset of movement disorders at maximal severity is also commonly seen in functional movement disorders, where patients will often present to emergency departments from the start. Most hypokinetic, hyperkinetic, and ataxic movement disorders will slowly worsen over time. Disorders that improve over time are less common; for example, tic disorders will typically improve from childhood into adolescence and adulthood. Static movement disorders may occur with birth injury or some dystonic disorders.

3. Are the movements continuous or intermittent?

Although many movement disorders start out as intermittent or suppressible, they tend to become more continuous or constant when they progress over time. The rest tremor seen in parkinsonian disorders is a classic example, where the tremor starts intermittently in a limb before becoming more regular and spreading to other limbs. Early on, this type of tremor can be sometimes voluntarily suppressed or decreased with movement, but later the tremor is continuous. Episodic movement disorders are much less common. Paroxysmal disorders, which are typically choreic or dystonic in nature, can many times be diagnosed by history alone if specific triggers such as sudden movements cause the disorder to occur. Functional (psychogenic) movement disorders are also frequently episodic. The circumstances under which the movement occurs can be particularly helpful. For example, restless legs syndrome worsens at night when the patient is laying down.

4. Is there a family history?

All modes of inheritance patterns are seen in movement disorders and the genetic basis of these disorders is rapidly being discovered. It is not sufficient to inquire only about the particular movement disorder seen in the patient, since broadening the questioning to other biological family members may yield additional important clues. For example, patients with grandchildren with intellectual disabilities may be at risk for fragile X-associated disorders. Tic patients may have associated diagnoses in the family, such as attention deficit hyperactivity disorder.

5. Are there other medical illnesses?

The majority of movement disorders are restricted to the nervous system, but systemic organ involvement may provide diagnostic clues. For example, patients with underlying cancers may be at risk for paraneoplastic disorders and iron deficiency anemia or diabetes may predispose to restless legs syndrome. The presence of cardiomyopathy is associated with Friedreich ataxia or mitochondrial disorders. Enlargement of visceral organs (spleen, liver) may suggest a lysosomal storage disease.

6. Have the movements been treated in the past and what was the response to treatment?

A response to dopamine medications may facilitate diagnosis of dopa-response dystonia. Paroxysmal movement disorders may be exquisitely responsive to antiepileptic medications. Other substances may improve movements, such as the improvement of essential tremor, essential myoclonus, and myoclonus-dystonia with alcohol.

Examination

Depending on the movement disorder, abnormal movements may be present in focal or contiguous areas of the body or may be generalized. By determining the location and phenomenology of the movement, most patients can be placed into one of *seven distinct patterns* of abnormal movement.

Parkinsonism

The main features of parkinsonism are tremor at rest, bradykinesia or akinesia, rigidity, loss of postural reflexes, flexed posture, and freezing. Parkinsonism, in particular, Parkinson disease, is the most common disorder seen in movement disorder clinics and is covered by another volume of this series.

Tremor

This pattern is typically rhythmical and oscillatory and may affect more than one body part. Tremor should be classified on examination by the conditions under which it is activated: at rest, with posture, or with action. Tremor may be present in multiple conditions, for example, essential tremor, which is frequently seen with posture and action or intention. Tremors may also be task specific, such as the dystonic tremor of writer's cramp.

Chorea

Choreic movement is random in nature and is purposeless, non-rhythmic, and unsustained. It may appear to flow from one body part to another. Huntington disease is a frequent cause of chorea and manifests with brief, irregular movements. Chorea can be suppressed or camouflaged. It can be accompanied by "negative chorea" or motor impersistence.

Dystonia

In dystonia, agonist and antagonist muscles contract simultaneously causing twisting movements that are frequently sustained. The speed of the movement is variable and when sustained, can lead to abnormal postures and contractures. Dystonia is typically worsened with action, sometimes only occurring with specific actions. It can be classified by location, age of onset, and etiology, and the classification system has recently been revised.

Myoclonus

This pattern consists of brief, sudden, typically irregular jerks from muscle contraction. Myoclonus may be synchronized and triggered by action or startle. Negative myoclonus is caused by inhibition of the muscles, with the classic example being asterixis. Myoclonus can be rhythmic or oscillatory and occur in various parts of the body, either focally or generally.

Tics

Tics are abnormal movements (motor) or sounds (phonic) that are abrupt, usually transient, and can be simple or complex. Tics can vary over time and can be accompanied by an uncomfortable urge or feeling. Tics may be suppressible, although severe tics may be continuous. Gilles de la Tourette syndrome is characterized by the presence of both motor and phonic tics, present for more than one year, with young onset.

Ataxia

Lack of coordination of movement distinguishes ataxia from other movement disorders. The pattern of ataxic movement varies, but may include clumsy limb movements (dysmetria), dysarthria, ataxic eye findings such as abnormal pursuit, and uncoordinated walking. Kinetic tremor can also accompany ataxic signs. Ataxia can be localized to the peripheral or central nervous system so a thorough sensory and vestibular examination is necessary in these patients.

Other patterns of movements

There are several other types of abnormal movements that, despite being distinctly recognizable, do not fit well into the preceding patterns. These include stiff-muscles, akathetic movements, myokymia, paroxysmal dyskinesias, restless legs, and stereotypy. In addition, some movement disorders have more than one pattern of movement, such as in the myoclonus-dystonia disorders. Functional movement disorders frequently do not fit well into the above-described patterns, but caution must be maintained, since many unusual movement disorders can be labeled functional.

Diagnostic testing

Accurate description of the phenomenology of the abnormal movements as a result of the history and examination is the first and most fundamental step in diagnosis of movement disorders. Additional diagnostic testing is not warranted in many situations, for example, in the classic appearance of Tourette syndrome. However, there are some studies that may enhance or confirm clinical diagnosis. For example, laboratory studies can be useful particularly with tremor. Abnormalities of the thyroid, evidenced by elevated or low thyroid stimulating hormone (TSH), may cause or worsen tremor. Wilson disease, diagnosed by abnormal copper levels (in serum and/or urine), low ceruloplasmin, and the presence of Kaiser–Fleischer rings; should be considered in younger patients who present with bizarre tremors or other unusual movement patterns/combinations.

Genetic testing is available for many movement disorders and is driven by family history, age of the patient, and financial resources. For the more rare movement disorders, such as the inherited ataxias and Huntington disease, it may be the only testing that can give a definitive diagnosis. For individuals who are considering family planning, it may be necessary that genetic testing be accompanied by genetic counseling.

Neurophysiological assessment may be helpful in myoclonus, where myoclonic jerks show brief electromyography (EMG) bursts of 10–50 milliseconds. Rhythmicity in tremor can be demonstrated on EMG, but this is not frequently ordered by clinicians when evaluating a patient with tremor. Electromyography may also be helpful therapeutically in dystonic patients when used in conjunction with botulinum toxin treatment. Nerve conduction studies may be used to evaluate ataxic individuals for sensory abnormalities in peripheral nerves.

Imaging can be valuable in movement disorders that do not fit classic patterns or presentations. The most common movement disorders typically show normal basal ganglia structures on routine imaging, as in essential tremor, and dystonia. However, patients with movement disorders that are localized to one side of the body, that have abrupt stroke-like onset, or that include ataxia should be imaged with computed tomography or preferably, magnetic resonance imaging. Atrophy of specific structures, such as the striatum in Huntington disease, or the cerebellum in degenerative ataxias, may support the clinical diagnosis. Functional or nuclear medicine imaging is playing an increasingly important role in diagnostics.

Treatment

The majority of treatment options in movement disorders are symptomatic, not curative. However, in a few circumstances, early intervention of treatable forms of movement disorders may be curative or halt the progression of the disease. While rare, such conditions should be considered in patients with particular disease profiles; examples include patients with young onset tremor, dystonia or parkinsonism (Wilson disease), or fluctuating dystonic and parkinsonian features (dopa-responsive dystonia).

The approach described in this chapter offers a straightforward approach to evaluating a movement disorder patient. Questions about the movements, course, family history, medical illnesses, and medication response will help the clinician with the evaluation. Correctly describing the phenomenology is key to narrowing the list of diagnostic possibilities and guides the need for additional testing. The subsequent chapters will fill in the details, and with this framework, the reader will gain an ease of diagnosis and treatment of movement disorders.

Further Readings

Fahn S, Jankovic J, Hallett M. *Principles and Practice of Movement Disorders*, 2nd ed. Philadelphia: Saunders, 2007.

Fernandez HH, Rodriguez RL, Skidmore FM, Okun MS. *A Practical Approach to Movement Disorders: Diagnosis, Medical and Surgical Management*. New York: Demos Medical Publishing, 2007.

Part 1

Hypokinetic

2

Hypokinetic (Non-Parkinsonian) Movement Disorders

Shyamal H. Mehta, MD, PhD[1] and Alberto J. Espay, MD, MSc[2]

[1]Department of Neurology, Movement Disorders Division, Mayo Clinic, Phoenix, Arizona, USA
[2]Gardner Center for Parkinson's Disease and Movement Disorders, Department of Neurology, University of Cincinnati, Cincinnati, Ohio, USA

Introduction

Movement disorders can be broadly classified into two categories, based on the presence of excess movement or a deficiency of movement. Hyperkinetic movements involve the presence of excessive involuntary movements that may manifest as tremor, chorea-ballism, myoclonus, and tics, among other disorders. Hypokinetic movements show paucity of movement and are described with terms such as bradykinesia (slowness of movement) or akinesia (absence or extreme poverty of movement). The most common form of hypokinetic disorders are the parkinsonian syndromes, including idiopathic Parkinson Disease (PD), atypical parkinsonism, (multiple system atrophy, corticobasal syndrome, progressive supranuclear palsy, etc.), and secondary causes of parkinsonism (midbrain tumors, paraneoplastic disorders, etc.). These topics are covered in another book in this series. A different category of slowness comes from disorders that affect motor function to the extent of rendering it "parkinsonian" but that cannot be explained by traditional impairments in the basal ganglia circuitry. This chapter focuses on the *non-parkinsonian* causes of hypokinetic movement disorders, which may not be traditionally included in the differential diagnosis of parkinsonism.

This chapter aims to highlight some of the important and treatable causes of non-parkinsonian hypokinetic syndromes such as stiff person syndrome, primary lateral sclerosis, catatonia and psychomotor depression, hypothyroidism, and normal pressure hydrocephalus. These, along with other general causes, which can result in paucity or absence of movement, are listed in Table 2.1.

Stiff-person syndrome (SPS)

Moersch and Woltman described "stiff man syndrome" in 1956 in 14 patients who had progressively fluctuating rigidity and painful spasms affecting the muscles of the back and abdomen. An association between SPS and DM was established in the late 1980s; however, only a few of the originally reported patients had concomitant diabetes mellitus (DM). Solimena and colleagues later reported the presence of anti-glutamic acid decarboxylase (anti-GAD) antibodies in patients with SPS and DM. Since GAD is the rate-limiting enzyme for the synthesis of GABA, the major inhibitory neurotransmitter, in the central nervous system, GABAergic depletion at the cortical and spinal interneuronal level is central to the pathogenesis of SPS.

About 80% of SPS patients have a high titer of anti-GAD antibodies detectable in the serum or CSF.

Non-Parkinsonian Movement Disorders, First Edition. Edited by Deborah A. Hall and Brandon R. Barton.
© 2017 John Wiley & Sons, Ltd. Published 2017 by John Wiley & Sons, Ltd.
Companion website: www.wiley.com/go/hall/non-parkinsonian_movement_disorders

Table 2.1 Non-parkinsonian causes of hypokinesia

Stiff-person syndrome and related disorders

- Primary lateral sclerosis (PLM)
- Catatonia
- Neuromuscular causes: hypothyroidism, Brody syndrome, myotonia
- Akinetic mutism

Sequelae of vascular events (affecting anterior cerebral artery distribution)
Structural lesions: tumors, hydrocephalus, traumatic brain injury
Post-infectious: Creutzfeldt–Jakob disease, post-encephalitic parkinsonism

- Functional or psychogenic slowness

GAD is synthesized in the presynaptic GABAergic neurons in both the central nervous system and in the islet of Langerhans β-cells of the pancreas, hence the association with DM. There are two GAD isoforms—GAD65 and GAD67—but it is GAD65 that has been implicated in both SPS and DM. The GAD antibodies recognize different regions (epitopes) of the GAD molecule. The GAD antibodies in type 1 DM recognize the carboxy-terminal end or the center of the GAD molecule, while in SPS they recognize the amino-terminal fragment of GAD. Even though GAD antibodies are the most common antibodies associated with SPS, other proteins, both pre- and post-synaptic, in the GABAergic neuron have been implicated in the etiology of SPS or its variants (Box 2.1).

Clinical features

SPS disease is sporadic in nature, affecting women more often than men (in a recent series ~70% patients were women). Although the age of onset is variable, most of the afflicted adults are between 29 to 59 years of age. Symptoms start slowly and insidiously with episodic aching and stiffness of the axial musculature (paraspinal and abdominal muscles). Symptoms are usually symmetric and progress to involve the proximal muscles in all four extremities (Video 2.1). Typically the distal limb and facial

Box 2.1 Autoimmune antibodies in SPS and variants

Presynaptic: GAD and amphiphysin
Postsynaptic: GABA-A receptor associated protein, glycine and gephyrin

muscles are spared. Patients have a characteristic hyperlordosis of the spine, which makes it very difficult for them to bend over to touch their toes. The hyperlordosis persists even when they are laying down. The rigidity and stiffness may fluctuate on an hour-to-hour or daily basis. If it affects the neck, patients should be counseled not to drive until adequately treated, as it may significantly limit their ability to turn their heads.

Superimposed on the stiffness, patients also have intermittent severe spasms. These can be precipitated by various triggers, such as loud noise, sudden movement, touch, stress, and fatigue. Spasms usually last for minutes and abate once the offending stimuli are removed. However, during the spasms, patients can experience significant pain. The spasms can be variable in magnitude and severity, may occur in rapid succession, leading to a "spasmodic storm," and can be severe enough to cause fracture of the long bones.

The fear of precipitating the spasms causes patients to have anxiety and task-related phobias. More than 50% of patients fear open spaces. The presence of phobias, excessive startle, and exacerbation of symptoms when emotionally upset many times leads to an erroneous diagnosis of a functional or psychogenic disorder and, unfortunately, delays proper treatment.

Electromyography (EMG) studies show the presence of continuous motor unit activity at rest without any abnormality in the motor unit morphology. Reflex-induced spasms are short-latency (<80 ms), stereotyped motor responses to nerve stimulation. These are expressed as one or more hypersynchronous bursts of EMG activity followed by short pauses and then slow cessation.

Diagnosis of SPS variants and related conditions

SPS is a clinical diagnosis. Dalakas and colleagues have outlined criteria, which can assist the clinician in making the diagnosis (Box 2.2). However, there are patients who do not meet all of these criteria or have other additional features: they are often categorized as SPS variants, which we describe below (Box 2.3).

Progressive encephalomyelitis with rigidity and myoclonus

Progressive encephalomyelitis with rigidity and myoclonus (PERM) variant of SPS (formerly, "stiff-person plus syndrome") is a rare paraneoplastic

Box 2.2 Guidelines for diagnosis of SPS—Dalakas criteria

- Stiffness in axial muscles (abdominal and thoracolumbar) leading to hyperlordosis of the spine
- Superimposed painful spasms precipitated by sudden noise, stress, or tactile stimuli
- Confirmation of the continuous motor unit activity in agonist and antagonist muscles by electromyography
- Absence of other neurological findings that could explain the stiffness
- Positive serology for GAD65 (or amphiphysin) autoantibodies, assessed by immunocytochemistry, western blot, or radioimmunoassay
- Response to benzodiazepines*

* Not part of Dalakas's criteria, but commonly included in the diagnostic criteria.

Box 2.3 SPS variants and associated conditions

Stiff-person plus syndrome

- Stiff-limb syndrome
- Paraneoplastic SPS
- Progressive encephalomyelitis with rigidity and myoclonus (PERM)

disorder characterized by brainstem (cranial nerve) signs, long tract signs from spinal cord involvement, and myoclonus, in addition to the typical SPS signs/symptoms. Patients with PERM have symptoms atypical for SPS and poor response to medications. Imaging may show white matter hyperintensities in the brain and/or spinal cord. CSF studies show lymphocytic pleocytosis, elevated IgG, and oligoclonal bands. Recently, antibodies to glycine receptors have been detected in patients with PERM in addition to amphiphysin and GAD antibodies.

Stiff-limb syndrome

Some patients have focal onset of rigidity, affecting a single limb. This is descriptively termed "stiff-limb syndrome (SLS)." In this SPS variant, the symptoms remain most severe in the presenting limb, although eventually axial muscles may be affected as well.

However, spread to other areas is less common. Patients with stiff-limb syndrome are often anti-GAD-antibody negative, and in general, anti-GAD antibodies are less common in SLS as compared to SPS (15% vs. 88%). Also patients with SLS may not adequately respond to GABAergic medications such as benzodiazepines, which are very beneficial in classic SPS. Successful treatment with botulinum toxin type A has been reported, since the symptoms of SLS are focal in nature as compared to SPS.

Paraneoplastic SPS

SPS of paraneoplastic etiology (ca. 5% of the SPS patients) predominantly affects the neck and arms as opposed to the typical lower-body-predominant distribution of SPS. It is associated with malignancies of the breast, colon, lung, thymus, and Hodgkin's lymphoma. The antibodies involved are amphiphysin and gephyrin. If these antibodies are positive, a high degree of clinical suspicion for a covert malignancy is warranted.

Treatment

Benzodiazepines form the mainstay of treatment in SPS. Diazepam (10–100 mg/d) and clonazepam (4–6 mg/d) both have been used with considerable success. Patients tend to stabilize clinically and are able to function on this regimen, but they may continue to experience disability from residual stiffness. Baclofen, a $GABA_B$ receptor agonist, is the second drug of choice. Oral doses up to 100 mg/d and intrathecal pump infusion have been used. A practical approach is to use a combination of diazepam and baclofen, allowing lower doses than may be possible with each drug alone. Anticonvulsants that augment GABAergic transmission, such as valproic acid, gabapentin, vigabatrin, and levetiracetam, have been successfully used in selected cases.

Given the immunologic etiology of SPS, immunomodulatory therapy has also been considered. Anecdotal reports and a placebo-controlled trial with intravenous immunoglobulin (IVIg) have yielded promising results, and IVIg is the preferred immunotherapeutic option. Reports of benefit with plasmapheresis are also reported. Treatment with prednisone and other immunosuppressive agents are less promising. However, there are increasing reports of rituximab (a B-cell depleting monoclonal antibody) being successfully used in the treatment of benzodiazepine-refractory SPS and to treat the PERM variant. Treatment of paraneoplastic SPS also requires addressing the underlying malignancy. Botulinum toxin injections can be considered for targeted areas (paraspinal or thigh muscles) or in an affected extremity in stiff-limb syndrome, to supplement oral medications.

Primary lateral sclerosis

Primary lateral sclerosis (PLS) was a term coined in the nineteenth century by Erb to describe a disorder characterized by "spinobulbar" spasticity exclusively due to upper motor neuron degeneration. Some patients with PLS eventually develop lower motor neuron signs, meeting criteria for amyotrophic lateral sclerosis (ALS). Lower-extremity onset and slow progression increase confidence in the diagnosis of PLS and decrease the likelihood of later evolution into ALS. PLS affects equally both genders. The age of onset ranges from 30s to late 60s (Box 2.4). Although it is a sporadic disease with no family history in affected individuals, a rare hereditary variant affecting infants and children has been identified, called juvenile PLS. Mutations in the amyotrophic lateral sclerosis 2 (*ALS2*) gene coding for the protein Alsin or a loss of function mutation in *ERLIN2* gene (which codes for endoplasmic reticulum lipid raft protein that plays a role in ER associated degradation pathway) have been implicated in the etiology of juvenile PLS.

Box 2.4 Criteria for diagnosis of primary lateral sclerosis— Pringle criteria

Adult onset

- Spastic quadriparesis, spastic dysarthria, hyperreflexia, and bilateral Babinski signs with or without pseudobulbar affect for at least three years
- Absence of lower motor neuron signs
- Preservation of higher cognitive functions
- Magnetic resonance imaging demonstrates atrophy of the precentral gyrus
- Negative spinal cord MRI (to exclude cervical myelopathy)
- Negative family history
- Negative CSF studies (to exclude inflammatory, autoimmune and paraneoplastic processes)

PLS typically manifests with slowly progressive, lower extremity pain, weakness and spasticity (Video 2.2). Less commonly, upper extremity or bulbar symptoms can be presenting features. The spastic paresis tends to progress in a cephalad fashion to involve the axial musculature and upper extremities, eventually involving the bulbar musculature causing dysarthria and dysphagia. A diagnosis of PLS should not be made at the initial onset of symptoms unless at least three years have elapsed with slowly progressive upper motor neuron signs, in the absence of other motor, extrapyramidal, or cognitive impairments. Lower extremity onset, very slow progression, and absence of lower motor neuron signs at five years increases the diagnostic certainty of PLS.

Nerve conduction studies are normal in PLS and electromyography (EMG) studies may be normal or show mild denervation changes in the distal muscles (in stark contrast to ALS). However, repeat biannual testing for at least five years should be done to monitor for development of lower motor neuron involvement. MRI of the cervical spine is mandatory to exclude cervical myelopathy, which is the main PLS mimic. CSF studies may be considered to exclude inflammatory, post-infectious, or autoimmune encephalomyelopathies.

The treatment for PLS is symptomatic. Muscle relaxants (e.g., baclofen, tizanidine, and cyclobenzaprine) or benzodiazepines (diazepam or clonazepam) may help alleviate the spasticity. When oral medications do not provide adequate relief, intrathecal baclofen may be considered. Treatment of other comorbid infections such as respiratory tract and urinary tract infections are necessary to prevent exacerbation of spasticity. Physical therapy for muscle strengthening and stretching exercises may be beneficial. Physical therapy assessments of gait and balance and speech therapy evaluations of swallowing are crucial in tailoring management to minimize these complications. In later stages, when breathing is affected, non-invasive ventilatory support may be necessary. With appropriate care, the median survival of PLS of 20 years and is significantly longer than ALS.

Catatonia

Dr. Karl Kahlbaum (1828–1899) first described catatonia in his monograph published in 1874, wherein he published case histories of 28 patients with cata-

BOX 2.5 CAUSES OF CATATONIA

- Psychiatric Illness: schizophrenia, depression, obsessive-compulsive disease
- Drugs—dopamine receptor blocking drugs (antipsychotics and some antiemetics), selective serotonin reuptake inhibitors
- Post-encephalitic parkinsonism
- Tacrolimus-induced neurotoxicity in solid organ transplant patients
- Anti-NMDA receptor antibody-mediated encephalitis
- Some neurodevelopmental diseases such as autism and Tourette syndrome
- Post-anoxic brain injury

tonic episodes. Catatonia is a syndrome of excessive motor inhibition associated with disorders of mood, behavior, or thought. It is commonly encountered in the psychiatric inpatient setting, especially in patients with schizophrenia (Box 2.5). Although catatonia is not typically categorized as a movement disorder, it is characteristic for its extreme poverty of movement (akinetic form) and can sometimes be difficult to distinguish from parkinsonism. Other presentations include hyperexcitable and malignant forms associated with the neuroleptic malignant syndrome (NMS). The common signs in catatonia include mutism or echo phenomena (echolalia, echopraxia) cataplectic posturing, waxy flexibility, negativism, and staring (Video 2.3). Variable features include stereotypy, mannerisms, and automatic obedience. Catatonia may also occur in special populations such as children with developmental and neurological disorders, especially those with autism and related disorders, as well as geriatric patients with severe depression. Some other causes of catatonia include post-encephalitic parkinsonism, tacrolimus neurotoxicity in organ transplant patients, anti-NMDA receptor antibody-mediated encephalitis, post anoxic brain injury, and as a part of neurobehavioral disorders such as autism and Tourette's syndrome.

Treatment of catatonia should be done in concert with a psychiatrist. Identification of the syndrome and the underlying cause is key to its successful treatment. The motor manifestations of catatonia syndrome are exquisitely responsive to benzodiazepines and barbiturates. In fact, symptomatic improvement after the acute administration of a challenge with lorazepam is used as a confirmatory test of the diagnosis. Lorazepam 1–2 mg is administered sublingually or intramuscularly. If this is ineffective, it should be repeated again in three hours and then again in another three hours as an adequate treatment trial. Higher doses (4–12 mg/d) are rarely necessary. Also the presence of catatonia can increase the risk of NMS if antipsychotics are introduced prior to treatment of catatonia. Antipsychotics can be safely introduced once the patients are ambulatory and catatonia is resolved. There are data to support the use of electroconvulsive therapy (ECT) for the treatment of catatonia, regardless of various psychiatric disorders and organic causes, if symptoms do not improve with benzodiazepines.

Neuromuscular causes of hypokinesia

Hypothyroidism

Hypothyroidism is common in the elderly, affecting 5–20% of women and 3–8% of men. Common causes include autoimmune thyroiditis, previous thyroid surgery, and radioiodine therapy. Medications such as amiodarone and lithium, among others, can also cause hypothyroidism. Some of the common clinical signs, which can be mistaken for signs of PD, include changes in voice, fatigue, weakness/slowness of the extremities, and constipation. In addition, patients can have "hung-up" reflexes (delayed relaxation of the deep tendon reflexes) in hypothyroidism, which are not seen in PD. Hence screening and testing for thyroid dysfunction should always be done in elderly patients, especially if there are other signs or symptoms which might be atypical for PD.

Brody syndrome

This is an autosomal recessive, male-predominant disorder associated with impaired calcium uptake by the sarcoplasmic reticulum (Science Revisited). The characteristic clinical feature involves chronic difficulty in performing sustained muscular activities due to an exercise-induced failure in relaxation. A task may be feasible to perform initially, but with continued effort, significant slowing to the point of movement cessation occurs, requiring a period of rest for the movement to be restored. This may give the false appearance of bradykinesia, although amplitude decrement is not appreciated. Clinical

Genetics of Brody disease and syndrome

Brody disease—rare inherited myopathy due to mutations in *ATP2A1* gene (ATPase, Ca++ transporting, cardiac muscle, fast twitch 1) causing reduced sarcoplasmic reticulum Ca2+ ATPase (SERCA1) enzyme activity. Low SERCA1 activity leads to slow entrance of calcium ions into the sarcoplasmic reticulum, thus delaying muscle relaxation and causing muscle cramps.

Brody syndrome—similar phenotype except for prominent myalgias. Reduced SERCA1 enzyme activity occurs in the absence of *ATP2A1* gene mutations.

exam reveals normal strength with single effort, normal sensation, normal deep tendon reflexes, and the absence of percussion myotonia. EMG shows electrical silence in a contracted muscle after exercise. Dantrolene sodium and calcium channel blockers, such as verapamil and nifedipine, have been used successfully in the treatment of Brody syndrome.

Myotonia

Myotonia is the delayed relaxation of skeletal muscle fibers after voluntary muscle contraction. It manifests as painless muscle stiffness immediately on initiating activity. Patients may have difficulty relaxing their tight grip after a handshake or opening their eyes after tight eye closure, giving the appearance of slowness of movement. Percussion of the thenar eminence with a reflex hammer results in prolonged adduction or opposition of the thumb (percussion myotonia).

Myotonia improves after repeated effort and exercise (the "warm-up phenomenon"). EMG reveals motor unit potentials with a characteristic waxing and waning pattern—similar to the sound of a dive-bomber or motorcycle.

The two major categories of myotonia are dystrophic and non-dystrophic. Myotonic dystrophy is a common muscular dystrophy, involving progressive muscle weakness, myotonic discharges and multi-organ involvement. There are two genetically distinct types, both of which are autosomal dominant (Science Revisited). Adult-onset myotonic dystrophy type 1 is characterized by muscle weakness, myotonia, cataracts, cardiac conduction defects (a significant cause of early mortality), insulin resistance, male hypogonadism, and frontal baldness. In contrast, signs and symptoms in myotonic dystrophy type 2 can be variable, and myotonia may or may not be present. Muscle weakness in type 2 disease begins at a later stage than type 1, the clinical course is more favorable, and life expectancy is almost normal since fewer patients with type 2 disease have severe cardiac complications. However, myalgias can be quite severe in type 2 disease and patients may need round-the-clock pain medications.

Other disorders with clinical and electrical myotonia or paramyotonia include myotonia congenita: Becker and Thomsen, which are responsive to acetazolamide, paramyotonia congenita (sodium or chloride channelopathies) (Box 2.6); chondrodystrophic myotonia (Schwartz-Jampel syndrome); hyperkalemic periodic paralysis; myotonia fluctuans; and myotonia permanens. Mexiletine 200 mg tid is effective in improving the signs and symptoms of myotonia, as are other sodium channel blockers (phenytoin, procainamide, tocainide).

Genetics of myotonic dystrophy

	Type 1	Type 2
Inheritance	Autosomal Dominant	Autosomal Dominant
Chromosome	19Q13.3	3Q21.3
Abnormal Gene	Dystrophia-Myotonica Protein Kinase (*DMPK*)	Zinc-Finger-Protein-9 Gene (*ZNF9*)
Expansion	CTG Trinucleotide Repeat Expansion	CCTG Tetranucleotide Repeat Expansion
Anticipation	Common	Rare

Box 2.6 Important features of common non-dystrophic myotonias

	Recessive myotonia congenita (Becker)	Dominant myotonia congenital (Thomsen)	Paramyotonia congenital
Inheritance	Recessive	Dominant	Dominant
Causative gene	*CLCN-1*	*CLCN-1*	*SCN4A*
Myotonia distribution	Lower limbs more than upper limbs	Upper limbs more than lower limbs. Facial muscles may be involved	Facial, eyelid, and pharyngeal more than lower limbs
Trigger	Forceful muscle contraction after rest	Forceful muscle contraction after rest	Cold or exercise
Warm-up phenomenon*	Present	Present	Absent
Paradoxical myotonia†	Absent	Absent	Present
Episodic muscle weakness	Common, but transient	Uncommon	Common, prolonged for several hours
Eyelid myotonia	Absent	Infrequent	Common

* Warm-up phenomenon refers to the abatement of myotonia after repeated contractions.
† Paradoxical myotonia refers to the worsening of myotonia after repeated contractions.
Source: Adapted from Matthews 2010.

Functional slowness

Functional movement disorders can have a myriad of presentations including tremor, myoclonus, and dystonia. Patients can also present with excessive slowness of movement, whereby the "bradykinesia" is expressed as a breakdown of movements into small, individually normal, but overall slow movements, yielding an appearance of deliberate, effortful slowness (Video 2.4). Some additional clues to the functional etiology include: (1) sudden, abrupt onset of severe slowness of movement in the absence of weakness, (2) significant slowness during the exam and objective testing that is not evident during natural spontaneous movements involving the same body parts, (3) no evidence of slowness when the patient is being observed without his/her knowledge (in the rare cases of malingering), and (4) effortful, grimacing execution of movement in the absence of pain involving the body part being tested.

Treatment involves a compassionate debriefing of the diagnosis to the patient, then referral to a therapist or counselor to identifying underlying stressors and to provide cognitive behavioral therapy with or without adjunctive pharmacotherapy with antidepressants or antianxiety agents, if needed. Patients may also benefit from physical and/or occupational therapy.

Akinetic mutism

Cairns et al. first defined the term akinetic mutism in 1941 as a "condition of apparent alertness along with a lack of almost all motor functions including speech, gestures, and facial expression." This clinical picture of extreme akinesia results from various different pathologies either affecting bilateral mesial frontal lobes or the mesodiencephalic region. The patient described by Cairns et al. had akinetic mutism secondary to an epidermoid cyst in the third ventricle, which resolved upon the cyst being punctured. Akinetic mutism is most commonly encountered in the setting of anterior cerebral artery strokes, structural lesions such as tumors, Creutzfeldt–Jakob disease, hydrocephalus, and neurodegenerative dementias. Treatment of the underlying disorder, if possible, can sometimes reverse the symptoms.

Further Readings

Fink M. Catatonia: a syndrome appears, disappears, and is rediscovered. *Can J Psychiatry*, 2009; **54**(7): 437–445.

Gordon PH et al. Clinical features that distinguish PLS, upper motor neuron dominant ALS and typical ALS. *Neurology* 2009; **72**: 1948–1952.

Hadavi S et al. Stiff-person syndrome. *Practical Neurology* 2011; **11**: 272–282.

Lang AE et al. Psychogenic parkinsonism. *Arch Neurol*. 1995; **52**(8): 802–810.

Le Forestier N et al. Does primary lateral sclerosis exist? A study of 20 patients and a review of literature. *Brain* 2001; **124**: 1989–1999.

Mankodi A. Myotonic disorders. *Neurol India* 2008; **56**: 298–304.

Matthews E et al. The non-dystrophic myotonias: molecular pathogenesis, diagnosis and treatment. *Brain*. 2010; **133**(1): 9–22.

McKeon A et al. Stiff-man syndrome and variants: clinical course, treatments and outcomes. *Arch Neurol*. 2012; **69**(2): 230–238.

Otto A et al. Akinetic mutism as a classification criterion for the diagnosis of Creutzfeldt– Jakob disease. *J Neurol Neurosurg Psychiatry* 1998; **64**: 524–528.

Pringle CE et al. *Brain*. Apr 1992; **115**(Pt 2): 495–520.

Udd B et al. The myotonic dystrophies: molecular, clinical and therapeutic challenges. *Lancet Neurol* 2012; **11**: 891–905.

Voermans NC et al. Brody syndrome: a clinically heterogeneous entity distinct from Brody disease: a review of literature and a cross-sectional clinical study in 17 patients. *Neuromuscul Disord*. 2012; **22**(11): 944–954.

Part 2

Hyperkinetic

3

Common Types of Tremor

Jeff Kraakevik, MD[1] and Bernadette Schoneburg, MD[2]

[1]Oregon Health and Science University, Portland, Oregon, USA
[2]Northshore Medical Group, Glenview, Illinois, USA

Introduction

Tremor is defined as a rhythmic oscillation of a one or more body parts. Tremor is typically classified as resting or action tremor (Table 3.1). According to the consensus statement of the Movement Disorders Society on tremor, rest tremor is defined by its occurrence in a body part that is not voluntarily activated and is completely supported against gravity. *Action tremor*, also referred to as "kinetic tremor," is further subdivided into postural and intention tremor and is defined as any tremor that is produced by voluntary contraction of muscle. *Postural tremor* is present while voluntarily maintaining a position against gravity (i.e., holding up outstretched arms). *Intention tremor* occurs when tremor increases as one is approaching a target (i.e., with finger-to-nose movements).

Since the differential diagnosis for tremor is vast, a thorough medical and medication history must be obtained. The routine laboratory evaluation for tremor should include thyroid function and other labs as clinically appropriate (i.e., test to exclude Wilson disease in anyone under the age of 40 who presents with a movement disorder).

Table 3.1 Types of tremor

Type of tremor	Common diseases associated with tremor type
Rest tremor	Parkinson disease and other parkinsonian disorders, severe essential tremor
Action tremor (kinetic)	Essential tremor, cerebellar dysfunction
Postural tremor	Medication-induced tremor, enhanced physiologic tremor, dystonia, orthostatic tremor, Parkinson disease
Variable	Psychogenic tremor

> ★ **TIPS AND TRICKS**
>
> **Routine initial evaluation for tremor**
>
> **Key features of history**
> - Identify whether tremor is or is not interfering with daily activities
> - Screen for tremor-inducing social habits—such as caffeine consumption or tobacco products
> - Careful review of medication list for tremor-causing agents
>
> **Physical examination**
> - Assign tremor type as rest tremor, action tremor, or postural tremor
> - Complete neurological examination to look for other focal neurological deficits
>
> **Initial routine laboratory evaluation**
> - Thyroid function testing
> - IF patient <40 years old—screen for Wilson disease
>   - Slit-lamp examination, serum ceruloplasmin/copper, 24 hour urine collection for copper

Non-Parkinsonian Movement Disorders, First Edition. Edited by Deborah A. Hall and Brandon R. Barton.
© 2017 John Wiley & Sons, Ltd. Published 2017 by John Wiley & Sons, Ltd.
Companion website: www.wiley.com/go/hall/non-parkinsonian_movement_disorders

Potential additional testing depending on clinical suspicion
- Brain MRI—for potential structural abnormalities
- Dopamine transporter imaging—for Parkinson disease versus essential tremor
- Other functional imaging tests
- Neurophysiology (EMG)
  - Can help establish regularity of frequency if psychogenic tremor is suspected, or agonist/antagonist muscle co-contraction in dystonia, also has specific pattern for orthostatic tremor
- Fragile X gene testing—if cerebellar ataxia or imaging abnormalities (middle cerebellar peduncle sign) present as well

Although the differential diagnosis for tremor is potentially expansive, generally the disorders can be relatively easily arrived at by first categorizing tremor type and adding to that additional information from the physical examination. Indeed, much of the evaluation of tremor is accomplished with a thorough history and physical examination. Common disorders associated with tremor will be described below to outline both salient clinical features along with basic evaluation and treatment options.

Essential tremor (ET)

ET remains one of the most prevalent movement disorders and the most prevalent form of pathologic tremor. Worldwide prevalence estimate for all ages is 0.9% but increases to 4.6% in those over 65. One of the earliest descriptions of essential tremor dates back to 1887 when Dr. Charles Dana described the presence of tremor in several large New York families.

ET is alternatively referred to as benign essential tremor, and as familial, hereditary, idiopathic, or senile tremor. The older term "benign" essential tremor is no longer used, as the perception that ET does not significantly affect morbidity and mortality is inaccurate. Indeed, ET is a progressive disease that can be quite severe, significantly impairing someone's quality of life.

In most cases, ET clinically appears to have an autosomal dominant inheritance pattern; however,

no definitive causal single genetic mutations have been confirmed. Proposed genetic mechanisms include potential polygenetic or epigenetic interactions or mitochondrial disorders. Recent genome-wide association studies (GWAS) of large cohorts of patients with ET have shown some promise by identifying potential variant alleles.

Clinical characteristics of ET

ET is characterized by the predominance of bilateral postural and kinetic tremor. It is typically symmetric in nature and involves the hands and arms, becoming most apparent when holding arms in outstretched position. ET can also affect the head and/or voice. Leg tremor is uncommon. Isolated head tremor may occur but must be distinguished from dystonic head tremor (which is usually due to cervical dystonia). Head tremor in ET is typically vertical ("yes-yes" tremor) differentiating it from dystonic head tremor, which is more frequently a horizontal tremor ("no-no" tremor). Improvement of the tremor with alcohol is common in ET but is not diagnostic. ET increases with goal-directed activities and can be best visualized by the clinician during finger-to-nose movements, when drinking or pouring water from a cup, or when writing/drawing spirals. Vocal tremor is best assessed by having the patient sustain a vowel sound such as "Ah," and listening for variance in the pitch and amplitude of the sound. If you would like a good example of what that sounds like, it is recommended that you watch a movie featuring Katherine Hepburn later in her career. If a leg tremor is suspected, then having the patient hold the leg with the knee extended in a seated position will often produce a tremor. If the tremor is difficult to elicit, an effective strategy is to ask the patient what activity generally produces the tremor, and try to reproduce that activity in the room. Sometimes this may be better done by having the patient send a video of this activity later, or re-evaluating on a return visit where they bring the object that induces the tremor.

ET remains a clinical diagnosis based on a thorough history and neurological exam. The Movement Disorders Society has developed diagnostic criteria for ET (Table 3.2). In addition to the positive findings that suggest tremor, there are red flags that would make the diagnosis unlikely. This includes sudden onset, as ET is generally slowly progressive,

Methods to make a mild tremor more apparent on clinical exam

Clinical maneuvers to try:

- Observe rest tremor with limb fully supported
- Observe postural/action tremor with arms outstretched and on finger-to-nose maneuvers
- Perform repetitive movements with opposite hand
- Drinking or pouring water from a cup
- Spiral drawing
- Ask patient to perform task that typically brings out tremor (i.e., writing, or other). May require patient to bring in outside objects like a musical instrument.

Table 3.2 Movement Disorder Society Criteria for diagnosis essential tremor

Criteria	Description
Core	Bilateral, largely symmetric postural or kinetic tremor involving hand and forearms that is visible and persistent
	May have isolated head tremor (without abnormal posturing)
	Absence of other neurologic signs
Secondary	Duration >3 years
	Positive family history
	Positive response to alcohol
Red flags that diagnosis is not likely to be ET	Sudden onset
	Presence of tremorogenic drugs
	Withdrawal state
	Tremor at rest
	Bradykinesia, rigidity, unilateral tremor, dystonia, leg tremor, gait disturbance

presence of medications that may cause tremor, withdrawal from alcohol or illicit drugs, or parkinsonism on examination.

Recent work has found that patients with essential tremor are much more likely to have mild gait ataxia in the later stages of the disease. These clinical findings have come at the same time as pathology showing changes within the cerebellum with loss of Purkinje cells. This suggests that the pathological process leading to essential tremor may include cerebellar changes that create the initial insult and lead to the primary symptoms of essential tremor. There has been growing evidence as well that those patients with essential tremor for many years are much more likely to have mild to moderate cerebellar gait ataxia in addition to the tremor.

Pharmacologic treatment of ET

Propranolol and primidone are the commonly prescribed medications used to treat ET (Table 3.3). They are equally efficacious for the treatment of tremor, each reducing tremor magnitude by approximately 50%. When one of these two medications fails, they may be used in combination. It is estimated that approximately 30% of individuals will not respond to these first-line agents. The 2011 American Academy of Neurology (AAN) Practice Parameter guidelines for the treatment of ET outlines recent evidence for the treatment of ET. This review found level A evidence for propranolol, sustained-release propranolol, and primidone for use in limb tremor associated with ET. Of note, propranolol is the beta-blocker with the best evidence for effectiveness in ET as it has the best CNS penetrance. Sotalol and atenolol do have level B evidence as second-line agents, and metoprolol has not been sufficiently studied. Thus, if a beta-blocker is considered to be started solely for ET, propranolol would be the first choice based on the current evidence. Choice of which agent to start first will largely depend on patient's comorbidities. Propanolol's side-effect profile limits use in patients with diabetes, depression, and bradycardia. However, if a patient has concurrent hypertension, it may be preferred. Primidone can be sedating and caution should be used in elderly individuals as it is a barbiturate derivative and may cause confusion. Slow escalation of primidone in 25 mg increments is recommended.

Other second line agents, including gabapentin (monotherapy) and topiramate, were found to have level B evidence of effectiveness at treating limb tremor. Gabapentin is found to be effective in monotherapy, but not as an adjunct therapy for limb tremor. Benzodiazepines were considered potentially useful, but caution was recommended due to potential for abuse. This would include use of alprazolam (level B), and clonazepam (level C). Beyond these medications, there is weaker evidence for nadolol and nimodipine. Pregabalin, zonisamide,

Table 3.3 Medications for use in essential tremor

Medication	Suggested dosage and escalation*	Level of evidence per AAN guideline
First line		
Propranolol	Start 40 mg twice daily, titrate up to max of 320 mg in divided doses daily (if using sustained release formula—start at 80 mg once daily and escalate to 160 mg once daily).	Level A (limb tremor) Level B (head tremor)
Primidone	Start 12.5 to 25 mg once daily at bedtime (be aware smallest tab available is 50 mg, so will require splitting pills). Slowly escalate by 25 mg/d per week to effect. Max 750 mg per day. Typically divide dose to twice daily at 100 mg at bedtime.	Level A (limb tremor)
Second line		
Gabapentin	Start 100 mg three times daily. Escalate slowly to effect. Max dose 3600 mg per day.	Level B
Topiramate	Start 25 mg twice daily. Escalate slowly to effect with max dose of 100–200 mg twice daily.	Level B
Atenolol	Start 25–50 mg once daily, escalate to effect with max dose 200 mg/d.	Level B
Sotalol	80 mg every 12 hours, escalate to effect, max dose 480 mg/d.	Level B
Alprazolam	0.5–1.0 mg three times daily, may be used as needed. If scheduled, consider using extended-release form.	Level B
Third line		
Clonazepam	0.5–1.0 mg once daily at bedtime. Escalate by 0.5–1.0 mg/wk dividing dose twice daily to three times daily. Max dose 4 mg per day.	Level C

* Adjust dose accordingly depending on the patient.

and clozapine have insufficient evidence at present. Leviteracetam, trazodone, and 3,4-diaminopyridine were not effective, and the recommendation is that they should not be considered (level B evidence). For medically refractory tremor, botulinum toxin has Level C evidence for limb, head, and voice tremor. Medically refractory patients may also be considered for surgical options, which will be discussed below.

There are some patients with ET who do not feel the tremor is sufficiently bothersome to warrant pharmacologic therapy. A referral to occupational therapy is often useful in these patients as there are numerous products now available for tremor reduction. These include low-tech options such as adding weight to common household objects, and newer high-tech options that use accelerometer data and robotic motors to sense and counteract tremor frequency movements. See the Tips and Tricks box for further details; also more information about adaptive techniques can be found through contacting the International Essential Tremor Foundation.

> ★ **TIPS AND TRICKS**
>
> **Adaptive techniques and devices for tremor**
>
> - Weighted glasses and utensils
> - Wrist weights
> - Wide grip or weighted pens
> - Clothing with snap closure, Velcro, etc.
> - Mouse adapter to avoid multiple clicks or cursor tremor
> - Utensils with accelerometers and pivot motors that can cancel tremor frequency

Surgical treatment

Surgical intervention is an option for those individuals whose tremor remains disabling despite adequate trials of optimal pharmacologic therapy. Deep brain stimulation (DBS) and thalamotomy of the ventrointermedius nucleus (VIM) of the thalamus are effective surgical interventions for the treatment of tremor. Proponents of DBS argue for the reversible and nondestructive nature of this method. Although both procedures are equally effective for the suppression of drug-resistant tremor, DBS arguably has fewer side effects. Thalamotomy offers a safe alternative to those patients who are not optimal candidates for DBS, but bilateral thalamotomy is not recommended due to adverse side effects, particularly with speech and swallowing issues. Gamma knife surgery is available at some centers for treatment of ET, but there is currently insufficient evidence to determine if it is efficacious.

Surgical options for ET are very effective, and have revolutionized the treatment of medically refractory ET. As with any surgical procedure, care should be used in selecting a surgeon who has adequate procedural volume to maintain skills in these stereotactic surgical techniques. In addition, DBS treatment necessitates initial and ongoing programming with a qualified provider, typically found in a subspecialty neurology group focused on movement disorders. Thus adequate follow-up should be arranged prior to placement of the device.

☼ SCIENCE REVISITED

The target generally chosen for DBS highlights a neuroanatomical pathway which is associated with tremor. Stimulation of the VIM is thought at least partially to be working as it impacts the function of the cycle of structures joined by what is known as Guillian–Mollaret's triangle. Guilian–Mollaret's triangle includes a series of tracts connecting in a circular fashion the red nucleus, the Purkinje cell layer of the cerebellum, and the VIM nucleus of the thalamus. Other important fiber tracts in tremor production include thalamocortical loops and tracts from the brainstem to the basal ganglia. It is likely that these loops set up oscillations in motor control at varying frequencies, and theoretically these oscillations reverberate to create tremor. It is not entirely understood how DBS stimulation modulates this pathway, but it is thought to change oscillation patterns in fibers that are outgoing from the thalamus.

In summary, ET is typically a very rewarding condition to treat as the majority of patients will respond adequately to one of the two first-line agents, propranolol and primidone. Untreated essential tremor can be very disabling, so pharmacologic and, if needed, surgical intervention have very favorable outcomes that may justify risks of treatment.

Drug-induced tremor

Some degree of tremor occurs in all human beings and is commonly referred to as *physiologic tremor*. In clinical practice, the term *enhanced physiologic tremor* is frequently used to refer to tremor exacerbated by drugs or circumstances that increase adrenergic activity (i.e., caffeine, alcohol withdrawal, smoking, stress, anxiety). Enhanced physiologic tremor is the common form of drug-induced tremor. Differentiating drug-induced tremor from other causes of tremor requires a thorough history and physical examination of the patient. A temporal relationship to the initiation of pharmacologic therapy is very useful in making the diagnosis. Tremor severity is typically dose dependent and improves with cessation of the drug. Drug-induced tremor is usually symmetric in nature, predominantly occurs during posture and action, and is of low amplitude and high frequency (10–12 Hz). The exception is drug-induced parkinsonian tremor that occurs at rest and can be asymmetric in onset.

A list of substances and medications that are associated with tremor is provided in Table 3.4. A recent review by Morgan et al. reported that the most frequently encountered drug-induced tremor is due to lithium therapy. Because valproate is commonly prescribed for various neurologic disorders, including epilepsy, migraine prophylaxis, and mood stabilization, tremor due to this drug is also common. It is important to note that while alcohol improves some tremors, including ET, alcohol abuse is also a frequent cause of tremor. Alcohol withdrawal classically has an associated postural tremor, and alcoholism can cause tremor as a downstream effect of chronic liver disease.

Treatment of drug-induced tremor may not be necessary, as the majority of patients do not feel that the tremor interferes with their daily activity. This is because most patients with drug-induced tremor have low-amplitude postural tremor. If tremor is

Table 3.4 Drugs that commonly cause tremor[*]

Antiarrhythmics
- Amiodarone
- Procainamide

Antidepressants and mood stabilizers
- Tricyclic antidepressants (Amitriptyline)
- Selective serotonin reuptake inhibitors
- Lithium
- Valproate

Bronchodilators
- Salbutamol
- Salmeterol

Immunosuppressants
- Tacrolimus
- Cyclosporine

Neuroleptics
- Antiemetics
  - Metoclopramide
- Other
  - Caffeine
  - Ethanol
  - Nicotine
  - Levothyroxine

[*] Adapted from Morgan et al. (2005).

causing functional impairment, and it is a clinically viable option, the most efficacious response is generally to stop the causative medication. If this is not a viable option, and the medical condition requiring the tremorogenic drug requires treatment, switching to an equivalent non-tremor causing agent would be reasonable. An example of this would be a patient on valproate or lithium for mood stabilization purposes, who could be switched to lamotrigine, which is much less likely to cause tremor but is still an effective agent. If none of these are options, then use of a tremor-reducing agent such as propranolol or a benzodiazepine is a consideration.

Drug-induced parkinsonism (DIP) can cause a rest tremor. DIP was first described in the late 1970s when a designer drug contaminated with MPTP, which is toxic to dopaminergic neurons of the substantia nigra, caused acute parkinsonism in a number of patients. DIP due to dopamine-blocking agents (neuroleptics) affects 10–15% of patients on these drugs, depending on the type of neuroleptic used, and results in rest and action tremor that can be asymmetric in nature. The older, "typical" neuroleptics, including haloperidol, Fluphenazine, and thioridazine are more likely to cause DIP than the

newer, "atypical" antipsychotics like quetiapine or clozapine. It is important to note that dopamine-blocking agents also include antiemetic drugs such as metoclopramide. Treatment of DIP-related tremor includes switching to one of the newer "atypical" antipsychotics, with quetiapine and clozapine being the least likely to cause symptoms. If this is not an option clinically, then treatment is often initiated with an anticholinergic medication such as benztropine or trihexyphenidyl.

Parkinsonian tremor

Classic parkinsonian tremor is asymmetric in onset, occurs at rest, and becomes less prominent with posture and action. It has been described as a "pill-rolling" tremor as it typically affects the thumb and index finger, mimicking the action of rolling a pill between these two digits. Although usually rest tremor is predominant, tremor may be present with posture, and action; in this case, the clinician pays more attention to which tremor state has a greater degree of tremor than others. In Parkinson disease (PD), a postural tremor is much more likely to be "re-emergent," with a brief period where the hand is still when first held out in a static position. The tremor then slowly redevelops over several seconds. ET may be differentiated from PD tremor by noting that it is expressed primarily in a postural setting, seen immediately after holding the hands out.

Although it should not be difficult to differentiate the classic tremor of ET from classic PD rest tremor, a recent study reported that up to 20% of patients with ET may develop PD, and 10% report a family history of PD. Clinically, this distinction can be difficult at times as, when a tremor becomes more severe, it can move from a more pure rest tremor to be present with posture and intention. One key clinical point here is that the tremor will typically be more severe with one of these positions. However, it is well known that people may present with what looks like ET and over time develop a clinical picture that becomes more classic for PD. Whether ET is a risk factor for PD remains a controversial issue. At this point there is no definite pathologic link between the two entities.

In 2011, the United States Food and Drug Administration approved the use of DaTscans to detect dopamine transporters (DaT) in individuals with parkinsonian syndromes. This imaging modality

Table 3.5 How to differentiate ET from PD tremor

Clinical features	Essential tremor	Parkinson disease
Onset	Symmetric	Asymmetric but progresses to bilateral involvement
Tremor type	Posture/action	Resting and postural (re-emergent)
Response to alcohol	Yes	No
Head/neck tremor > chin tremor	Yes	No
Presence of bradykinesia or rigidity	No	Yes
Writing/spiral drawing	Large and tremulous loops	Small print (micrographia)

cannot diagnose PD and should be used as an adjunct to confirm a diagnosis, especially in individuals where there is some uncertainty (Table 3.5). For example, DaTscans may help clinicians differentiate between ET and tremor caused by PD.

Parkinsonian tremor is primarily treated with dopaminergic medications typically used in PD, such as carbidopa/levodopa or a dopamine agonist. Although the majority of parkinsonian tremor cases will respond to dopaminergic medications, not all patients will respond; some parkinsonian tremors can be very resistant to treatment. In these cases, one option is to use an anticholinergic medication such as trihexyphendyl or benztropine. These must be used carefully in elderly patients due to the potential side effects of anticholinergic medications. Deep brain stimulation may also be useful in the treatment of tremor for PD as well.

✋ CAUTION

Meds to avoid in Parkinson disease
- Dopamine D2 receptor blockers (typical worse than atypical). Also included in this category are antiemetics like metoclopramide, promethazine, prochlorperazine.
- Dopamine depleters—Tetrabenazine, reserpine

Functional tremor

Functional (psychogenic) movement disorders can manifest as any abnormal movement; however, functional tremor is the common presentation. The diagnosis of functional tremor can be challenging,

and often will require referral to a movement disorders specialist. Diagnosis is based on exclusion of organic causes of tremor and supported by acute onset and resistance to treatment. The diagnosis is also supported by variability of symptoms over time, and if the tremor comes and goes in discrete paroxysmal episodes that last for hours to days. In some cases, a precipitating event such as a personal life stressor, trauma, or major illness can be identified. On examination, functional tremor will vary in its appearance throughout the course of the clinic visit. It will often migrate from one limb to another. The amplitude and the frequency of functional tremor are highly variable and diminish with mental distraction maneuvers (e.g., having the patient perform serial 7 s or name the months of the years in reverse order). Another characteristic feature of functional movement disorders is "entrainment" and can be evaluated by having the patient tap his fingers with the contralateral (non-affected) hand. If the tremor of the affected hand then shifts to match the frequency of tapping hand, this is entrainment and is suspicious of functional tremor.

Treatment of functional tremor has variable results. Evidence for effective therapy is conflicting at best. In general, clear communication that the tremor is not due to a life-threatening disease, and that this may potentially resolve with time is essential. It is important to remain empathetic when expressing this information, and also to clarify that the functional movements are not considered to be under voluntary control of the affected individual. Pyschotherapy has been found to have a variable response, as has use of physical therapy. Specific medication treatment and ordering of diagnostic studies that are not absolutely necessary is not generally helpful.

Clinical distinction between functional and organic tremor

	Functional tremor	Organic tremor
Onset of symptoms	Can be abrupt	Typically slowly progressive
Clinical course over time	Non-progressive with potential for spontaneous remissions	Progressively worsens over time
Frequency	Relatively stable	Variable and will change with distraction and entrainment maneuvers.
Amplitude	Increases in size with distraction	Decreases in size with distractibility
Location of tremor (i.e., head, hand, trunk, feet)	Stable over the course of the clinic visit	Variable and will often move from one side of the body to the other

Brainstem/cerebellar tremor

Even though the typical sign associated with a cerebellar lesion is ataxia, tremor is also a very common presentation of cerebellar disease. The cerebellar tremor clinically appears as an intention tremor. It may also appear as a proximal tremor in the arm. This type of tremor is also referred to as a Holmes tremor or a rubral tremor. The name rubral tremor comes from the fact that lesions of the red nucleus in the midbrain can cause this clinical sign. Cerebellar tremors can be associated with any fiber tracts or structures that send close connections to the cerebellum. The potential causes of a cerebellar tremor mirror the potential causes of cerebellar ataxia, which are described in a separate chapter. The common causes of cerebellar tremor include multiple sclerosis, cerebrovascular disease, autoimmune encephalitides, and a host of other potential etiologies.

An important consideration is Wilson disease as it is potentially treatable. The tremor in Wilson disease is classically described as "wing-beating." Wilson disease is often accompanied by psychiatric disturbances and can present with other movement disorders like dystonia, parkinsonism, and ataxia. Wilson disease is caused by mutations in copper metabolism causing abnormal accumulation of copper. This disease is usually diagnosed by testing for serum ceruloplasmin, serum copper, and a 24-hour urine test for copper levels. The 24-hour urine copper levels will be abnormally high in Wilson disease. Slit-lamp examination will reveal Kayser–Fleisher rings in the cornea of nearly all patients with neurological symptoms. A liver biopsy can be also diagnostic as there is copper accumulation in the liver. Genetic testing for a mutation of the *ATP7B* gene is also available. Treatment is copper chelation therapy with penacillamine or trientine. Once copper levels have been decreased, dietary copper restriction and treatment with zinc to compete with copper for gut absorption are also used.

Dystonic tremor

Tremor can often be a presenting symptom of dystonia of any part of the body. The tremor shares some common phenomenology with functional tremor, and this may delay diagnosis of a dystonic tremor. Both of these tremor types will have variable frequencies and amplitudes. However, the dystonic tremor will be more predictable as to when it worsens in that it is always going to get worse with a consistent direction of the movement. For example, in a cervical dystonia, as the neck is turned away from the overactive muscle group, the tremor will increase in amplitude. Turning the head toward the overactive muscle group will dampen the amplitude. Dystonic tremor may also reliably respond to a

Dystonic tremor is often difficult to diagnose. Patients with cervical dystonia may take four to five years to properly diagnose. The presence of a sensory trick, and the irregular nature of the tremor coupled with chronic pain complaints make some physicians call this a functional disorder.

sensory trick. The differential diagnosis for dystonia is dealt with in a separate chapter. The treatment is primarily botulinum toxin injections.

There is some controversy about tremors that primarily occur in a task-specific manner. The common condition in this group of tremors is called primary writing tremor. In this condition, there is a rhythmic tremor that only occurs when the patient writes. Interestingly, when the patient uses the same hand to do other activities, like typing, the tremor may not be present at all. The controversy with this condition corresponds to disagreement among movement disorders experts as to whether this pathologically is related to ET or dystonia. Treatment options for dystonic tremor consist of medications typically used for ET or botulinum toxin injections. Occupational therapy can also be an option as retraining writing style can help.

Orthostatic tremor

Orthostatic tremor (OT) is a rare disorder that is characterized by a high-frequency tremor involving the legs that occurs upon standing, resulting in subjective postural instability. Symptoms improve with sitting, lying down, or walking. Due to its high frequency (13–18 Hz), the tremor may not be visible to the patient or clinician. The clinician may feel for the tremor by placing his or her hand or stethoscope on the patient's leg. EMG is often necessary to confirm the diagnosis in cases where the tremor is not immediately able to be visualized. The classic surface EMG finding is a very rapid, thumping sound much like a helicopter.

Treatment of OT is not always necessary. Some people are able to adequately treat the symptoms by simply bringing along with them a portable seat so that they can sit down any time they have to stand for a long time. A wheeled walker with a seat or a portable stool is ideal for this purpose. Some medications may be effective for OT, with clonazepam typically used as a first-line agent. Other treatment options include gabapentin, primidone, and dopaminergic medications. As OT is relatively rare, good clinical trial data on treatments is lacking, even for clonazepam.

Conclusion

Tremor is the common movement disorder, and careful attention by the clinician can lead to a definitive diagnosis. Categorizing the tremor as rest, postural, or intention will aid in the differential diagnosis. Tremor as a whole is responsive to medication, and when medications are refractory, tremors due to ET or PD are amenable to surgical therapies.

Further Readings

Deuschl G, Bain P, Brin M. Ad hoc Scientific Committee. Consensus statement of the Movement Disorder Society on Tremor. *Mov Disord* 1998; **13** (suppl 3): 2–23.

Elble RK. What is essential tremor? *Curr Neurol Neurosci Rep* 2013; **13**: 353.

Ferreira JJ, Costa J, Coelho M, Sampaio C. The management of cervical dystonia. *Expert Opin Pharmacother*. 2007; **8**(2): 129–240.

la Fuente-Fernández de R. Role of DaTSCAN and clinical diagnosis in Parkinson disease. *Neurology* 2010; **78**(10): 696–701.

Jones L, Bain PG. Orthostatic tremor. *Pract Neurol* 2011; **11**(4): 240–243.

Koch M, Mostert J, Heersema D, DeKeyser J. Tremor in multiple sclerosis. *J Neurol* 2007; **254**(2): 133–145. Epub 2007 Feb 21.

Limousin P, Speelman JD, Gielen F, Janssens M. Multicentre European study of thalamic stimulation in parkinsonian and essential tremor. *JNNP* 1999; **66**(3): 289–296.

Lyons KE, Pahwa R. Deep brain stimulation and tremor. *Neurotherapeutics*. 2008; **5**(2): 331–338.

Morgan JC, Sethi KD. Drug-induced tremors. The lancet. *Lancet Neurol* 2005; **4**(12): 866–876.

Rana AQ, Vaid HM. A review of primary writing tremor. *Int J Neurosci* 2012; **122**(3): 114–118.

Zesiewicz TA, Elble RJ, Louis ED, et al. Evidence-based guideline update: treatment of essential tremor. Report of the Quality Standards Subcommittee of the American Academy of Neurology. *Neurology* 2011; **77**: 1752.

Zeuner KE, Deuschl G. An update on tremors. *Curr Opin Neurol* 2012; **25**(4): 475–482.

4

Myoclonus

Daniel Burdick, MD and Pinky Agarwal, MD

Movement Disorders Center, Evergreen Health Neuroscience Institute, Kirkland, Washington, USA

Introduction

Myoclonus can be one of the most difficult movement disorders to diagnose and treat, as its localization is often unclear and the differential diagnosis is vast. In his 2007 review, Mark Hallett emphasized the breadth of causes, writing that a classification of etiologies of myoclonus "runs to a textbook of neurology." However, a systematic approach to the diagnosis can lead to etiologic clarity and a direction for treatment.

Definition

Myoclonus is defined as a sudden, brief, shock-like, involuntary movement. This can be further divided into positive myoclonus, which is active contraction of the muscle, and negative myoclonus or asterixis, defined as sudden loss of tone in the muscle.

Differential diagnosis of myoclonus

Myoclonus is generally distinguishable from other hyperkinetic movement disorders by its velocity and amplitude, although at times it may be difficult to distinguish from tremor, chorea, dystonia, or tics.

- *Tremor* is by definition rhythmic, while myoclonus may be rhythmic or non-rhythmic. Tremor is an oscillatory movement, whereas myoclonus has a more rapid acceleration and deceleration. The maximum velocity of a tremor is usually slower than myoclonus. However, on rare occasions, myoclonus may suggest a superficial similarity to tremor, and electromyography may be needed to differentiate them.
- *Chorea* is a rapid, random, flowing, dance-like movement, taking its name from the ancient Greek for dance, *choréia*. Although components of chorea may resemble myoclonus, the movements in chorea flow from one body part to another with a random distribution in space and time, whereas the movements of myoclonus are much simpler.
- In *dystonia*, there may be brief muscle spasms. However, these produce the twisting and turning postures characteristic of dystonia. Myoclonus, by contrast, produces only simple muscle contraction, without sustained posturing.
- *Tics* are characterized by their semi-volitional or "unvoluntary" nature. The movements in a tic disorder are frequently preceded by a conscious urge to move, and are followed by a release of tension. In addition, tics can, if only temporarily, be consciously suppressed. Myoclonus shares none of these characteristics.

Physiologic myoclonus

Before going further, it must be noted that a number of physiologic causes of myoclonus exist, which do not require further evaluation or treatment. These include hiccups, myoclonus induced by exercise or by anxiety, and sleep myoclonus (hypnic jerks). All are spontaneous, non-rhythmic, and in general short-lived. Hypnic jerks are a multifocal or generalized myoclonus occurring specifically at the sleep-wake transition. Movements that persist into sleep should

Non-Parkinsonian Movement Disorders, First Edition. Edited by Deborah A. Hall and Brandon R. Barton.
© 2017 John Wiley & Sons, Ltd. Published 2017 by John Wiley & Sons, Ltd.
Companion website: www.wiley.com/go/hall/non-parkinsonian_movement_disorders

prompt consideration of other disorders, such as periodic limb movements during sleep (PLMS).

Clinical Localization

Once it has been established that the movement phenomenology is myoclonus, a consideration of the cause and appropriate treatment may be undertaken. Myoclonus can be classified on the basis of either clinical features or anatomic localization, which can in turn help identify etiology and treatment choices.

Clinical features

In describing the clinical features of myoclonus, four elements must be considered: distribution, effect of provocation, rhythmicity, and the effect of sleep. *Distribution* can be described as (1) generalized, involving most or all of the body, (2) axial, involving all muscles of the trunk, (3) multifocal, with several noncontiguous muscles involved, or (4) focal or segmental, involving a single muscle or a few contiguous muscles. The effect of *provocation* is divided into spontaneous myoclonus, occurring at rest; action myoclonus, occurring only when the muscles are activated; and reflex myoclonus, occurring as a response to a sensory input, usually tactile or auditory. *Rhythmicity* refers to whether the pattern of myoclonus occurs regularly or irregularly. Finally, myoclonus can either persist or cease during *sleep*.

Anatomic localization

Myoclonus may be generated by the cortex or subcortical structures, brainstem, spinal cord, or, rarely, a peripheral lesion. Cortical myoclonus is either epileptic (e.g., epilepsia partialis continua) or non-epileptic. Myoclonus may be reticular (brainstem), palatal, or startle (e.g., hyperekplexia). Spinal myoclonus is classified as either propriospinal or spinal segmental. Peripheral myoclonus may be further localized to lesions of the root, plexus, or nerve.

Table 4.1 serves as a quick reference guide to turn clinical observation into possible localization,

Table 4.1A Clinical localization of non-rhythmic myoclonus*

Non-Rhythmic	Spontaneous	Action	Reflex
Focal/segmental	Cortical, spinal segmental, peripheral	Cortical, spinal segmental	Cortical, spinal segmental
Axial	Cortical	Cortical Cortical, brainstem	Cortical
Multifocal	Cortical	Cortical (Lance–Adams)	Cortical (Lance–Adams)
Generalized	Cortical, brainstem reticular, propriospinal	Cortical, brainstem reticular (if post-anoxic)	Cortical, brainstem startle

*Subcortical myoclonus shares clinical features of cortical myoclonus, and evaluation and treatment is essentially the same.

Table 4.1B Clinical localization of rhythmic myoclonus*

Rhythmic	Spontaneous	Action	Reflex
Focal/segmental	Cortical (EPC), brainstem palatal, spinal segmental	Cortical, spinal segmental	
Axial		Cortical	
Multifocal	Cortical	Cortical	
Generalized	Cortical		

*Subcortical myoclonus shares clinical features of cortical myoclonus, and evaluation and treatment is essentially the same.

leading to the appropriate evaluation and treatment considerations. Cortical myoclonus has the greatest variability in its clinical features. Its distribution may be any of the above, though it is rarely purely axial. It may be spontaneous, present with action or reflex. It may or may not be rhythmic. However, although the possibilities are broad, the common pattern for cortical myoclonus is to be focal or multifocal, present as action or reflex, and to be non-rhythmic, with the notable exception of epilepsia partialis continua, which is spontaneous and rhythmic.

Subcortical myoclonus has as much clinical variability as cortical myoclonus and differs only in the absence of identifiable EEG discharges. For the ensuing discussion of etiology and treatment, subcortical myoclonus is considered together with non-epileptic cortical myoclonus. One important exception is thalamic myoclonus, which produces a unilateral negative myoclonus, rarely seen with cortical lesions. A thalamic lesion is an important consideration when presented with unilateral asterixis.

Brainstem myoclonus, with the specific exception of palatal myoclonus, is generalized. Brainstem reticular myoclonus is either spontaneous or action, while hyperekplexia or startle myoclonus is always a reflex. From the cord, propriospinal myoclonus is generalized, spontaneous, and non-rhythmic. Spinal segmental myoclonus has slightly more variability. While it is by definition focal or segmental, it may be spontaneous, present as action or reflex, and be rhythmic or non-rhythmic. Peripheral myoclonus, with hemifacial spasm being the common example, is focal, spontaneous, and non-rhythmic.

Diagnostic approach and etiology

Cortical and subcortical myoclonus

After a reasonable attempt at localization is made, a further diagnostic evaluation can be undertaken. If the myoclonus is thought to be cortical, or if the localization is uncertain, an electroencephalogram (EEG) is a reasonable starting point. Definitive localization requires time-locked back-averaged EEG, but this is rarely available clinically. Nonetheless, a routine EEG is often helpful in determining whether the myoclonus is epileptic, which will guide treatment decisions.

Whether or not the cortical myoclonus is found to be epileptic, the next step is to obtain a magnetic resonance imaging (MRI) of the brain. Focal lesions of the brain, such as stroke, tumor, or demyelination, may cause either epileptic or non-epileptic cortical or subcortical myoclonus. If a focal lesion is not found on imaging but epileptic discharges are seen on EEG, the myoclonus is classified as a primary epileptic myoclonus, and treated with anti-epileptic medication. A complete description of myoclonic epilepsy is outside the scope of this review, but includes syndromes such as infantile spasms, Lennox–Gastaut syndrome, progressive myoclonic epilepsy (Unverricht–Lundborg syndrome), and juvenile myoclonic epilepsy.

If neither EEG nor brain MRI reveals a finding in cortical or subcortical myoclonus, the next consideration is whether the myoclonus is syndromic or non-syndromic. Syndromic cortical or subcortical myoclonus includes myoclonus with dementia and/or parkinsonism, progressive myoclonic ataxia (Ramsay Hunt syndrome type I), opsoclonus-myoclonus, and post-hypoxic myoclonus (Lance–Adams syndrome), among others. Myoclonus with dementia and/or parkinsonism is seen in the later stages of these diseases, with the notable exceptions of corticobasal degeneration (CBD), Creutzfeld–Jakob disease (CJD), and neurodegeneration with brain iron accumulation (NBIA), all of which could have myoclonus as an early sign. Although these syndromes may be apparent even before a diagnostic workup is undertaken, it is still important to exclude alternative causes with EEG and MRI.

If there are no associated neurological signs to suggest one of these syndromes, then further diagnostic steps are necessary. A complete metabolic evaluation should be undertaken, with particular attention to renal or hepatic failure. A lumbar puncture should be considered to evaluate for an infectious or inflammatory cause. In addition to the routine protein, glucose, and cell count, the CSF should be evaluated for viral polymerase chain reactions (PCRs), since a number of viral encephalopathies (e.g., herpes simplex virus, cytomegalovirus, arbor viruses, subacute sclerosing panencephalitis) may cause myoclonus. Human immunodeficiency virus testing may be indicated. Paraneoplastic antibodies may be associated with myoclonus and can be evaluated in both serum and CSF.

Myoclonus has been specifically linked to the anti-neuronal nuclear antibody-2 (ANNA-2, a.k.a. anti-Ri), occurring with breast, small-cell lung, and gynecologic cancers, and to the anti-NMDA receptor antibody, occurring with teratomas or spontaneously. In theory, though, any paraneoplastic antibody that produces an encephalomyelitis (ANNA-1/anti-Hu, anti-CRMP5/CV2, anti-Ma1, anti-Ma2, anti-amphiphysin, ANNA-3, anti-Purkinje cell antibody-2/PCA2, anti-AMPA receptor, and anti-Ta) may cause myoclonus, and investigation of a complete panel is prudent.

Additionally, a thorough medication review is necessary, as a number of medications, including narcotics, anti-epileptics, and antidepressants (particularly SSRIs), may produce iatrogenic myoclonus. Finally, potential toxin exposures, such as heavy metals and organochlorine pesticides, should be considered. (For a list of causes of non-epileptic cortical or subcortical myoclonus, see Table 4.2.)

Brainstem myoclonus

Brainstem myoclonus is often easy to recognize. The exaggerated startle syndromes (hereditary hyperekplexia, Latah, and related syndromes) are generalized brainstem reflexes, usually in response to auditory stimuli. Hereditary hyperekplexia is identified by family history, as its inheritance is typically autosomal dominant, though rarely it may be autosomal recessive or X-linked. It is characterized by an exaggerated startle response followed quickly by stiffening that may produce falls. The Latah syndrome of Malaysia shares the exaggerated startle reflex but is followed by an emotional and behavioral response rather than stiffening. This syndrome is seen across many cultures, including the "Jumping Frenchmen of Maine," the "Ragin' Cajuns" of Louisiana, the Imu of Japan, and "Lapp panic" in Lapland (northern Finland and Sweden). Some authors have argued that these are culture-bound syndromes rather than biologic, although it must be noted that the characteristics of these startle syndromes bear remarkable resemblance across these many cultures.

Hyperekplexia may also be idiopathic or symptomatic. In cases where a family history is not apparent, MRI with and without contrast should be performed to evaluate for brainstem lesions, such as tumor, stroke, demyelination, or encephalomyelitis (infectious or inflammatory). Exaggerated startle may also be seen in post-anoxic or post-traumatic encephalopathy.

Brainstem (reticular) myoclonus, also generalized but independent of the startle reflex, is most often the result of anoxic injury or toxic/metabolic derangement. In cases where there is no preceding anoxia, a brainstem MRI and complete metabolic workup are indicated.

Palatal myoclonus, the only focal myoclonus arising from the brainstem, can be essential or symptomatic. Essential palatal myoclonus, sometimes called palatal tremor because of the rhymicity of the movements, is characterized by its "ear click," a sound produced by the repeated opening of the pharyngotympanic (Eustachian) tube due to rhythmic contraction of the tensor veli palatini, innervated by the trigeminal nerve. The combination of an ear click, cessation during sleep, and the absence of other brainstem signs makes the diagnosis of essential palatal myoclonus possible without imaging.

Unlike the essential form, symptomatic palatal myoclonus will be accompanied by other brainstem signs. These may include pendular vertical nystagmus or facial myoclonus. MRI is indicated to identify the lesion responsible for the damage, often stroke, trauma, tumor, or demyelination; encephalitis is a rare cause.

Symptomatic palatal myoclonus is due to damage in the Guillain–Mollaret triangle: defined by the red nucleus, the inferior olive ipsilateral to the red nucleus, and the contralateral dentate nucleus. The damage is often to the central tegmental tract, connecting the red nucleus to the ipsilateral inferior olive and producing visible (on MRI) hypertrophy of the inferior olive, which is not seen in essential palatal myoclonus. In essential palatal myoclonus, the palatal movement is due to contraction of the levator veli palatini, innervated by the vagus nerve from the nucleus ambiguus.

Table 4.2 Etiologies of non-epileptic cortical myoclonus

Lesion on MRI	Focal	Stroke
		Tumor
		Abscess
		Demyelination
		Trauma
		Post-thalamotomy (Iatrogenic)
	Diffuse/multifocal*	Post-hypoxic (Lance–Adams)
		Post-traumatic
		Infectious/post-infectious — SSPE, Encephalitis Lethargica, Arbor virus, HSV, Whipple, HIV/AIDS
		Other inflammatory
		Paraneoplastic
		Electric shock
		Heat stroke
No lesion on MRI	Syndromic	Basal ganglia degeneration — CBD, NBIA, MSA, DLB, PSP, Huntington disease, Wilson disease, Parkinson disease
		Dementia — CJD, Alzheimer disease
		Ataxia — Friedreich ataxia, Ataxia-telangiectasia, SCAs, DRPLA, Celiac disease
		Inborn errors of metabolism — Lafora body Disease, Neuronal ceroid Lipofuscinosis, Lipidoses, Sialidosis

Non-syndromic		
	Metabolic encephalopathy	Liver failure
		Renal failure
		Hyponatremia
		Hypoglycemia
		Nonketotic hyperglycemia
		Dialysis disequilibrium syndrome
		Vitamin E deficiency
		Biotin (vitamin B7) deficiency
		Multiple carboxylase deficiency
	Toxic encephalopathy	Mercury
		Bismuth
		Aluminum
		Other heavy metals
		Organochlorine insecticides
		Dichloroethane (DDT)
		Toluene
	Prescription drugs (partial list)	Levodopa
		SSRIs
		Narcotics
		Anti-epileptics (esp. gabapentin and lamotrigine)
		Lithium
		Buspirone
		Neuroleptics
		Anesthetics
		Calcium-channel blockers
		Anti-arrhythmics
	Recreational drugs	Marijuana
		Cocaine
		MDMA (Ecstasy)

*Most of the conditions listed under "Lesion on MRI → Diffuse/multifocal" may also produce myoclonus in the absence of imaging findings.

Abbreviations: SSPE = Subacute sclerosing pan-encephalitis; HSV = Herpes Simplex Virus; HIV = Human Immunodeficiency Virus; AIDS = Acquired Immune Deficiency Syndrome; CBD = Corticobasal Degeneration; NBIA = Neurodegeneration with Brain Iron Accumulation; DLB = Dementia with Lewy Bodies; PSP = Progressive Supranuclear Palsy; MSA = Multiple Systems Atrophy; CJD = Creutzfeld-Jakob Disease; SCAs = Spinocerebellar Ataxias; DRPLA = Dentatorubropallidoluysian Atrophy.

Sources: Fahn et al. (1986), Fahn (2002), Hallett et al. (1987), Hallett (2007).

Spinal myoclonus

Both propriospinal myoclonus and spinal segmental myoclonus may be the result of a spinal cord lesion, although propriospinal myoclonus is thought to be most often the result of trauma, tumor, or idiopathic causes. Some authors have proposed that many suspected cases of propriospinal myoclonus are functional in etiology. Spinal segmental myoclonus may be produced by trauma, tumor, demyelination, infection, arteriovenous malformation, spondylosis, spinal ischemia, spinal anesthesia, or idiopathic causes. MRI with and without contrast of the appropriate cord level is usually sufficient, but if no lesion is identified, a lumbar puncture should be considered. If clinically available, MRI with diffusion tensor imaging may be more sensitive in identifying white matter lesions producing spinal myoclonus.

Peripheral myoclonus

The quintessential peripheral myoclonus is hemifacial spasm. This is a non-rhythmic, spontaneous myoclonus producing rapid eyelid closure and/or pulling of the lips unilaterally. It is either idiopathic or due to vascular or neoplastic compression of the facial nerve. In theory, any lesion of a root, plexus, or nerve may produce myoclonus, although in practice this is rare. The myoclonus is focal or segmental, spontaneous, and non-rhythmic. In the case of such clinical features, cortical, sub-cortical, and spinal myoclonus typically have to be ruled out first, and in the absence of findings in these regions, a peripheral investigation, including structural imaging and electromyography/nerve conduction studies, may be undertaken. In the specific case of hemifacial spasm, the clinical features are sufficiently recognizable that EMG/NCS is not necessary. Brainstem imaging serves only to evaluate for possible compression of the ipsilateral facial nerve; other imaging is not necessary.

Uncertain localization

In clinical practice, localization is often difficult because of the overlapping clinical features. In such cases, a systematic investigation of the entire neuraxis is necessary. Because of the clinical significance of central lesions, it is best to begin with EEG and MRI with and without contrast of the brain and spinal cord. If the myoclonus is focal or segmental,

imaging of the appropriate peripheral root, plexus, or nerve may then be done. In the case in which imaging is not revealing, a lumbar puncture should be considered to investigate infectious or inflammatory causes. Finally, if the myoclonus is peripheral, electromyography and nerve conduction studies may be useful.

Treatment

Treatment of myoclonus is often difficult, requiring multiple medications and producing an incomplete resolution. Of course, if the myoclonus is found to be symptomatic, then the underlying pathology must be addressed. To the extent that treatment for myoclonus is still required after resolving the underlying pathology, or in the case of idiopathic myoclonus, drugs with anti-seizure properties are generally used. A complete review of treatments for myoclonic epilepsy is deferred to a textbook of epilepsy; however, even in the case of non-epileptic cortical or subcortical myoclonus, anti-epileptics are first-line therapy. Sodium valproate, piracetam, and levetiracetam are the commonly used drugs and have the best evidence for improving myoclonus (Table 4.3). If one of these drugs in monotherapy is not sufficient, a benzodiazepine, typically clonazepam, is added, followed by addition of one of the other first-line drugs. Second-line anti-epileptics can be added after that, including zonisamide, topiramate, gabapentin, and lamotrigine. Notably, gabapentin and lamotrigine may each paradoxically worsen (or primarily cause) myoclonus. Serotonergic treatments, namely the selective serotonin reuptake inhibitors (SSRIs), may be used for post-anoxic (Lance–Adams) myoclonus, but they often worsen myoclonus in other cases.

For brainstem or spinal myoclonus, it is conventional to start with benzodiazepines (clonazepam) and then add other anti-epileptics (valproate, levetiracetam, or one of the others mentioned above), although evidence to support this convention is scant. Palatal myoclonus, being focal, may be treated with botulinum toxin into the tensor veli palatini for essential palatal myoclonus or the levator veli palatini for symptomatic. There are also case reports or small series to suggest benefit from tetrabenazine, baclofen, and tizanidine, and one published case report supports the use of gamma hydroxybutyrate (GHB) in alcohol-responsive myoclonus associated

Table 4.3 Pharmaceutical treatment of myoclonus

Localization	First-line treatment	Second-line treatment	Third-line treatment
Cortical or subcortical	Sodium valproate, piracetam, levetiracetam	Benzodiazepines, e.g., clonazepam	Zonisamide, topiramate, gabapentin, and lamotrigine
Brainstem	Benzodiazepines, e.g., clonazepam	Sodium valproate, piracetam, levetiracetam	Zonisamide, topiramate, gabapentin, and lamotrigine
Spinal	Benzodiazepines, e.g., clonazepam	Sodium valproate, piracetam, levetiracetam	Zonisamide, topiramate, gabapentin, and lamotrigine
Peripheral	Botulinum toxin (first- line for any focal myoclonus)	Gabapentin, pregabalin, carbamazepine, oxcarbazepine, topiramate	Benzodiazepines, e.g., clonazepam

with myoclonus-dystonia (DYT-11) or post-anoxic myoclonus. Myoclonus-dystonia is most often due to mutations in the epsilon sarcoglycan gene and presents with myoclonus and dystonia of the neck and upper limbs (e.g., myoclonus with cervical dystonia and/or writer's cramp). The myoclonus, but not the dystonia, is highly responsive to alcohol, and thus also to gamma-hydroxybutyric acid.

Peripheral myoclonus can be effectively treated with botulinum toxin, as can any focal myoclonus. Indeed, because of its limited systemic effects and greater efficacy, botulinum toxin is considered first-line for focal myoclonus. Alternatively, anti-epileptics such as gabapentin, pregabalin, carbamazepine, oxcarbazepine, and topiramate may be tried, along with benzodiazepines. Again, combination therapy is often necessary to produce a clinically meaningful response.

Conclusion

Myoclonus may appear to be a clinically daunting challenge because of the extensive differential diagnosis and the difficulty of treatment. However, with a systematic approach to its localization and diagnosis, it can be a treatable problem. In using a combination of anti-epileptics, benzodiazepines, and, in the case of focal myoclonus, botulinum toxin, clinical improvement can be achieved.

Further Readings

Agarwal P, Frucht SJ. Myoclonus. *Curr Opin Neurol* 2003; **16**: 515–521.

Bakker MJ, van Dijk JG, van den Maagdenberg AM, Tijssen MA. Startle syndromes. *Lancet Neurol* 2006; **5**(6): 513–524.

Brown P. Myoclonus: a practical guide to drug therapy. *CNS Drugs* 1995; **3**: 22–29.

Fahn S. Overview, history and classification of myoclonus. In Myoclonus and Paroxysmal Dyskinesias: Advances in Neurology, vol. **89**, pp. 13–17. Fahn S, Frucht S, Hallett M, Truong DD, eds. Philadelphia: Lippincott Williams Wilkins; 2002.

Fahn S, Marsden CD, Van Woert MH. Definition and classification of myoclonus. *Adv Neurol* 1986; **43**: 1–6.

Frucht S. Myoclonus. *Curr Treatment Options Neurol* 2000; **2**(3): 231–242.

Gordon MF. Toxin and drug-induced myoclonus. *Adv Neurol* 2002; **89**: 49–76.

Hallett M. Myoclonus: phenomenology, etiology, physiology, and treatment. In Principles and Practice of Movement Disorders, pp. 519–540. Fahn S, Jankovic J, eds. Amsterdam: Elsevier; 2007.

Hallett M, Marsden CD, Fahn S. Myoclonus. In Handbook of Clinical Neurology, pp. 609–625. Vinken PJ, Bruyn GW, Klawans HL, eds. Amsterdam: Elsevier Science; 1987.

Hallett M, Shibasaki H. Myoclonus and myoclonic syndromes. In Epilepsy: A Comprehensive Textbook, pp. 2765–2770. Engel J, Jr, Pedley TA, eds. Philadelphia: Lippincott Williams Wilkins; 2008.

Marsden CD, Hallett M, Fahn S. The nosology and pathophysiology of myoclonus. In Movement Disorders, pp. 196–248. Marsden CD, Fahn S, eds. London: Butterworth Scientific; 1982.

Matsumoto J, Hallett M. Startle syndromes. In Movement Disorders, vol. 3, pp. 418–433. Marsden CD, Fahn S, eds. Oxford: Butterworth-Heinemann; 1994.

Monday K, Jankovic J. Psychogenic myoclonus. *Neurol* 1993; **43**: 349–352.

Obeso JA. Therapy of myoclonus. *Clin Neurosci* 1995; **3**(4): 253–257.

Shibasaki H, Hallett M. Electrophysiological studies of myoclonus. *Muscle Nerve* 2005; **31**(2): 157–174.

5

Tics and Tourette Syndrome

David Shprecher, DO, MSc

Cleo Roberts Center, Banner Sun Health Research Institute in Sun City, Arizona, USA

Introduction

Tics are stereotyped, non-rhythmic, repetitive movements (motor tics) or sounds (phonic tics) characterized by premonitory urges and suppressibility. Tourette syndrome is a primary mixed (motor and phonic) tic disorder characterized by childhood onset, an evolving tic repertoire, and intermittent waxing and waning of symptoms. Initial history should focus on ruling out secondary causes of tics and identifying the primary source of disability, including commonly comorbid conditions such as attention deficit disorder, obsessive compulsive disorder, mood disorders, impulsivity, and rage attacks. First-line therapy may include education, behavioral therapies, alpha-2-agonists, topiramate, and tetrabenazine. Antipsychotics are appropriate second line therapies that can to be used even early in the course when severe or self-injurious tics are present. In select cases, botulinum toxin or deep brain stimulation (DBS) may be considered.

Phenomenology and definitions

Tics are stereotyped, repetitive movements or sounds. Motor tics can involve any voluntary muscle group but do not cause vocalizations. Phonic (also known as vocal) tics create an audible sound using orobuccolingual, pharyngeal, or diaphragmatic muscles. Simple motor or phonic tics are brief and involve a single movement or sound. Complex motor tics involve a series of movements and may resemble purposeful movement. Complex phonic tics have linguistic meaning. In contrast to the image portrayed in movies and television, coprolalia (complex phonic tics with profanity) is rare and occurs in a minority of patients. Tics are frequently accompanied by echolalia and echopraxia.

Tics are referred to as "unvoluntary" because the vast majority (90% or more) of affected individuals over the age of 10 report a premonitory urge and can suppress the tic (sometimes for prolonged periods of time). Descriptions in the history may include "building up of tension" or "an irresistible feeling" that occurs if the movement is suppressed. These phenomena are less frequent in younger children, possibly due to an inability of the child to articulate these feelings. Tics may be suggestible, meaning the urge and/or tic are exacerbated by talking about the tics, witnessing similar movements or other people with tics. Tics can persist during all stages of sleep, a feature that is absent in most other hyperkinetic movement disorders.

History and diagnosis

The goals of the history and examination are to rule out secondary causes of tics, identify comorbidities, and clarify the patient's primary sources of concern or disability. It is also useful to clarify up front whether a child is bothered by the tics or whether a parent, educator, or another healthcare provider is initiating the consultation for treatment. While parents' concerns need to be addressed, children should contribute to the history and participate in discussion of the treatment plan.

Non-Parkinsonian Movement Disorders, First Edition. Edited by Deborah A. Hall and Brandon R. Barton.
© 2017 John Wiley & Sons, Ltd. Published 2017 by John Wiley & Sons, Ltd.
Companion website: www.wiley.com/go/hall/non-parkinsonian_movement_disorders

Primary versus secondary tic disorders

A primary tic disorder is a condition where there is no underlying medical condition or pharmacological trigger that explains the presence of tics. Primary tic disorders are categorized based on duration, age of onset, and the presence of motor or phonic tics (Table 5.1). Tics that last less than one year are classified as transient tic disorder (with childhood onset) or tic disorder not otherwise specified (with onset in adulthood). Chronic motor tic disorder, chronic phonic tic disorder, and Tourette syndrome (TS) each last at least one year. TS begins in childhood (before age 18 by DSM-IV criteria or before age 21 by TS study group criteria). It is characterized by multiple motor and phonic tics. Tic severity waxes and wanes, and new tics appear over time.

SCIENCE REVISITED

Pathophysiology of TS

Evidence for TS as a neurodevelopmental disorder:

Epidemiological	Transient tics and OCS are common in childhood
Genetic	Bilineal inheritance of TS, OCS, and ADHD
Neuropathological	Abnormal density of basal ganglia GABAergic neurons
MRI	Reduced caudate volumes
rs-f-MRI	Immature functional connectivity patterns

Evidence for TS as a neurotransmitter disorder of dopamine and GABA systems:

PET	Excessive dopamine release in response to amphetamine challenge
	Increased striatal dopaminergic nerve terminals (DAT and VMAT2)
	Abnormal basal ganglia/limbic circuit GABA receptor densities

ADHD = Attention deficit hyperactivity disorder; OCS = Obsessive compulsive symptoms; DAT = dopamine transporter; GABA = gama-amino-butyric acid; Rs-f-MRI = resting state functional MRI; VMAT2 = type 2 vesicular monoamine transporter.

Patients with secondary tics often have a more limited tic repertoire, may not evolve into new tics over time, and are less likely to endorse premonitory urge or suppressibility. Secondary causes of tics are outlined in Table 5.2. Tics are more common in the setting of autistic spectrum disorders and pervasive developmental delay, and are therefore considered by some experts to be secondary in this situation. However, according to the Diagnostic Statistical Manual-IV-Text Revision (DSM-IV-TR) criteria, a separate diagnosis for a primary tic disorder should still be rendered. Antipsychotic medications can rarely cause tardive tics. Commonly, exacerbation of an underlying tic disorder is seen if the drug is withdrawn too quickly. Such withdrawal-emergent tics can be mitigated by reintroduction and more gradual weaning of the antipsychotic. Stimulants including cocaine and amphetamine can transiently induce tics. Because they may also precipitate or exacerbate tics in a primary tic disorder, parents may mistakenly assume that the tic disorder was caused by the drug. It is important to emphasize that methylphenidate has been shown to improve symptoms (and not precipitate tics) in those patients with Tourette syndrome and comorbid ADHD. Therefore, it should not be withheld from those requiring ADHD treatment. Traumatic brain injury or stroke (commonly involving the caudate nucleus) can cause adult-onset tic disorders. When a primary tic disorder begins in adulthood, there is usually a personal or family history of obsessive compulsive disorder (OCD), attention deficit disorder (ADD), or tic disorders. When such history is absent, adult-onset tics should prompt additional investigation (including neuroimaging) to consider secondary causes.

Tic subtypes

Motor tics need to be distinguished from other hyperkinetic movement disorders (see Tips and Tricks). Motor tic subtyping may seem confusing at first but can guide therapy. Rapid or ballistic tics are sometimes referred to as "myoclonic tics." Tics with sustained postures (commonly of neck or facial muscles) are referred to as "dystonic tics." When painful or socially disfiguring, myoclonic and dystonic tics may respond to botulinum toxin injection of the muscles involved. Tics with compulsive qualities (a need to even things out, touch a certain number of times, or get a "just right" feeling to the movement) are called "compulsive tics." These may require use of serotonergic drugs or atypical

Table 5.1 Primary tic disorders*

DSM-IV-TR diagnostic criteria for Tourette syndrome
Multiple motor and one or more phonic tics have been present for at least some of the time.
Tics occur many times a day, nearly every day or intermittently for a period of more than 1 year, and during this period there was never a tic-free period of more than three consecutive months
Onset is before age 18
Tics are not due to the direct physiological effects of a substance or general medical condition
DSM-IV-TR diagnostic criteria for chronic motor or phonic tic disorder
Single or multiple motor or phonic tics, but not both, have been present at some time
Tics occur many times a day, nearly every day or intermittently for a period of more than 1 year, and during this period there was never a tic-free period of more than three consecutive months
Remaining above criteria for Tourette syndrome are met
DSM-IV-TR diagnostic criteria for transient tic disorder
Single or multiple motor or phonic tics, but not both, have been present at some time
Tics occur many times a day, nearly every day for at least 4 weeks, but for no longer than 12 consecutive months
Remaining above criteria for Tourette syndrome are met

*If none of the criteria are met (as in case of an adult onset primary tic disorder), a diagnosis of *tic disorder* NOS (not otherwise specified) is rendered.
Source: Diagnostic and Statistical Manual of Mental Disorders, 2013. Reproduced with permission of APA.

Table 5.2 Secondary Tic Disorders

Disease Category	Differential Diagnosis
Autoimmune	Demyelinating disease
Developmental	Autistic spectrum disorders, pervasive developmental delay
Drug-induced	Antipsychotics (tardive/withdrawal-emergent), amphetamines, cocaine, lamotrigine
Chromosomal disorders	Beckwith-Weidemann, Down or Klinefelter syndromes, Fragile X syndrome
CAG repeat disorders	Dentatorubral pallidoluysian atrophy, Huntington disease
Genetic mutations	Lesch–Nyhan syndrome, mitochondrial disorders, neuroacanthocytosis, neurodegeneration with brain iron accumulation, tuberous sclerosis, Wilson disease
Infectious (encephalitis)	Mycoplasma pneumonia, Lyme disease, rubella, syphilis, herpes simplex virus (HSV)
Post-infectious	Post-HSV, Sydenham chorea (post-streptococcal)
Trauma/vascular	Traumatic brain injury, stroke
Toxic	Carbon monoxide

antipsychotics similar to those used for classic OCD. Those tics that involve an irresistible urge to complete an inappropriate or destructive act (shouting a racial slur, breaking things, hitting or stabbing self or others) are called "impulsive tics." Such impulsive tics, or ballistic tics, may lead to cervical injury (particularly radiculopathy or myelopathy) and need to be addressed as a medically urgent or emergent condition. In such cases, more aggressive use of antipsychotics, dopamine depletors, and nonmedical (behavioral) therapies is indicated and inpatient treatment may be necessary.

★ TIPS AND TRICKS

Key features differentiating tics from other hyperkinetic disorders

Hyperkinetic movement	Stereotyped?	Rhythmic?	Premonitory sensations?	Suppressible?	Continuous?	Persistence in sleep
Tic	Yes	No	Yes	Yes	No	Often
Myoclonus	Often	Rarely	Sometimes	No	No	Sometimes
Dystonia	Sometimes	No	No	No	Sometimes	No
Chorea	No	No	No	No	Yes	No
Stereotypy	Yes	Yes	No	Yes	Sometimes	No
Tremor	Yes	Yes	No	No	Often	No
Psychogenic	Sometimes	Rarely	Sometimes	Sometimes	Sometimes	Sometimes

Comorbidities and heredity

Obsessive compulsive behaviors (OCB) or frank OCD and ADD are seen much more frequently in primary tic disorders than in the general population. A bilineal inheritance pattern has been described, where 25% of individuals with TS have two parents with OCB, ADD, and/or tics (and 80% have at least one parent with one of more of these symptoms). Therefore, OCB/ADD/tics are frequently referred to as "TS spectrum" disorders or the "TS triad." In addition to this triad, history should also cover other common comorbidities including anxiety disorders, depression, impulsivity, and rage attacks.

Prognosis

Several prospective studies have reported that a majority of children with TS will experience considerable improvement in tic symptoms by late adolescence and early adulthood. However, tics can still be recognized by an experienced clinician in half of young adults who feel they are "tic free." Furthermore, recrudescence of symptoms may occur in adulthood, even after long intervals of apparent remission. ADD is frequently a lifelong disorder, and prognosis of OCD in TS is still unclear.

Key predictors of persistent disability or poor quality of life in adulthood may include global tic severity, severity of phonic tics, presence of copralalia, and severity of comorbidities. Discussions about prognosis should emphasize that TS is a lifelong disorder, which can be managed with a good outcome in the majority of patients. It is important to avoid appearing too dismissive ("don't worry, you'll grow out of it") in these discussions, and to arrange clinical follow-up on at least an annual basis.

Management

Initial treatment decisions are guided by the primary source of disability or concern to the patient. If the child is not impacted by the tics or comorbidities, and neurological evaluation is not suggestive of other secondary causes, then counseling should focus on education and prognosis. Video 5.3 demonstrates a child with a simple motor tic (wrinkling the nose) whose treatment was simple reassurance of the parent.

Education

The Tourette Syndrome Association (TSA), http://tsa-usa.org/, is a valuable source of educational resources and support for individuals with primary tic disorders (as well as schools and healthcare providers). Social stigma, bullying, and need for school or workplace accommodations must be addressed through education. TSA youth ambassadors are also available to speak at a child's school on these topics. Typical accommodations at school include seating toward the back of the room (to make tics less noticeable to others) and a separate room for testing (so the patient is not distracted by trying to suppress tics). Individuals can also request equal opportunity and workplace accommodations under the United States Individuals with Disabilities Act.

Treatment of OCD

Obsessions and compulsions in TS are usually more egosyntonic than pure OCD (i.e., they are more consistent with the individual's personality and preferences); this fact can guide non-medication insight-oriented therapy. They often involve obsessive fears that something bad will happen to the patient or to others, which may lead to secondary insomnia. While cognitive behavioral therapy (CBT) can be effective for OCD in this context, it is important to emphasize that serotonin reuptake inhibitors (SSRIs) are often effective, but the tricylcic antidepressant (TCA) clomipramine may be necessary for severe cases. If OCD remits with treatment, some individuals are eventually able to wean successfully off medication. In cases refractory to first-line treatments, atypical antipsychotics or the TCA clomipramine can be considered.

Treatment ADD/ADHD

In mild cases, behavioral interventions or the use of alpha-2-agonists can be helpful. Methylphenidate has been shown to be safe, well tolerated, and effective in TS with comorbid ADHD. While amphetamine salts can lead to tic exacerbation in some patients, they are often well tolerated and effective in those who do not respond to methylphenidate. Atomoxetine and buproprion can also be considered for individuals who do not tolerate stimulants. TCAs can improve both tics and ADHD. However, given reports of desipramine-associated pediatric sudden cardiac death, children must be screened according to American Heart Association guidelines before initiating treatment, with dose changes, and periodically thereafter. Any cardiac disorder, family history of long QT syndrome or sudden cardiac death, electrocardiogram abnormalities, or new symptoms of potential cardiogenic origin should preclude its use or warrant discontinuation and pediatric cardiology consultation.

Treatment of tics

The goal of tic management is to mitigate the impact of tics on a patient's quality of life and chances of academic or vocational success. It is important to emphasize that treatment will lessen tic severity or impact but is unlikely to abolish tics (Table 5.3). For patients who are self-conscious about even mild tics, CBT to address self-image (and, if present, OCD or personality disorders) must be considered.

Habit reversal therapy (HRT) is a non-medical approach that focuses on identification of premonitory urge and substitution of a more subtle competing movement or sound. This approach can be considered when certain tics in an individual's repertoire are disruptive or painful. Video 5.2 shows an individual with a painful complex motor tic of the right arm, and failure to respond to oral medications, where non-medical approaches were indicated. Comprehensive behavioral interventional therapy (CBIT) is a nonmedical therapy that combines HRT with individualized coping strategies. These include mitigation of factors that exacerbate tics and education of family members in order to minimize impact of tics on home life. CBIT can be effective for children and adults, but the benefit is less clear for those with ADHD. Lack of trained personnel and failure of insurance to cover psychological treatments for TS both pose barriers to this type of therapy. The TSA offers courses and educational materials to clinicians interested in learning to administer CBIT.

The alpha-2-agonists can have limited benefit for mild tics, and can also have mild benefit for comorbid ADHD and impulsivity. Of these, clonidine and guanfacine are commonly used. Clonidine, which may be associated with weight gain, usually requires dosing three to four times per day. Guanfacine may be started with bedtime dosing and titrated to twice per day in those who experience daytime wearing off. Main side effects leading to discontinuation of either drug are irritability or sedation. Long-acting oral guanfacine and clonidine patch are available, but it remains unclear whether they have specific advantages in tic treatment given their cost.

Topiramate has emerged as a potential treatment for tic suppression, which can also be a good choice for those with comorbid headaches. It is important to warn about risk of heat stroke due to reduced sweating, and to avoid topiramate in those with personal/family history of nephrolithiasis or glaucoma.

Tetrabenazine is a dopamine depletor that may be considered when moderate to severe tics are the primary problem. It generally lacks the weight gain associated with antipsychotics. It requires careful monitoring during titration for sedation, depression, anxiety, or akathisia. Neuroleptic malignant syndrome is extremely rare with dopamine depletors, but is still considered a serious potential side effect.

Table 5.3 Treatment options for tic disorders

Class	Preferred agents	Special indications	Common side effects	Rare/serious side effects
Education	Clinician counseling, TSA materials	Always indicated	—	—
Nonmedical	HRT, CBIT	Appropriate targets for therapy	—	—
Alpha-2-agonists	Guanfacine	Mild tics, Comorbid ADHD	Sedation, dizziness	Irritability, hypotension, mania
Tricyclic	Desipramine	Comorbid ADHD, mood disorder, OCD	Sedation, constipation	Sudden death
Antiepileptics	Topiramate	Comorbid headache or neck tics	Hypohydrosis, sedation, weight loss	Acute angle closure glaucoma nephrolithiasis
Dopamine depletors	Tetrabenazine	Moderate to severe tics	Fatigue, Sedation	Akathisia, depression, NMS
Typical antipsychotics	Risperidone, Fluphenazine	Severe tics, impulticis, rage attacks, tic status	Sedation, weight gain	Tardive dyskinesia, NMS
Atypical antipsychotics	Aripiprazole	Severe tics, refractory mood disorder/OCD	Sedation, weight gain	Tardive dyskinesia, NMS
Benzodiazepines	Clonazepam	Comorbid anxiety	Sedation	Addiction
Botulinum toxin	Type A	Dystonic/myoclonic tics; severe complex phonic tics	Dry eyes, dry mouth, focal weakness	Botulism
Surgical	DBS	Refractory to all other measures	Anxiety, apathy, depression, nausea, paresthesias.	Infection, hemorrhage

CBIT: cognitive behavioral intervention therapy; DBS: deep brain stimulation; HRT: habit reversal therapy; NMS: neuroleptic malignant syndrome; OCD: obsessive compulsive disorder; TSA: Tourette Syndrome Association.
Source: Shprecher 2014. Reproduced with permission of Wolters Kluwer Health.

Antipsychotics can be considered when first-line therapies fail, but may need to be used urgently in cases of "malignant TS."

⚠ CAUTION

Malignant TS is a condition where frequency or severity of the tics puts the patient at serious risk of harming oneself, others, or property. Examples include ballistic neck tics (which can cause myelopathy or radiculopathy); tics that involve injury to self or others (hitting, stabbing, eye gouging); impulsive tics (requiring the individual to break things or utter contextually offensive words or phrases); or severe copralalia. Stronger agents including antipsychotics (and botulinum toxin where appropriate) must be considered early in this context, and there should be low threshold to hospitalize the patient to ensure rapid optimization of therapy.

Though tardive dyskinesia is rare, it has been reported in TS, making appropriate counseling and monitoring mandatory. Neuroleptic malignant syndrome is also a serious potential side effect of all antipsychotics. Haloperidol and pimozide are the only FDA approved treatments for Tourette syndrome, but they should generally be avoided. Risperidone and Fluphenazine are better tolerated, equally effective, and do not prolong QT interval to the extent of pimozide. For those who fail to respond to these typical antipsychotics, or those requiring second-line treatments for OCD or depression, aripiprazole can be considered.

Benzodiazepines such as clonazepam have been used with some success in open label reports. They can be considered when anxiety is a factor precipitating tic exacerbations. Counseling and monitoring for dependence and sedation are mandatory with this class. While there are some data to suggesting that tetra-hydrocannabinol may reduce tics or comorbid anxiety, the safety and legality of regular marijuana use remains unclear. Other agents including baclofen, dopamine agonists (ropinirole or pramipexole), and levetiracetam have conflicting data and generally do not perform better than a placebo.

Botulinum toxin injections can be effective for simple motor or even complex phonic tics. The benefit may last longer than typically seen for dystonia (where average duration is three months), and in some cases the tic may not return (but new ones may evolve over time). Case examples of successful treatment include sustained eye closure, facial grimacing ("dystonic" tic), or painful, rapid ("myoclonic") neck tics. One report showed improvement of phonic tics with coprolalia following laryngeal muscle injections. Most neurologists do not have sufficient training to inject these muscles, and should refer to an otolaryngologist for the procedure.

When all other treatment approaches fail, deep brain stimulation may be considered as a promising, but still experimental, therapy. Consensus criteria from a TSA expert panel recommend that (1) DBS only be performed in adults, (2) tic severity remain elevated (at least 35/100 on the Yale global tic severity score) for a minimum of one year, (3) the patient have received optimized treatment for at least six months and failed all relevant conventional medical and non-medical/behavioral treatments, (4) the patient has a primary tic disorder, (5) the patient does not have comorbidities that make DBS unsafe, and (6) psychosocial factors must not preclude likelihood of close follow-up. Ideal target, predictors of outcome, and impact on comorbidities from DBS still remain unclear. In order to answer these questions, the TSA has created an International Registry for DBS Research in Tourette Syndrome (http://dbs.tsa-usa.org/).

Individualized therapy and the art of medicine

Tics are far more common than was once thought, with between 0.5% and 1% of the population meeting diagnostic criteria for TS, and up to 20% of children having at least transient tics. There are now extensive legal, educational, behavioral, and medical options for TS management, but none is curative. Because TS is a lifelong condition, individual self-image and acceptance of differences ("not being normal") are necessary components to successfully coping with the disorder. Once an individual moves beyond the personal stigma of the disorder, he or she can then become empowered to partner with their clinicians in living with TS.

Further Readings

Cavanna AE, Servo S, Monaco F, Robertson MM. The behavioral spectrum of Gilles de la Tourette syndrome. *J Neuropsy Clin Neurosci* 2009; **21**: 1; 13–23.

Cheung MY, Shahed BS, Jankovic J. Malignant Tourette syndrome. *Mov Disord* 2007; **22** (12): 1743–1750.

Felling RJ, Singer HS. Neurobiology of Tourette syndrome: current status and need for further investigation. *J Neurosci* 2011; **31**(35): 12387–12395.

Hanna PA, Janjua FN, Contant CF, Jankovic J. Bilineal transmission in Tourette syndrome. *Neurology* 1999; **53**; 813.

Hassan N, Cavanna AE. The prognosis of Tourette syndrome: implications for clinical practice. *Func Neurol* 2012; **27**(1): 23–27.

Jankovic J, Kurlan R. Tourette syndrome: evolving concepts. *Mov Disord* 2011; **26**(6): 1149–1156.

Lerner A, Bagic A, Simmons JM, Mari Z, Bonne O, Xu B, Kazuba D, Herscovitch P, Carson RE, Murphy DL, Drevets WC, Hallett M. Widespread abnormality of the gamma-aminobutyric acid-ergic system in Tourette syndrome. *Brain* 2012; **135**: 1926–1936.

McNaught KS, Mink JW. Advances in understanding and treatment of Tourette syndrome. *Nat Rev Neurol* 2011; **7**: 667–676.

Mink JD, Walkup J, Frey KA, Como P, Cath D, DeLong MR, Erenberg G, Jankovic J, Juncos J, Leckman JF, Swerdlow N, Visser-Vandewalle V, Vitek JL. Patient selection and assessment recommendations for deep brain stimulation in Tourette syndrome. *Mov Disord* 2006: **21**(11): 1831–1838.

Piacentini J, Woods DW, Scahill L, Wilhelm S, Peterson AL, Chang S, Ginsburg GS, Deckersbach T, Dziura J, Levi-Pearl S, Walkup JT. Behavior therapy for children with Tourette disorder: a randomized controlled trial. *JAMA* 2010; **303**(19): 1929–1937.

Robinson MM. The Gilles de la Tourette syndrome: the current status. *Arch Dis Child Educ Pract Ed* 2012; **97** (5): 166–175.

Viswanathan A, Jimenez-Shahed J, Carvallo JF, Jankovic J. Deep brain stimulation for Tourette syndrome: target selection. *Stereotact Func Neurosurg* 2012; **90**: 213–224.

6

Chorea, Athetosis, and Ballism

Rohit Dhall, MBBS, MSPH

Parkinson's Institute and Clinical Center, Sunnyvale, California, USA

Introduction

The term "chorea" is derived from the Greek word *choreomania*, which was coined by Paracelsus to describe what was believed to be a curse sent by Saint John the Baptist, or Saint Vitus. Choreomania was documented to have affected thousands of individuals between the fourteenth and seventeenth centuries. The affected individuals would dance wildly (often in large groups) until they collapsed from exhaustion. It is now thought that this dancing mania was a form of mass hysteria. Thomas Sydenham used the term "St. Vitus dance" to describe chorea seen in what is now his eponymous disease, although this is unrelated to the original use of the term.

Chorea is defined as involuntary, irregular, arrhythmic, non-patterned, purposeless movements that flow randomly from one body part to another. It is the hallmark movement disorder present in Huntington disease but can also be seen in several other inherited neurodegenerative disorders, as well as in acquired disorders from a myriad of causes, whether structural, immune-mediated, or metabolic. When chorea affects the proximal extremities, choreic movements assume a higher amplitude, violent look, and are termed ballism. Non-patterned, writhing movements generally affecting the distal extremities are called athetosis. Ballism can occur secondary to stroke or from damage to pallido-subthalamic pathways from other causes. Athetosis is commonly seen in cerebral palsy, but can be seen in the setting of primary dystonia as well as in combination with choreic disorders.

Chorea

Definition

The term "chorea" is used to describe involuntary movements that are irregular and unpredictable in temporal and anatomic distribution. Patients with chorea commonly demonstrate other features including motor impersistence (the inability to sustain voluntary muscle contraction), exaggerated gestures that are caused by superimposition of chorea onto voluntary movements, and an irregular, dance-like gait. Patients can usually temporarily and partially consciously suppress chorea, and choreic movements in one body part can be brought out by asking the patient to perform complex motor tasks elsewhere in the body. Although tone can be hard to test, it is usually reduced. Tendon jerks may assume a "hung up" characteristic (prolonged relaxation of the limb to neutral position after reflex testing).

Pathophysiology

The pathophysiology of chorea is not well understood and may differ between Huntington disease (HD) and other choreic syndromes. Evaluation of spinal cord function in HD reveals reduced reciprocal inhibition between agonist and antagonistic muscles, likely due to abnormalities in descending control of the cord by the basal ganglia. In HD there is a reduction in cortical somatosensory evoked potential (SEP) amplitude, but this reduction is not seen in Sydenham chorea (SC). There is also a

Non-Parkinsonian Movement Disorders, First Edition. Edited by Deborah A. Hall and Brandon R. Barton.
© 2017 John Wiley & Sons, Ltd. Published 2017 by John Wiley & Sons, Ltd.
Companion website: www.wiley.com/go/hall/non-parkinsonian_movement_disorders

reduction in amplitude of movement-related cortical potentials in HD, but not in chorea due to neuroacanthocytosis. These differences suggest that in HD the cortical activity needed to produce volitional movements is abnormal, while in other choreas it may be preserved. Additionally, impaired activity of primary and non-primary motor cortices may be responsible for the comorbid bradykinesia in HD.

In the neurologist's office, choreiform movements are commonly observed as levodopa-induced dyskinesias in Parkinson disease patients.

HD is the most common cause of inherited chorea, but when considering the differential diagnosis of slowly progressive adult-onset chorea, it is useful to separate potential diagnoses into autosomal dominant disorders, autosomal recessive disorders, X-linked disorders, and acquired conditions. Table 6.1 provides differential diagnosis of chorea. In the setting of HD, neuroacanthocytosis syndromes, and SC, similar principles may be applied to the management of other causes of autoimmune or acquired chorea.

Table 6.1 Differential diagnosis of chorea

Inherited causes	Vascular/metabolic/endocrine/immunological causes	Other acquired causes
Autosomal dominant: Progressive: • Huntington disease (HD) • Dentatorubro-pallidoluysian atrophy (DRPLA) • Huntington disease like syndrome type 1 (HDL1) • HDL2 • Spinocerebellar ataxia type 17 (SCA 17) (aka HDL 4) • SCA 1, 2, and 3 • Neuroferritinopathy • Fahr disease Non-progressive: • Benign hereditary chorea • Paroxysmal kinesigenic chorea **Autosomal recessive:** • Chorea-acanthocytosis • Pantothenate kinase associated neurodegeneration (PKAN) • Ataxia telangiectasia • Wilson disease • HDL 3 **X-Linked** • McLeod syndrome	**Vascular** (50% non-inherited chorea): • Infarction or hemorrhage (basal ganglia, subthalamic nucleus, posterior cerebral artery territory) • Arteriovenous malformations • Epidural or subdural hematoma • Polycythemia vera • Migraine **Metabolic:** Inherited: • Lesch–Nyhan syndrome • Aminoacidopathies • Porphyria • Lysosomal storage disorders Acquired: • Renal failure • Hepatic disease • Kernicterus • Hyponatremia **Endocrine:** • Chorea gravidarum • Hyperthyroidism • Hyperglycemia/hypoglycemia • Hypocalcemia • Hypomagnesemia • Hypo/hyperparathyroidism **Immunological:** • Systemic lupus erythematosus (SLE) • Antiphospholipid syndrome • Polyarteritis nodosa • Behcet's disease • Churg-Strauss syndrome • Henoch–Schonlein purpura	**Drug induced:** Dopaminergic modulation: • Levodopa and dopamine agonists • Neuroleptics Steroids: • Oral contraceptives • Anabolic steroids Noradrenergic modulation: • Cocaine • Amphetamines • Theophyline and aminophyline Anticonvulsants: • Dilantin • Valproate • Carbamazepine Others: • Thyroid replacement **Infectious:** • Human immunodeficiency virus • Viral (various viral encephalitides) • Neurosyphilis • Borreliosis • Tuberculosis **Post-infectious:** • Sydenham chorea (post-streptococcal) • Post-encephalitic

Huntington disease

Definition

HD is an autosomal dominant neurodegenerative disorder that usually presents in adulthood with abnormal movements, cognitive decline, behavioral disturbances, and progressive functional decline. The HD gene is located near the telomere of the short arm of chromosome 4 with the mutant gene containing an excess of CAG repeats that code for a polyglutamine stretch in the product, huntingtin. It is thought that the HD phenotype is a result of an abnormal gain of function.

Epidemiology

HD is seen throughout the world, with a prevalence rate of 2 to 10 per 100,000. There are considerable geographical differences in prevalence, with a much lower prevalence in Japan and among South African blacks and a much higher prevalence in the Lake Maracaibo region in Venezuela. Age at onset is distributed normally around 40 years for the majority, with juvenile HD (onset before age 20) accounting for 5–10% cases. It may be difficult to date the onset of adult HD, with some subtle signs seen up to five years or more before clinical diagnosis in frequently followed high-risk cohorts. Age of onset is inversely related to CAG repeat length, with repeat lengths over age 60 associated with disease onset before age 21. Age at onset in families is characterized by the phenomenon of anticipation, where the CAG repeat length expands during transmission and may lead to an earlier onset of symptoms (and higher symptom severity) in offspring who inherited the mutant gene through paternal lineage. The relationship between CAG repeat length and the clinical progression of the illness remains inconclusive, and there is poor correlation between the phenotype and CAG repeat length, except for juvenile-onset HD where it often exceeds 55 repeats. Duration of disease varies around a mean of age 19.

Pathophysiology

The characteristic neuropathological features of HD include atrophy of the caudate and neuronal loss and astrocytosis in the striatum. The neuronal loss is selective for medium-sized spiny neurons containing GABA/enkephalin and GABA/substance P. The expanded polyglutamine (CAG) stretch leads to a conformational change and abnormal protein-protein interactions. The N-terminal of mutant huntingtin can bind to transcription factors and lead to a reduction in acetylated histones and decreased gene expression, which may adversely affect neuronal survival. Other mechanisms may include altered excitotoxicity, impaired mitochondrial function, and abnormalities in gene transcription (Figure 6.1)

Clinical features

Chorea is the prototypical movement disorder of HD, and initially may pass for fidgetiness. People often try to blend their chorea into purposeful movements, which is termed "parakinesis." Later in the disease, these continuous, irregular, and fleeting movements may change into severe, uncontrollable flailing movements (ballism) of extremities, interfering with feeding, sitting, or sleeping. However, chorea is not usually disabling to the individual. With progression of HD, progressive parkinsonian signs such as bradykinesia, rigidity, and postural instability develop. Mild dystonia, in addition to chorea, gives rise to choreoathetosis, and use of antidopaminergic drugs may increase the likelihood of dystonia. Sustained dystonic posturing may cause contractures and immobility. Bradykinesia and dystonia are the heralding features of juvenile-onset HD (Westphal variant of HD). Rigidity and tremor may be seen early in the juvenile-onset variant, with epilepsy, conspicuous cerebellar dysfunction, and early dementia being more common than in adult HD.

Eye movement abnormalities are among the earliest motor signs, with slow, uncoordinated voluntary initiation of saccades, disrupted smooth pursuit and impersistence. Initiation of internally generated saccades is harder than that of externally triggered ones, suggesting relative sparing of parietal lobe-superior collicular pathways in the setting of extensive frontostriatal circuit dysfunction. Optokinetic nystagmus is impaired in both vertical and horizontal directions, with vertical movements impaired earlier in the course. Dysarthria may occur at any stage and may severely limit communication. Dysphagia tends to be prominent in the terminal stages and aspiration is a common cause of death.

Cognitive impairment occurs in all patients, but the rate of progression varies considerably. Dementia in HD has been characterized as a "subcortical dementia" and features of bradyphrenia, attentional and sequencing impairments, occur in the absence of cortical deficits (at least early in

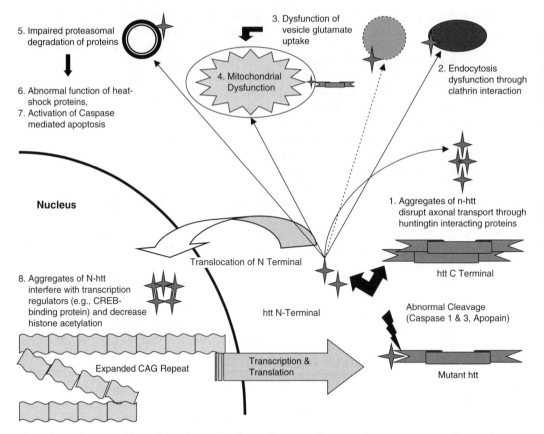

Figure 6.1 Science revisited: Possible mechanisms of neuronal injury in HD and therapeutic targets.
Wild-type huntingtin protein (htt) is predominantly cytoplasmic and probably subserves multiple functions including vesicle transport, cytoskeletal anchoring, endocytosis mediated by clathrin, and axonal transport. Htt may be transported into the nucleus and have a role in transcriptional regulation. Misfolded htt from the HD mutation accumulates in the cytoplasm. Ultimately, toxicity may be caused by mutant full-length htt or by cleaved N-terminal fragments, which may form soluble monomers, oligomers, or large insoluble aggregates. Therapeutic targets include: (1) treatment with brain-derived neurotrophic factor (BDNF) may improve trophic support and help rescue neurons, (3) N-methyl-D-aspartate (NMDA) receptor antagonists may exert protective effect by reducing excitotoxicity, (4) coenzyme Q10 (CoQ10) and nicotinamide may improve energy metabolism (although CoQ10 has not shown clinical benefit or disease modification) and cell survival, (5) rapamycin may enhance clearance of abnormal protein fragments, (7) Caspase inhibitors may improve cell survival, and (8) histone deacetylase (HDAC) inhibitors like sodium butyrate may slow neurodegeneration.

the course) such as aphasia, apraxia, and agnosia. Cognitive inflexibility and loss of executive function may be related to frontostriatal circuit dysfunction. Insight and central language function may remain preserved, even in the advanced stages.

A wide range of behavioral and psychiatric problems have been recognized in patients with HD, with affective disorders and frequent personality changes. Aggression and irritability are the common

behavioral changes seen, along with anxiety and apathy. Depression is an important and potentially treatable problem and can be seen in up to 50% of patients, with an additional 5–10% having mania as well. There is an increased rate of suicide in individuals with HD and their asymptomatic siblings. Psychosis is also more common in HD than in the general population, and there appears to be a familial influence on the incidence of psychosis.

Box 6.1 Clinical features of HD*

Motor	Cognitive	Psychiatric
• Chorea • Motor impersistence • Trouble with generating saccades and fine movements • Dysarthria/dysphagia • Bradykinesia and rigidity • Postural instability and ataxia • Dystonia • Tourettism and tics • Myoclonus • Weight loss	• Attentional disturbances • Impaired judgment • Executive dysfunction • Personality changes • Memory impairment (recent) • Apraxia • Impaired visuospatial processing • Dementia	• Dysphoria/depression • Agitation and Irritability • Obsessive compulsive behavior • Anxiety • Apathy • Disinhibition • Euphoria • Hallucinations and delusions

* See the Video 6.1 and Video 6.2 for several characteristic motor features.

Diagnosis

HD diagnosis should be considered in anyone presenting with (adult-onset) chorea, or juvenile-onset dystonia or parkinsonism. Diagnostic suspicion is increased by the presence of behavioral and psychiatric disturbances, which may be subtle at onset, and may need to be elicited by direct questioning (see Box 6.1 for a list of symptoms). Patients may be unaware of these symptoms and information should be corroborated by interviewing family members if possible. A psychiatric family history, including history of psychotic disorder, dementia, and suicide should also be obtained. Routine laboratory tests are unrevealing, and neuroimaging may be normal early in the course, or may show striatal or cortical atrophy (Figure 6.2).

Diagnosis is established by DNA testing, which has been available since 1993. The testing can identify gene carriers before or after the onset of clinically manifest disease. Pre-symptomatic gene testing should only be carried out in association with genetic counseling, preferably also in combination with a psychologist and a neurologist with supportive care and counseling before and after testing.

☆ TIPS AND TRICKS

Gene testing in HD

In HD, the CAG repeat length in the huntingtin gene is ≥36. Intermediate repeat lengths of 27–35 repeats (with normal being <27 repeats) do not cause HD, but they can undergo expansion during meiosis, especially with paternal transmission. Tests for CAG repeat length in HD are commercially available in the US. Testing is appropriate for establishing diagnosis in symptomatic patients.

Management of HD includes counseling patients and their families as well as at-risk individuals about undergoing gene testing. A valid reason for pre-symptomatic testing includes family planning, but testing merely out of curiosity should not be done casually. Pre-symptomatic and at-risk individuals should be given the opportunity to discuss the risks and benefits of testing and be provided psychological and social support in the context of genetic testing. CAG repeat length should be disclosed to patients (if requested) only after appropriate counseling. The availability of pre-implantation diagnosis with in vitro fertilization (IVF) and embryo selection methods may also inform the decisions of couples at-risk wanting to undergo pre-symptomatic testing. Recommended guidelines for genetic testing are available through the World Federation of Neurology and the International Huntington Association and through the Huntington Disease Society of America (HDSA).

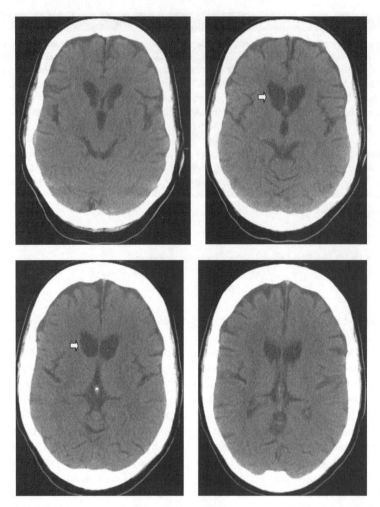

Figure 6.2 Characteristic caudate atrophy in HD. Serial 5 mm computed tomography (CT) sections through the midbrain and level of diencephalon showing prominent atrophy of the caudate nucleus. Cortical atrophy is also appreciated. This CT was obtained six years after initial presentation of HD.

Therapeutic strategies

There are no therapies that delay onset or slow progression of HD, and treatment remains symptomatic.

1) *Treatment of motor impairment:* It is important to remember that chorea may not cause serious disability and that anti-choreic therapy (especially when aggressive) may have adverse effects. Hence, in general, it is not recommended to treat chorea unless it is causing disabling functional and social impairment. Dopamine receptor blockers and dopamine-depleting medications are the mainstay of treatment of chorea in HD. Tetrabenazine reversibly binds to type-2 vesicular monoamine transporter and causes central monoamine depletion. It is the only agent approved by the FDA to treat chorea in HD. Commonly reported adverse effects include sedation, depression, anxiety, insomnia and akathisia. Additionally, function may worsen from worsening parkinsonism and dysphagia. Neuroleptics are used frequently: atypical antipsychotics may reduce chorea with fewer extrapyramidal side effects than typical antipsychotics. Amantadine (300–400 mg/d) and remacemide, both NMDA blockers, and riluzole (at a 200 mg/d dose), a corticostriate glutamate release inhibitor, may

also improve chorea. The recent AAN guidelines for management of chorea are summarized in Table 6.2.

Pharmacological management of HD chorea
The decision to treat HD chorea with dopamine receptor blocking or dopamine depleting medications should largely be based on functional disability from choreiform movements. Social embarrassment is also a consideration. It is advisable to use the lowest effective doses of tetrabenazine or antipsychotics for chorea management. Tetrabenazine is started at 12.5 mg once daily, and increased gradually to 3 times a day, with a maximum dose of 100 mg/d over 8 to 12 weeks. When using tetrabenazine doses above 50 mg/d, consider genotyping for cytochrome P450 family 2, subfamily D, polypeptide 6 (CYP2D6) activity, and avoid doses >50 mg/d in poor metabolizers. Paroxetine and fluoxetine inhibit CYP2D6 and may necessitate tetrabenazine dose reduction with concomitant use. Periodically reassess (and if necessary, reduce) therapy with these agents, since parkinsonism, dysphagia, and gait impairment may evolve and become prominent with advancing disease, with less chorea, and tetrabenazine may worsen these symptoms.

2) *Symptomatic treatment of cognitive/behavioral impairment:* Cholinesterase inhibitors have been studied with the hopes of improving cognitive function in HD and results for studies using rivastigmine and donepezil have been disappointing.

Venlafaxine, a mixed serotonergic and noradrenergic reuptake inhibitor (SNRI), was found to be effective in improving depression in 26 HD subjects, but similar small studies evaluating selective serotonin reuptake inhibitors (SSRIs) have failed to show clinical benefit. In the absence of supporting data from controlled human trials, SSRIs have remained the agents of choice for management of depression and aggression. Episodic or situational anxiety may warrant a short course of benzodiazepines. Valproic acid, benzodiazepines, and propranolol have all been reported to reduce aggression in HD. Psychosis is uncommon but disabling, and newer antipsychotics are the mainstay of treatment, with clozapine, quetiapine, and olanzapine thought to have the fewest neurological side effects.

3) *Neuroprotective strategies:* Currently there are no neuroprotective agents for HD. Coenzyme Q-10 was the first agent tested for a potential neuroprotective effect in HD and did not reach statistical significance. Several compounds with beneficial effects in animal models like riluzole (which reduced excitotoxicity and striatal degeneration and increased brain derived neurotrophic factor BDNF serum levels), minocycline (which delays mortality in mouse model), and creatine (which improves survival of striatal neurons in rodent HD model) have been tested in human clinical trials without success. Another therapeutic prospect is histone deacetylase (HDAC) inhibitor medication, which proved to arrest neurodegeneration in the drosophila model. Although some HDAC inhibitors are in use in cancer therapy, their safety and tolerability in HD has not been evaluated (except for valproic acid, which also inhibits HDAC). The potential targets for neuroprotection are summarized in the Science Revisited box.

Other inherited choreas

Chorea may result from several other inherited neurodegenerative disorders. Table 6.3 summarizes the characteristic clinical, laboratory, and imaging features of several non-HD inherited chorea syndromes. Of these, neuroacanthocytosis syndromes will be discussed in more detail below. Chorea may infrequently be seen in Wilson disease; therefore anyone younger than 50 presenting with chorea, tremor, or dystonia should be screened using urine copper, serum ceruloplasmin, and slit-lamp examination, since copper chelation may halt the progression and even improve motor function in this otherwise devastating disorder.

Neuroacanthocytosis syndromes

Neuroacanthocytosis (NA) syndromes are a group of disorders characterized by acanthocytosis (spike-like protrusions from red blood cell membranes

Table 6.2 HD management: Evidence at a glance

Source Agent	American Academy of Neurology			Cochrane Database review		
	Type of study	Conclusion	Comments	Number of studies	Intervention effects	Adverse effects (where discussed)
Tetrabenazine	1 Class I, 1 Class II	Likely effective in chorea	Monitor adverse events	5 Studies	Improved maximal chorea (UHDRS) and CGI	Worse functional score, sleepiness and reading
Clozapine	1 Class III	Insufficient evidence		1 Study	Improved chorea in neuroleptic naïve patients, not in neuroleptic treated	Worse self evaluated disability
Amantadine	1 Class I, 1 Class II	Beneficial per patient reported outcome & class II	Class I study video ratings: No benefit	2 Studies	In one, (100–400 mg/d) improved max and rest chorea, in other (300 mg/d) no change.	
Riluzole	1 Class I, 1 Class II	200 mg/d effective, 100 mg/d not at 8 wk, or 3 yr	100 mg/d modest benefit can't be excluded	1 Study	200 mg/d improved total chorea, but not Dystonia, or independence score	Persistent elevation of liver function tests
Ethyl-eicosapentaenoic acid	1 Class I, 1 Class II	Likely ineffective	Moderate benefit can't be excluded	2 Studies	No improvement of UHDRS total motor score (TMS-4)	
Creatine	1 Class I, 1 Class II	Probably ineffective	Moderate benefit can't be excluded	1 Study	No difference in secondary measures including chorea	
Coenzyme Q-10	1 Class I, 1 Class II	Likely ineffective	Modest benefit can't be excluded	Not discussed	—	—

Donepezil	1 Class I, 1 Class II	Insufficient evidence	—	Not discussed	—	—
Minocycline	1 Class I, 1 Class II	Likely ineffective	Moderate benefit can't be excluded	Not discussed	—	—
Nabilone	1 Class I, 1 Class II	Possibly modest improvement	Safety, addiction potential unknown	Not discussed	—	—
Sulpiride (300–1200 mg/d)	Not discussed	—	—	1 Trial (300–1200 mg/d)	Improved median movement count and chorea severity	No corresponding functional improvement
Tiapride	Not discussed	—	—	2 Studies, different doses	@ 3 g/d dose: improvement in chorea and motor skills, @ 300 mg/d: no difference	—
Ketamine	Not discussed	—	—	1 Study	No improvement	Worse total motor score, memory and behavior scores.
Remacemide	Not discussed	—	—	1 Study	Trend to improved maximal chorea, verbal learning and Stroop color naming	—

Table 6.3 Summary of non-HD inherited choreas*

Disorder (mode of inheritance)	Age at onset	Clinical characteristics	Imaging characteristics	Laboratory findings	Genetic abnormality
HDL1 (AD)	3rd–5th decade	Similar to HD, prominent psychiatric features, myoclonus	None characteristic, *BG, F, T, Ce* atrophy	No characteristic	Octopeptide repeat expansion in prion protein gene (PRNP)
HDL2 (AD)	3rd–4th Decade	Black Africans Similar to HD; dystonia and parkinsonism	None characteristic, *St, Co* atrophy	Occasional acanthocytes	CTG-CAG expansion in JPH (junctophilin) 3
HDL4 (*SCA17*) (AD)	3rd–5th decade	Ataxia pronounced, pyramidal signs, epilepsy	None characteristic, *Ce, Co* atrophy	No characteristic	CAG expansion TATA-binding protein (*TBP*) gene
DRPLA (AD)	4th decade	Frequent in Japan 3 phenotypes prominent: 1. chorea 2. ataxia 3. myoclonus	*Co, Ce,* and *Br* atrophy, ↑T2WI in *WM*	No characteristic	CAG expansion in atrophin 1 (*ATN1*)
Neuroferritinopathy (AD)	4th decade (some in 2nd)	Chorea + prominent oromandibular dyskinesias, parkinsonism, dystonia	↓T2*WI in *Co, BG, Ce* ↑T2WI in *BG, Th, Ce* nuclei ↓T1WI+↑T2WI in *GP, Put*	Low serum ferritin	Ferritin light chain gene (*FTL*) mutation
Benign hereditary chorea (AD)	1st decade	Mild chorea in arms, face, tongue, slow progression. No dementia.	Imaging generally normal	Abnormal thyroid functions	Thyroid transcription factor 1 (*TITF1*) mutation
Chorea-acanthocytosis (AR)	3rd–4th decade	Prominent orofacial dystonia, self-mutilation, neuropathy, myopathy	None characteristic, *Ca* atrophy	Elevated CPK, abnormal LFTs Acanthocytes	Vacuolar protein sorting 13 A (*VPS13A*) mutation
McLeod syndrome (AR)	4th – 6th decade	Chorea (legs), dystonia, neuropathy, myopathy, seizures, dementia, cardiomyopathy	*Ca, Ce* atrophy, rim of ↑T2WI in lateral *put*	Elevated CPK, abnormal LFTs Hemolytic anemia	Mutation of *XK* gene
PKAN (AR)	1st decade	Orofacial, limb and lingual dystonia, chorea, parkinsonism/spasticity, pigmentary retinopathy; no neuropathy or myopathy.	"Eye of the tiger" sign	Acanthocytes in 10%.	Pantothenate kinase 2 (*PANK2*) mutation
HDL3 (AR)	3–4 years	Parkinsonism, dystonia, ataxia, spasticity, dementia	None characteristic, *F, Ca* atrophy	No characteristic	Unknown, 4p15.3

* *Br* = Brainstem, *BG* = Basal Ganglia, *Ca* = Caudate, *Ce* = Cerebellar, *Co* = Cortical, *F* = Frontal, GP = Pallidum, *P* = Parietal, Put = Putamen, *T* = Temporal, *St* = Striatal, *WM* = White matter, ↓ = Hypointense signal, ↑ = Hyperintense signal, T1WI = T1 weighted imaging, T2WI = T2 weighted imaging, T2*WI = T2* weighted imaging.

seen on microscopic exam) and neurological dysfunction. Acanthocytes may arise due to altered lipoprotein metabolism, or as a result of the "core" NA syndromes, where there is progressive degeneration of the basal ganglia. We will discuss only the latter group, which includes choreoacanthocytosis (ChAc), McLeod syndrome (MLS), and pantothenate kinase associated neurodegeneration (PKAN). (See Table 6.2 in Chapter 16 on heavy metals.)

Although these disorders are all rare, when progressive chorea presents without a history suggestive of autosomal dominant inheritance, NA should be the first syndrome to consider in the differential diagnosis. Ch-Ac and MLS are both HD phenocopies: with onset in adulthood, a progressive hyperkinetic disorder associated with cognitive impairment, and behavioral/psychiatric features that progress at a slow rate. In addition, both of these disorders have neuromuscular involvement and might have hepatosplenomegaly, which can help narrow the differential.

In Ch-Ac, the motor phenotype includes limb and orolingual dystonia including the characteristic "feeding dystonia," where the tongue protrudes and pushes food out of the mouth. Chorea, orofacial dyskinesias, and dysarthria may also be present. In addition, there may be prominent self-mutilation in the form of tongue biting and lip-biting. Seizures may be the first manifestation of the disease, and psychiatric manifestations including psychosis and obsessive-compulsive behaviors are also common. Mild axonal neuropathy and myopathy with elevated creatine phosphokinase (CPK) may be seen, but weakness and muscle atrophy are not common. Progression is slow, over decades.

MLS is defined by the absence of Kx antigen and weak expression of Kell erythrocyte antigens in blood. Carriers of the MLS blood group generally develop a progressive neurological syndrome in the third to sixth decades, with chorea, facial dyskinesias, and involuntary vocalizations. Unlike Ch-Ac, self-mutilation, dysphagia, and dystonia are infrequent. Psychosis, obsessive-compulsive disorder, and depression are common, and may predate the movement abnormalities. Generalized seizures are also common. There is prominent myopathy with muscle atrophy, and cardiomyopathy with conduction abnormalities and life-threatening arrhythmias can occur.

PKAN is a disorder with abnormal accumulation of iron in the brain as well as the presence of acanthocytosis on blood smear. Onset of neurological symptoms is in the first decade, with orofacial and limb dystonia, spasticity, and chorea. Dysarthria, and lingual dystonia are also common; but the "feeding dystonia" seen in Ch-Ac is not observed in PKAN. This is the common NBIA disorder with an "eye of the tiger" sign on MRI.

Management of chorea in NA disorders is similar to HD. Lingual dystonias, including the feeding dystonia seen with Ch-Ac, may respond to some degree to botulinum toxin injections in the genioglossus. Anticonvulsants, such as valproate, used to treat seizures may help the involuntary movements as well. However, lamotrigine and carbamazepine may worsen these movements. Supportive care, including speech therapy, to help with dysphagia and physical/occupational therapies to improve gait impairment are generally required.

Acquired choreas

Chorea may also present as a symptom of metabolic and endocrine disorders, vascular disorders (including inflammatory vasculitides), infectious or parainfectious processes, and toxicity related to medications or other agents (Table 6.1). Box 6.2 provides the recommended investigations in the evaluation of chorea, with a focus on treatable etiologies. The investigations should be guided by a careful history and physical exam. For many acquired choreas, removal of the inciting cause may help alleviate chorea. When the cause is a structural lesion, the abnormal movements generally improve with time, although symptomatic treatment may be helpful in the acute stages or with disabling movements.

Sydenham chorea

SC was first described by Thomas Sydenham and is the common cause of childhood-onset chorea, although the prevalence is decreasing. SC develops in association with group A beta-hemolytic streptococcal (GABHS) infection and the neuropsychiatric manifestations are thought to be mediated by antibodies against GABHS that cross-react with neuronal epitopes.

Clinical features of SC include the neurological manifestations of chorea, incoordination, hypotonia, and muscle weakness, which can be severe and cause a stroke-like appearance, termed chorea paralytica. Behavioral and psychiatric abnormalities

Box 6.2 Suggested investigations in chorea

Careful and thorough history, including psychiatric, drug, and family history and physical examination.

1. **CBC, Metabolic profile, B12 levels, LFTs, CPK:** lipid profile and peripheral smear if appropriate.
2. **RPR/VDRL and HIV ELISA.**
3. **Thyroid function tests.**
4. **Sedimentation Rate and ANA, anticardiolipin antibodies and lupus anticoagulant:** if autoimmune disorders suspected.
5. **Antistreptolysin O (ASLO) or anti-DNase-B titer:** in cases with suspected streptococcal infection.
6. **Serum ceruloplasmin and 24 hour urine copper:** if Wilson disease suspected.
7. **Ophthalmologic exam:** including fundus exam.
8. **MRI:** Evaluate for intracranial structural lesions for acute ballistic or choreiform movements or evaluate for typical abnormalities seen with several heredodegenerative etiologies.
9. **Genetic testing:** when appropriate and after counseling.
10. **EEG:** With history suspicious for paroxysmal movement disorder or seizures.

CBC = complete blood count; LFT = liver function tests; CPK = creatine phosphokinase; RPR = rapid plasma reagent; VDRL = venereal disease research laboratory; HIV = human immunodeficiency virus; ANA = anti-nuclear antibody; EEG = electroencephalogram.

include hyperactivity, anxiety, depression, obsessive-compulsive behaviors, emotional lability, impaired verbal fluency, and executive dysfunction. Other features of acute rheumatic fever, such as carditis and arthritis, may also be present. There may be discordance between the extent of psychiatric and neurological involvement. Although classically described as a benign and self-limiting condition, SC generally lasts for several months and may have a relapsing course. Further, impairment in quality of life may occur from the neuropsychiatric features as well as evolution of SC into a chronic movement disorder.

Diagnosis is made by history and supported by the presence of elevated anti-streptolysin O (ASLO) titer, elevated anti-DNA-ase B titers, or positive throat culture for streptococcus pyogenes. With the diagnosis of SC, the physician should implement strategies to prevent rheumatic heart disease, since a sizable but modifiable proportion of patients diagnosed with SC will later develop rheumatic heart disease. Treatment with penicillin (penicillin 500 mg twice a day for 10 days) is mandatory to eliminate GABHS. Secondary prophylaxis with long-term penicillin therapy (intramuscular benzylpenicillin every 4 weeks, or daily oral administration of penicillin VK) is required to minimize development of rheumatic heart disease. Patients should also be advised to seek primary treatment for future streptococcal pharyngitis.

Other than elimination of the streptococcal infection, the major principles of management include symptomatic treatment of abnormal movements and behavioral and psychiatric features, in addition to treating the inflammatory/immune response. There are no universally accepted protocols for managing SC. Dopamine receptor blockers and drugs facilitating GABA, along with restriction of physical activity are commonly used as first-line treatment. Typical neuroleptics like haloperidol control chorea effectively but are commonly associated with adverse effects including drug-induced parkinsonism. These agents should be started at low doses (0.025 mg/kg/d in divided doses for haloperidol), with slow dose escalation to maximal benefit or to a maximum dose (0.05 mg/kg/d for haloperidol). Tetrabenazine may also be useful and does not have the potential side effect of tardive dyskinesia. Valproic acid (20 mg/kg/d) and carbamazepine (at 10–15 mg/kg/d) are alternative first line agents, or may be used if neuroleptics are ineffective or poorly tolerated.

Immunomodulatory therapies, including steroids, IVIG, and plasma exchange, have all been used to decrease immune response with the hope of ameliorating symptoms and shortening the course of the disease. Steroids (prednisone at 2 mg/kg/d) may decrease the severity of chorea, as well as time to remission, but may not decrease the rate of symptom recurrence. Plasma exchange and IVIG may have benefits comparable to steroids. Supportive measures, including managing the comorbid behavioral and psychiatric issues with psychotherapy, patient and family education, as well as early diagnosis and treatment of SC and streptococcal pharyngitis may improve outcomes and decrease the risk of rheumatic heart disease.

Ballism

When choreic movements affect the proximal limbs, they appear as large amplitude, repetitive, but constantly varying involuntary movements termed ballism. Ballism, which is Greek and means "to throw," often affects only one side of the body, and is then termed hemiballism. Rarely, it can occur bilaterally (biballism) or affect both legs (paraballism).

Clinico-pathological and imaging studies have described injury to several basal ganglia structures, including the subthalamic nucleus, corpus striatum, and thalamus. The injury may occur from vascular insults, including ischemic or hemorrhagic strokes, intracranial space-occupying lesions including arteriovenous malformations, tumors, abscesses, and demyelination from multiple sclerosis. The subthalamic nucleus and its connections appear to be commonly damaged and may play an important role in the emergence of ballism. A subset of cases described showed no lesions on MRI or CT scans.

Hemiballism due to a vascular etiology has a sudden onset, unlike that from a tumor or intracranial space-occupying lesion. With tumors and intracranial space-occupying lesions, onset may be gradual and severity of movements may increase over several weeks. Generally, these large-amplitude, ballistic proximal movements are associated with distal choreic movements in the same limb. In vascular hemiballism, ballistic movements emerge as the hemiparesis starts to improve. Cranial imaging is advised for all patients experiencing hemi-ballistic movements. Additionally, since hemiballism may be associated with hyperglycemia, blood sugar should be tested.

Since hemiballism is usually associated with significant disability, treatment is necessary in the acute stage. For the management of ballism in the acute stage, non-pharmaceutical interventions like padding the limb or hard surfaces that may injure the limb are important. Limb restraint may be required to prevent injury. Pharmacological management of ballism is similar to management of other choreas. The commonly used medications include dopamine receptor blockers and atypical neuroleptics. Dopamine-depleting medications, such as tetrabenazine, may also be successful. If dopamine receptor blocking medications or dopamine-depleting medications are associated with excessive sedation or other adverse effects, sodium valproate may be tried.

In general, it is advisable to taper the medications off after weeks or months of treatment, once there is improvement of the hemiballistic movements, since in the long-term, spontaneous remissions are common. After the remission of hemiballism, mild chorea may persist as a milder manifestation of the movement disorder. If hemiballism persists and remains disabling, surgical interventions, including stereotactic thalamotomy or deep brain stimulation surgery of the ventral intermediate (VIM) nucleus of thalamus have been shown to be effective.

Athetosis

Athetosis refers to slow, writhing, continuous movements predominantly affecting the distal limbs. These movements resemble dystonia and may indeed be a manifestation of dystonia in the distal extremities in some patients. Athetosis is grouped in this text along with chorea, since these movements are non-patterned, unsustained, and not painful (unlike dystonia). Further, athetosis and chorea may coexist or evolve from one to the other. Dystonia may also accompany athetosis, especially in cerebral palsy, where there are athetotic movements of distal extremities as well as facial grimacing. The facial spasms may be especially pronounced with bulbar tasks like eating or talking.

Cerebral palsy is the common disorder in which athetosis is encountered in the clinic, although athetosis can be seen with metabolic abnormalities, including Lesch–Nyhan syndrome and aminoacidurias. Additionally, patients with large fiber neuropathy and severe proprioceptive impairment may have writhing, continuous movements involving fingers or even toes, termed "pseudo-athetosis" (see Video 6.3). When athetosis is a prominent feature of cerebral palsy, neuroimaging may not show any evidence of basal ganglia injury, and cognition may be relatively preserved, although communication may be impaired because of severe dysarthria and impaired dexterity.

Several pharmacological agents have been tried for the management of athetosis, but response is generally less than satisfactory. Anticholinergics, especially at high doses, and benzodiazepines have been used with modest benefits. Levodopa should be tried because of the possibility of dopa-responsive dystonia, but also because some patients with athetotic cerebral palsy may have significant improvement with levodopa. Response to medications is unpredictable, and adverse effects need to be monitored carefully, especially since communication challenges in patients with cerebral palsy may preclude the patients from reporting these. cBotulinum toxin and intrathecal baclofen mainly help with spasticity and may also help dystonia in athetotic cerebral palsy. Neuroleptics can also be tried although success is generally limited.

Further Readings

Armstrong MJ, Miyasaki JM. Evidence-based guideline: pharmacologic pharmacologic treatment of chorea in Huntington disease. Report of the Guideline Development Subcommittee of the American Academy of Neurology. *Neurology* 2012; **79**(6): 597–603. doi: 10.1212/WNL.0b013e318263c443.

Berardelli A, and Curra A. Choreas, Athetosis athetosis, dyskinesias, hemiballismus. In Hallett M, ed. Handbook of Clinical Neurophysiology, Vol. 1: Movement Disorders, 571–582. Amsterdam: Elsevier, 2003.

Bhidayasiri R, Truong DD. Chorea and related disorders. *Postgrad Med J* 2004; **80**: 527–534.

Donaldson IM, Marsden CD, Schneider SA, Bhatia KP, eds. Other idiopathic choreic syndromes. Marsden's Book of Movement Disorders, 785–815. New York: Oxford University Press, 2012.

Donaldson IM, Marsden CD, Schneider SA, Bhatia KP, eds. Ballism. Marsden's Book of Movement Disorders, 881–888. New York: Oxford University Press, 2012.

Fahn S, Jankovic J, eds. Huntington disease. Principles and Practice of Movement Disorders, 369–392. Philadelphia: Churchill Livingstone Elsevier. 2007

HORIZON Investigators of the Huntington Disease Study Group and European Huntington's Disease Network. A randomized double-blind, placebo-controlled study of Latrepiridine in patients with mild to moderate Huntington disease. *Arch Neurol* 2012; **1**: 1–9. doi: 10.1001/2013. jamaneurol.382.

Jung HH, Danek A, Walker RH. Neuroacanthocytosis syndromes. *Orphanet J Rare Disord* 2011; **6**: 68. doi: 10.1186/1750-1172-6-68.

Mestre T, Ferreira J, Coelho MM, Rosa M, Sampaio C. Therapeutic interventions for symptomatic treatment in Huntington's disease. *Cochrane Database of Systematic Reviews* 2009; **3**: art. no.: CD006456. doi: 10.1002/14651858.CD006456.pub2.

Ross CA, Poirier MA. Protein aggregation and neurodegenerative disease. *Neurodegeneration* 2004; **10**(suppl. on *Nature Medicine*): S10–S17.

Schneider SA, Walker RH, Bhatia KP. The Huntington's disease-like syndromes: what to consider in patients with a negative Huntington's disease gene test. *Nat Clin Pract Neurol.* 2007; **3**(9): 517–525.

Shannon KM. Treatment of chorea. In A Miller, ed. Continuum: Lifelong Learning in Neurology (R): Movement Disorders, 72–93. Philadelphia, PA: Lippincott Williams and Wilkins; 2007. Copyright © 2011, American Academy of Neurology. http://aan.com/go/elibrary/continuum

Venuto CS, McGarry A, Ma Q, Kieburtz K. Pharmacologic approaches to the treatment of Huntington's disease. *Mov Disord* 2012; **27**(1): 31–41. doi: 10.1002/mds.23953.

Walker KG, Wilmshurst JM. An update on the treatments of Sydenham's chorea: the evidence for established and evolving interventions. *Ther Adv Neurol Disord* 2010; **3**(5): 301–309. doi: 10.1177/1756285610382063.

7

Dystonia

Lauren Schrock, MD[1], Tao Xie[2] and Brandon R. Barton, MD, MS[3,4]

[1]University of Utah, Department of Neurology, Salt Lake City, Utah, USA
[2]Department of Neurology, University of Chicago Medical Center, Chicago, Illinois, USA
[3]Department of Neurological Sciences, Section of Movement Disorders, Rush University Medical Center, Chicago, Illinois, USA
[4]Department of Neurological Sciences, Rush University Medical Center; Neurology Section, Jesse Brown VA Medical Center, Chicago, Illinois, USA

Introduction

Hermann Oppenheim first introduced the term dystonia (i.e., dystonia musculorum deformans) in 1911 to describe a progressive disorder affecting Jewish children, which caused muscle spasms, rapid or sometimes rhythmic jerking movements, and bizarre walking patterns with bending and twisting of the torso. The progression of symptoms led eventually to sustained fixed postural deformities. This case series is now thought to represent one of the first phenotypic descriptions of the dystonia-1 (*DYT1*) gene, which is characterized by a generalized dystonia phenotype. It was not until the 1970s, however, that a connection was made between generalized dystonia and the clinical features of adult-onset focal dystonias, and the nosological entity that we recognize today as dystonia was established.

Definition

A formal definition of dystonia was codified in 1984 by a committee assembled by the Dystonia Medical Research Foundation. The committee defined dystonia as a syndrome of involuntary, sustained muscle contractions affecting one or more sites of the body, frequently causing twisting and repetitive movements, or abnormal postures.

This definition was recently revised by a Consensus Committee of experts in 2013. Dystonia is now defined as a movement disorder characterized by sustained or intermittent muscle contractions, causing abnormal, often repetitive, movements, postures, or both. Dystonic movements are typically patterned, twisting, and may be tremulous. Dystonia is often initiated or worsened by voluntary action and associated with overflow muscle activation.

Classification of dystonia

Proper classification has real clinical implications for evaluation strategy, diagnosis, treatment, genetic counseling, prognosis, and research. In the past, the classification of dystonia has traditionally been organized along three parallel axes: (1) age of onset, (2) distribution, and (3) etiology. In the 2013 revisions, the methodology was simplified to include only two classification axes: (1) clinical characteristics and (2) etiology, as detailed below.

The term *primary dystonia* is used to describe the phenotype of pure dystonia syndromes, which is when dystonia is the only symptom, with the exception of tremor, and when there is no evidence of pathological abnormalities. However, many genetic causes for primary dystonias have now been discovered, yet they are still designated as "primary." *Secondary dystonia* has historically had various meanings, including any dystonia that is not "primary," dystonia that has a known underlying

Non-Parkinsonian Movement Disorders, First Edition. Edited by Deborah A. Hall and Brandon R. Barton.
© 2017 John Wiley & Sons, Ltd. Published 2017 by John Wiley & Sons, Ltd.
Companion website: www.wiley.com/go/hall/non-parkinsonian_movement_disorders

cause, dystonias that are due to an acquired insult, or dystonias secondary to a defined pathology. *Dystonia-plus* is a term whose creation is reflective of the weaknesses of previous classification systems, and refers to specific syndromes in which dystonia predominates, is combined with other neurological features such as parkinsonism or myoclonus, and in which there is no evidence of neurodegeneration. The *heredodegenerative* dystonia category was introduced to incorporate a mixed class of disorders, namely dystonia due to neurodegenerative disease or to disorders that are inherited. However, this category contained widely varied disorders that could be neurodegenerative, inherited, or both. The 2013 consensus committee has therefore recommended that all these terms be retired, due to lack of clarity, but they will likely continue to be used for many years to come.

Axis I: Clinical characteristics

The diagnosis of dystonia is clinical, and the diagnosis can be aided by the recognition of the following features unique to the dystonias:

Sensory tricks

A sensory trick (historically called a "geste antagoniste") is clinical feature that is unique to the dystonias, and reflects the sensorimotor integration abnormalities that underlie dystonia. A sensory trick is a method that patients often use to temporarily suppress dystonic movements. This usually will involve touching body parts that are either affected by or adjacent to those affected by dystonia. A classic example would be the person with cervical dystonia who holds their hand on their chin or cheek. Up to 84% of patients with dystonia are reported to respond to a sensory trick.

Overflow

Overflow is an unintentional muscle contraction that accompanies, but is anatomically distinct from, the primary dystonic movement. Overflow often results in the involvement of muscles not normally used for the intended task of movement and commonly occurs at the peak of dystonic movements

Mirror movements

Dystonic movements may be triggered in the affected limb when the unaffected limb performs a task (e.g., writing with the unaffected hand induces dystonic posturing in the affected hand).

Null point

This is defined as a position where dystonic movements abate (e.g., a patient with cervical dystonia whose dystonic tremor improves when he turns his head to one side). The position that produces the null point is usually in the direction of the "preferred" abnormal posture assumed by the patient when dystonia is not being consciously suppressed.

Tremor

Dystonic tremor is a spontaneous, oscillatory, "rhythmical," although often inconstant, patterned movement produced by contractions of dystonic muscles and may be exacerbated by an attempt to maintain "normal" posture. It may or may not be relieved by allowing the abnormal dystonic posture to reach the null point by fully developing without resistance (where it reaches a "null point"). Dystonic tremor may be difficult to distinguish from a tremor similar to that seen in essential tremor, although dystonic tremor can by more irregular or jerky.

Clinical classification

Five descriptors are used to specify clinical characteristics of dystonia: age of onset, body distribution, temporal pattern, coexistence of other movement disorders, and other neurological manifestations.

Age of onset

Classification by age of onset is of particular importance as it may be the strongest predictive factor for prognosis. There are two basic rules that hold true with regard to age of primary dystonia onset and its relation to both bodily distribution of dystonia and likelihood of spread. First, age of onset follows a caudal-to-rostral pattern, with lower extremity onset common in children but rare in adults. Cranial onset is common in adults but rare in children. Lower extremity onset is common in children but rare in adults. With increasing age dystonia is less likely to spread to become either generalized or segmental; for example, dystonia commonly affects the legs first in children, less commonly in adolescence, and rarely in adults. Primary dystonia in adults nearly always begins in the head (cranial dystonia), neck (cervical dystonia), or arm (writer's cramp), and the dystonia remains focal or segmental. Second, age of dystonia onset correlates strongly with the likelihood that dystonia will spread to involve multiple parts of the body. Dystonia that begins in childhood has a high likelihood of progressing to generalized or multifocal dystonia (approximately 60%). With onset in adolescence (age >12), progression to generalized or multifocal dystonia is less common (35%), but it is very rare (3%) when dystonia begins in adulthood.

Historically, dystonia has been dichotomously classified into childhood-onset and adult-onset forms, with the discriminating age of 26 years, However, it may be more useful for both the formulation of a diagnostic approach and prognostic counseling to separate age of dystonia onset into more stratified age groups.

1) Infancy (birth to 2 years)
   - Onset at this age is most likely to be related to an inherited metabolic disorder with specific diagnostic implications and prognosis is likely to be poor.
2) Childhood (3–12 years)
   - Onset of dystonia between ages 2 and 6 years should raise suspicion for dystonic cerebral palsy, especially in the context of developmental delay.
   - Dopa-responsive dystonia and other generalized isolated or pure dystonia syndromes are likely to develop between ages 6 and 14 years.
   - Dystonia is most likely to start in the foot or leg, and has a high probability of becoming generalized.
3) Adolescence (13–20 years)
   - Age of onset of some of the generalized isolated dystonia syndromes.
   - Dystonia can have onset in the leg but also is more likely to have onset in the trunk or arm.
   - Less likely to become generalized than with childhood-onset dystonia, but still much more likely than in adults.
4) Early adulthood (21–40 years)
   - Most likely to remain focal or segmental.
   - Onset in leg is uncommon.
5) Late adulthood (>40 years)
   - Likely to remain focal or segmental; generalized dystonia is extremely rare.
   - Typically will involve cervical or cranial dystonia (e.g., blepharospasm, oromandibular dystonia); onset in leg is rare.

Body distribution

Classification by the body region affected is clinically relevant because it also has implications for both diagnostic strategy and therapy. The treatment of choice for focal and segmental dystonias typically involves botulinum toxin injections, whereas treatment of generalized dystonias more often involve medications or surgery.

In most cases, the part of the body affected by dystonia is inextricably intertwined with the age of onset. In fact, if dystonia develops in a body distribution not typical for the patient's age, it suggests that either a different diagnostic approach or an alternative diagnosis should be pursued.

Classification of dystonia by body region

1) *Focal:* Dystonia affects only one body region. Examples include blepharospasm, oromandibular dystonia, cervical dystonia, laryngeal dystonia, and writer's cramp.
2) *Segmental:* Dystonia affects two or more continuous body regions. Examples include cranial dystonia (blepharospasm with lower facial and jaw or tongue involvement) or bibrachial dystonia.
3) *Multifocal:* Dystonia affects two noncontiguous or more (contiguous or not) body regions.
4) *Generalized:* Dystonia affects the trunk and at least two other sites. Generalized forms with leg involvement are distinguished from those without leg involvement.
5) *Hemidystonia:* Dystonia affecting one side of the body (e.g., unilateral arm and leg). Hemidystonia is almost always due to an acquired brain lesion in the contralateral hemisphere.

Temporal pattern

Characterizing the temporal pattern of dystonia can facilitate both diagnosis and treatment options. There are two important temporal domains that can aid in clinical classification: *disease course* and *variability*.

The disease course of dystonia may be static or progressive. *Static dystonia* refer to cases where the dystonia does not worsen over time, whereas with *progressive dystonia* a pattern of clinical worsening is observed over time and may suggest an underlying metabolic or neurodegenerative disorder.

Dystonia often has some daily variability that can be activity or context dependent. Dystonia can be elicited or suppressed by specific activities or external triggers, and may be affected by psychological state. Thus characterizing the pattern of daily variability can be very useful in teasing out the diagnosis and etiology.

Four patterns of variability have been recognized:

1) *Action-specific:* Dystonia that occurs only during a particular task or activity (e.g., writer's cramp), and is no longer present when the specific task is completed.
2) *Persistent:* Dystonia that persists to approximately the same extent throughout the day.
3) *Diurnal fluctuations:* Dystonia fluctuates during the day, with recognizable circadian variations in occurrence, severity, and phenomenology. Dopa-responsive dystonia often follows this pattern.
4) *Paroxysmal:* Sudden self-limited episodes of dystonia usually induced by a trigger with return to preexisting neurological state. The dystonia typically persists for a short time after the trigger.

It is not uncommon for dystonia to begin as a task-specific dystonia (e.g., lower limb dystonia that occurs with walking only but that is not present when walking backward or running). Then, as symptoms progress, the dystonia is present during more actions (e.g., limb dystonia now occurs with both walking forward and backward) and eventually may be persistent during rest and be complicated by fixed contractures.

Associated features

Dystonia may occur in isolation or in association with other movement disorders. One important caveat to recognize when classifying dystonia is that tremor that occurs in the context of dystonia is necessarily considered to be a separate movement disorder. Instead of the clinical terms "primary" or "pure" to refer to dystonia that is the only phenotypic manifestation (with or without dystonic tremor), it is more straightforward to characterize dystonia as *isolated* or *combined with another movement disorder*:

Isolated dystonia: Dystonia is the only motor feature (with the exception of tremor). Historically, isolated dystonia has been referred to as primary dystonia.

Combined dystonia: Dystonia is combined with another movement disorder (myoclonus, parkinsonism, etc.).

Some forms of combined dystonia have also been referred to as "dystonia-plus" syndromes (myoclonus dystonia syndrome, dopa-responsive dystonia, etc.) or "heredodegenerative" disorders (Parkinson disease, X-linked dystonia-parkinsonism/*DYT3*, etc.).

Occurrence of other neurological or systemic manifestations

Examples of associated neurological or systemic features that are important for determination of diagnosis and etiology are as follows:

- Cognitive decline (seen commonly in degenerative or progressive dystonia syndromes).
- Psychiatric symptoms and liver disease raise suspicion for Wilson disease.
- Vertical supranuclear gaze palsy, ataxia, dysarthria, or psychiatric presentations in middle childhood to adulthood can be seen in Niemann Pick type C.

Classification along this Axis I (clinical characteristics) facilitates the recognition of and assembly of dystonia syndromes into diagnostically useful phenomenological categories.

Axis II: Etiology

The second axis of dystonia classification strictly addresses etiology. Due to the continued advancement of our understanding of the causes and risk factors for the development of dystonia, this is an evolving area and will need further revisions as new discoveries are made.

Two complementary aspects of etiology are helpful for classification: (1) identifiable anatomical changes and (2) patterns of inheritance. These two aspects should not be considered mutually exclusive. Anatomical causes of dystonia can be identified either on brain imaging or by pathology. Imaging, metabolic, genetic, or other tests may be helpful to distinguish inherited, acquired, and idiopathic causes of dystonia. It is now recommended that, rather than use the term "primary," etiological classification by nervous system pathology and pattern of inheritance be considered separately, as detailed below:

Nervous system pathology

Nervous system pathology (or lack thereof) can divide dystonia into three etiological subgroups:

1) *Degeneration:* There is evidence of progressive structural abnormalities such as neuronal loss (at the gross, microscopic, or molecular level).
2) *Static lesions:* Presence of non-developmental neurodevelopmental anomalies or acquired lesions. Examples would include perinatal stroke/hypoxia causing dystonia.
3) *No evidence of degeneration or structural lesion:* Several of the genetic or idiopathic isolated dystonia syndromes currently fit under this category (e.g., isolated generalized *DYT1* dystonia).

Inherited, acquired, or idiopathic

Recognition of patterns of disease inheritance can significantly narrow the etiological differential diagnosis of dystonia and guide diagnostic evaluation, treatment options, and counseling regarding prognosis and risk of genetic transmission to offspring. Identifying where dystonia is inherited, acquired, or idiopathic may not only be helpful for diagnosis and prognosis but also highlight the evolving nature of etiological classification. Idiopathic forms will undoubtedly be reclassified as inherited as new dystonia genes are discovered. Examples of each classification include the following:

1) Inherited (see Table 7.1)
   - *Autosomal dominant* DYT1, DYT5, DYT6, DYT11, rapid-onset dystonia-parkinsonism (*DYT12*), dentatorubral-pallidoluysian atrophy, Huntington disease, and neuroferritinopathy (*NBIA3*).
   - *Autosomal recessive* Wilson disease, type 2 juvenile Parkinson disease (*PARK2*), pantothenate kinase associated neurodegeneration (*PKAN*), and numerous metabolic disorders.
   - *X-linked recessive* Lubag (*DYT3*), Lesch–Nyhan syndrome, Mohr–Tranebjaerg syndrome.
   - *Mitochondrial* Leigh syndrome, Leber optic atrophy, and dystonia.
2) Acquired (i.e., dystonia due to a known specific cause)
   - *Perinatal injury* Dystonic cerebral palsy, delayed-onset dystonia.
   - *Infection* Viral encephalitis, encephalitis lethargica, subacute sclerosing panencephalitis, HIV, tuberculosis, syphilis.
   - *Drug* Levodopa and dopamine agonists, neuroleptics (dopamine receptor blocking drugs), anticonvulsants, and calcium channel blockers.
   - *Toxic* Manganese, cobalt, carbon disulfide, cyanide, methanol, disulfiram, and 3-nitropropionic acid.
   - *Vascular* Ischemic, hemorrhage, arteriovenous malformation, aneurysm.
   - *Neoplastic* Brain tumor, paraneoplastic encephalitis.
   - *Brain injury* Head trauma, brain surgery (including stereotactic ablations), electrical injury.
   - *Psychogenic* (functional).

Table 7.1 Classification of the common genetic dystonias

Genet	Inheritance pattern	Gene/chromosome	Clinical features
DYT1	AD	TOR1A	Young onset, limb onset, generalized
DYT3	X-linked	Xq13.1	Lubag in Filipino males (X-linked dystonia-parkinsonism)
DYT4	AD	TUBB4A	Whispering dysphonia
DYT5	AD	GCH1	Dopa-responsive dystonia
DTY6	AD	THAP1	Mixed, cervical/oromandibular dystonia
DYT11	AD	SGCE	Myoclonus-dystonia
DYT12	AD	ATP1A3	Rapid-onset dystonia-parkinsonism

3) *Idiopathic* Many cases of focal or segmental isolated dystonia with onset in adulthood fall in this category.
   - Sporadic
   - Familial

Common dystonia syndromes

Isolated (i.e., primary) dystonia accounts for approximately three-fourths of dystonia cases and has a broad clinical spectrum and age of onset. Familiarity with the typical presentations of isolated dystonia is important, so that atypical cases are recognized as potential harbingers of a combined dystonia syndrome or neurodegenerative disease, and so that the appropriate further investigations are pursued.

Early-onset generalized isolated (primary) dystonia

Dystonia that begins in childhood commonly will have onset in a limb (e.g., equinovarus posturing of an ankle with walking) and often progresses to generalized involvement. The most well characterized genetic cause is due to a founder mutation in the *DYT1* gene that encodes the TorsinA protein. *DYT1* dystonia has autosomal dominant inheritance with reduced penetrance (30%). This 3-bp deletion in the *TOR1A* gene accounts for 80% of early-onset generalized dystonia in the Ashkenazi Jewish population and <50% of cases in the non-Jewish population. The typical phenotype of *DYT1* dystonia is characterized by a mean age of onset is 13 years (with the majority before 26 years), with limb onset (arm or leg is affected first in 90%), and progression to generalized or multifocal involvement in 65%. It is not common for the dystonia to spread to cranial muscles (only seen in 15–20%).

More recently another autosomal dominantly inherited form of early-onset dystonia (*DYT6* dystonia) was discovered to be caused by mutations in the *THAP1* gene. It also has reduced penetrance (60%) and has been reported in primarily patients of European ancestry, including Amish-Mennonite families. The *DYT6* phenotype has a mean age of onset of 16 years (range 5–62 years), and starts in an arm in 50% of cases. However, uniquely for early-onset dystonias, onset of dystonia in the leg is rare (4%), whereas it may start in cranial muscles (25%) or the neck (25%) in a significant proportion of cases. The dystonia will spread to a generalized or multifocal distribution in >50%, and there is prominent speech involvement (e.g., spasmodic dysphonia or oromandibular dystonia) in more than two-thirds of cases.

While these are the two commonly identified genetic causes of early-onset generalized dystonia, there are many cases of childhood-onset dystonia, both familial and sporadic, that may have similar presentations but whose etiology remains undefined.

Focal or segmental isolated (primary) dystonia with onset in adulthood

Focal and segmental dystonias present about 8 to 10 times more often than generalized dystonia, nearly always have onset in adulthood, and they usually involve the craniocervical muscles or arms. Adult-onset focal dystonias rarely generalize but may become segmental in approximately 30%. Most adult-onset isolated dystonias present about twice as often in women as in men, with the exception of writer's cramp, which presents more in men.

Cervical dystonia (i.e., spasmodic torticollis) is a common form of focal dystonia with the usual onset in the fifth decade. It presents with variable involvement of cervical muscles, and results in abnormal head, neck, and shoulder positions. Initial symptoms often include neck stiffness, pain, and limited head mobility. Sensory tricks (e.g., placing a hand on the side of face) may temporarily relieve the dystonic spasms and are very common. Unlike many types of dystonia, pain frequently accompanies cervical dystonia and may be a major contributor to disability. Torticollis (horizontal head turning) and laterocollis (lateral flexion toward the shoulder) are the common abnormal head postures, but most patients show a combination of these head postures (torticollis, laterocollis, retrocollis, and anterocollis). Associated dystonic head tremor may be present in less than a third of patients. Isolated anterocollis or retrocollis is rare, and may suggest specific etiologies. For example, isolated anterocollis is commonly seen in the context of multiple system atrophy, whereas when isolated or predominant retrocollis is seen, progressive supranuclear palsy, tardive dystonia, or an acute dystonic reaction induced by medication should be considered.

Blepharospasm

Blepharospasm is a focal dystonia caused by dystonic contractions of the orbicularis oculi, presenting as intermittent or sustained bilateral eye closure. Without treatment, blepharospasm may cause functional blindness despite normal vision. Onset is typically insidious in the sixth decade, with eye irritation and dryness followed by excessive blinking. Bright light, reading, or driving commonly aggravates symptoms. More than half of cases may spread to become segmental dystonia within five years.

Oromandibular dystonia (OMD)

OMD affects the jaw muscles, with involuntary jaw opening, jaw deviation, or jaw closing. Commonly there is also involvement of tongue, facial, and pharyngeal muscles. Eating or talking may exacerbate symptoms.

Laryngeal dystonia (spasmodic dysphonia)

This task-specific dystonia has usual onset in the fourth and fifth decades, in which attempts at speaking causes involuntary adduction or abduction of the vocal cords. Initial symptoms include increased effort during speech, or loss of voice control that occurs with emotional stress.

Myoclonus-dystonia

Myoclonus-dystonia is a syndrome descriptively characterized by the presence of both a focal or segmental dystonia (typically of the neck or hand) along with myoclonic jerks (usually occurring in the upper body). Onset is typically in childhood or early adolescence, and in most cases are familial. Mutations in DYT-11 (SCGE) leads to an autosomal dominant inherency pattern, although some cases are the result of a de novo mutation. Other cases have been associated with DRD2 and DYT-1 mutations. Treatment with benzodiazepines, antiepileptic drugs, levodopa, sodium oxybate, and deep brain stimulation (DBS) have been reported as effective.

Task-specific dystonia: Writer's cramp

A task-specific dystonia is a form of dystonia that is mainly or only manifest with performance of a particular task. The common form is writer's cramp, in which there is dystonic posturing (flexion and/or extension) of the fingers, wrist, or forearm that interferes with proper execution of writing. Any activity that requires fine motor control may be associated with a focal dystonia, and the condition has also affected musicians (embouchure dystonia, hand dystonia, etc.), and athletes (golf, billiards, tennis, darts, etc.). Genetic susceptibility to dystonia is likely involved in the genesis of these cases.

Diagnostic evaluation

The challenge for the physician evaluating a patient with dystonia is determining which patients require further investigation and what diagnostic tests are indicated. There are currently no widely accepted guidelines for choosing which tests to do and in what order. A shotgun approach to diagnostic evaluation is neither desirable nor feasible. The recognition of dystonia syndromes, which is facilitated by detailed clinical classification allows the clinician to limit the list of etiological differential diagnoses and provides a rationale by which to tailor diagnostic studies.

For progressive disorders repeated clinical evaluations are often necessary to narrow down the diagnosis because some symptoms and signs may only present with time. In fact, the temporal evolution of neurological features in a progressive disorder can have diagnostic and etiological significance. For example, a degenerative disorder that primarily affects gray matter is likely to manifest with dystonia, dementia, and epilepsy earlier, whereas disease primarily affecting white matter would more likely present with spasticity or ataxia.

Some syndromes, based on the movement disorder, or the presence of other neurological or systemic features, will require extensive investigation regardless of age. However, where the presentation of dystonia is pure and follows a typical pattern with regard to age of onset and body distribution, there may little need for investigation beyond the history and clinical exam.

Evaluation

With childhood- or young adult-onset isolated (primary) dystonia, at least a three-week trial of levodopa should always be done to rule out levodopa-responsive dystonia, an exquisitely treatable disorder. Genetic testing for DYT1 mutations (and

DYT6 if the dystonia distribution is suggestive) should be considered. If the cause of dystonia remains unknown, then Wilson disease, another treatable disorder, should always be excluded (see Tips and Tricks).

☆ TIPS AND TRICKS

The possibility of Wilson disease should be considered in any patient presenting with dystonia. Since this is a treatable neurological disorder, it cannot be missed. An initial screen should include serum copper and ceruloplasmin, and ophthalmological slit-lamp examination to look for Kayser–Fleischer rings. Since on occasion these tests may be normal in the context of Wilson disease, with any significant degree of clinical suspicion it is important to do a 24 hour urine copper excretion as well as a brain MRI, which may not specific but are unlikely to be normal in patients with neurological Wilson disease. The specific tests are liver biopsy with measurement of hepatic copper content and genetic analysis of the ATP7B gene.

Taking careful birth, developmental, medication, toxin, trauma, and family histories are important. If the history and exam suggests a metabolic or other inherited form of a combined dystonia syndrome, the diagnostic evaluation will need to be more extensive but will vary depending on the presentation and associated signs. Potential diagnostic evaluations to consider may include serum and urine amino acids, urine organic acids, CSF analysis, lactate-pyruvate ratio, alpha-fetoprotein, lysosomal analysis, skin, muscle, nerve, or bone marrow biopsy, electromyography and nerve conduction study, blood smear for acanthocytes, or genetic testing.

Adult-onset focal or segmental dystonia with a typical clinical presentation may require no further testing beyond the history and clinical exam. However, when dystonia presents in with atypical distribution for adult-onset dystonia (e.g., focal leg dystonia, generalized dystonia), or whenever dystonia is combined with another movement disorder or neurological signs, then further investigations to uncover an underlying neurodegenerative disease, acquired, or inherited etiology should be pursued.

Imaging

A brain MRI should be considered in all early onset cases of dystonia and in all cases in which dystonia is combined with other neurological features. There are many findings on brain MRI that can further define the dystonia syndrome and narrow down the potential diagnosis. If there is suspicion of basal ganglia calcification, then a head CT is more sensitive. Imaging in adult-onset cervical dystonia has a very low diagnostic yield. However, if there is anything atypical about the presentation of cervical dystonia (e.g., abrupt onset, early fixed abnormal head posture without the presence of sensory tricks), MRI of the brain and cervical spine is recommended.

Bloodwork

In patients with combined dystonia syndromes, routine investigations should include complete blood count and at least an automated blood film to look for acanthocytes (although repeated wet smears may be required if there is a strong suspicion of neuroacanthocytosis). Iron studies, levels of calcium, parathyroid hormone, and manganese can be useful, particularly in patients with basal ganglia abnormalities on MRI.

A high serum uric acid can point to Lesch–Nyhan disease, but it does not have a high enough sensitivity or specificity to be a diagnostic test.

Treatment

There are few types of dystonia for which there are pathogenesis-targeted therapy (e.g., Wilson disease), therefore the primary goal of therapy for dystonia is to provide symptomatic relief of involuntary movements, abnormal postures, pain, and other comorbidities (e.g., depression, orthopedic complications). Treatment should be personalized to the individual, and should take into account the age of the patient, the anatomic distribution of dystonia, and the risk of adverse effects of therapy. Unfortunately, few randomized, double-blind, placebo-controlled trials do not exist for dystonia therapies, so any treatment algorithm will be primarily guided by the personal experience of the physician and empiric trials.

Although there are no robust evidence-based guidelines for a standardized approach to the treatment of dystonia, there are many therapeutic interventions that can significantly improve the quality of life of patients with dystonia. This includes, but is not limited to, patient education, physical therapy, medications, botulinum toxin injections, surgical therapy, and treatment of comorbidities.

Guiding principles in the treatment of dystonia
- Identify specifically treatable causes of dystonia (Wilson disease, drugs, structural lesions, metabolic abnormalities).
- Educate patient and family (genetic counseling).
- Address comorbidities (depression, orthopedic complications).
- Explain that therapy for dystonia is symptomatic not protective.
- Select treatment according to severity, age, type, and distribution.
- Encourage and guide patients to discover sensory tricks.
- Range of motion exercises to prevent contractures.
- L-dopa in childhood-onset and young-onset dystonia.
- Many treatments are based on empirical observation and experience (DBPC studies are needed).
- Surgical therapy should be reserved for patients with disabling dystonia resistant to pharmacological and/or BoNT therapy.

Pharmacologic treatment

Dopaminergic therapy

Pharmacologic therapy of dystonia is primarily based on empirical evidence rather than a scientific rationale. However, one exception is in the case of dopa-responsive dystonia (DRD), where the underlying pathophysiology has been clearly defined as a defect in dopamine synthesis. Some experts suggest a trial of levodopa in nearly all patients with dystonia, regardless of age or distribution, since the clinical spectrum of dopa-responsive dystonia has broadened with the advent of genetic testing. However, a common recommendation is that a levodopa trial is imperative in any case of dystonia presenting with childhood or young adult onset. In addition, a trial of levodopa should also be given any child with the diagnosis of cerebral palsy, since many cases of DRD (an exquisitely treatable disorder) are misdiagnosed as cerebral palsy. An additional group of patients that should always receive a levodopa trial is the adult who presents with focal leg dystonia because this is commonly a presenting symptom of a neurodegenerative disorder such as Parkinson disease.

Antidopaminergic therapy

Although dopamine receptor-blocking medications (neuroleptics) were commonly used in the past, the use of these drugs for the treatment of dystonia is discouraged due to a risk of significant side effects, including sedation, parkinsonism, and tardive dyskinesia.

Dopamine-depleting drugs, such as tetrabenazine, have been found to be helpful in some patients with dystonia, particularly tardive dystonia, and due to its presynaptic mechanism (inhibition of vesicular monoamine transporter 2; VMAT2), does not cause tardive dyskinesia. However, it can cause side effects of drowsiness, depression, insomnia, akathisia, or a transient acute dystonic reaction.

Anticholinergic therapy

Anticholinergic medications have the potential to be helpful in all types of dystonias, although their use in the treatment of focal and segmental dystonias has been largely surpassed by botulinum toxin therapy. Because of their potential for undesirable side effects, this class of drugs is now usually reserved only for treatment of generalized dystonia. Trihexyphenidyl, the primary anticholinergic used to treat dystonia in the United States, is actually one of only a few oral medications that was tested for the treatment of dystonia using a double-blind placebo-controlled trial. Children generally tolerate *much* higher doses than adults.

Baclofen

After trihexyphenidyl, high doses of oral baclofen are likely to be the next most effective drug for dystonia. Baclofen is a $GABA_a$ autoreceptor agonist that is commonly used to treat spasticity. Daily doses of 60–120 mg has been found to be helpful for some patients with segmental, generalized, and oromandibular dystonia. In addition, baclofen may be helpful for wearing off foot dystonia in Parkinson disease.

Intrathecal baclofen pump therapy has shown promise as a treatment for dystonia in small open-label studies, and it may particularly be a reasonable therapeutic option in patients with "spastic" dystonia involving the legs and trunk associated with cerebral palsy or other acquired forms of dystonia.

Other pharmacologic therapies

It is not uncommon for patients with dystonia to require a combination of several medications and treatments to achieve satisfactory control of their symptoms. In addition to the above-described classes of medications for dystonia, several other classes of medications have been used with some benefit. Benzodiazepines (e.g., clonazepam, lorazepam, diazepam) can provide additional benefit for patients who have not tolerated or satisfactorily responded to anticholinergics. Other muscle relaxants that can be useful for dystonia include cyclobenzapreine, carisoprodaol, methocarbamol, metaxalone, and tizanidine. Sodium oxybate has also been reported to be in the myoclonus-dystonic syndrome. Paroxysmal dystonia can respond effectively to medication (e.g., kinesigenic paroxysmal dystonia is usually well-controlled with anti-convulsants carbamazepine or phenytoin).

Botulinum toxin

A major breakthrough in the treatment of focal and segmental dystonia was the discovery that botulinum toxin (BoNT), the most potent biologic toxin known to humans, could be used in a controlled fashion for the treatment the involuntary, excessive muscle contractions associated with dystonia. Botulinum toxin serotypes A and B inhibit the release of acetylcholine into the neuromuscular junction. Injection into dystonic muscles reduces muscle spasm without systemic side effects. Botulinum toxin injections are the treatment of choice for cervical dystonia, blepharospasm, spasmodic dysphonia, oromandibular dystonia, and limb dystonia, providing long-term benefit (with repeated injections) in 70-90% of patients. BoNT can also be used in patients with generalized or multifocal dystonia to treat selected muscles.

⚜ SCIENCE REVISITED

Mechanism of botulinum toxin
Botulinum toxin is a toxic protein produced by the bacterium *Clostridium botulinum*. There are seven structurally and immunologically distinct forms, types A–G. These neurotoxins block the release of acetylcholine at the neuromuscular junction by cleaving peptides required for vesicular membrane fusion, which selectively blocks cholinergic neurotransmission to striate and smooth muscles and temporarily paralyzes the injected muscles.

✋ CAUTION AND WARNING

Contraindications for botulinum toxin
Use of botulinum toxin is contraindicated in patients with a history of neuromuscular junction diseases such as myasthenia gravis and Lambert–Eaton syndrome, and motor neuron diseases such as amyotrophic lateral sclerosis because of its anticholinergic effects. Injections are also contraindicated in patients with a history of hypersensitivity to botulinum toxin and albumin. Botulinum toxin should not be used in conjunction with medications such as aminoglycosides, penicillamine, quinine, and calcium-channel blockers because of the risk of potentiating these drugs. Additionally, the teratogenicity of botulinum toxin has not been established, thus use in pregnant or lactating women is discouraged.

Two of the seven serotypes found in nature are currently available commercially: type A—onabotulinumtoxinA (Botox®), abobotulinumtoxinA (Dysport®), incobotulinumtoxinA (Xeomin®); and type B (Myobloc®/NeuroBloc®). When switching from one to another preparation of botulinum toxin, one should reference the product insert for typical conversion ratios. Botulinum toxin is a toxic protein produced by the bacterium *Clostridium botulinum*. There are seven structurally and immunologically distinct forms, types A-G. These neurotoxins block the release of acetylcholine at the neuromuscular junction by cleaving peptides required for vesicular membrane fusion, which selectively blocks cholinergic neurotransmission to striate and smooth muscles and temporarily paralyzes the injected muscles. Endocrine glands are also affected, decreasing signals for secretion of stored products.

Deep brain stimulation (DBS)

Patients with dystonia experiencing progressive disability or pain, having failed reasonable medication treatments including trihexyphenidyl, baclofen, and a benzodiazepine alone or in combination, may be candidates for DBS. Patients should also have a negative trial of levodopa, in order to rule out possibility of dopa-responsive dystonia (DRD), and have failed treatment of focal dystonia with botulinum toxin injections. Ideal patients are those for whom expected benefits will outlast the inherent risks of the surgical procedure. The common surgical site is the globus pallidus internus (GPi).

★ TIPS AND TRICKS

- Dystonia can be missed on exam when patients try to control the involuntary movements. Patients should be instructed to allow the involuntary movements to occur freely. For example, a latent abnormal posture underlying a tremor-dominant cervical dystonia may be revealed by asking the patient to relax with eyes close and let the head drift to the position that feels most comfortable, which often demonstrates unrecognized torticollis or laterocollis.
- Dystonic tremor is often more irregular in timing and amplitude than non-dystonic tremor.
- In differentiating dystonic from spastic gait, dystonic spasms and posturing of the legs often may improve significantly or may even be absent during different walking tasks, such as walking backward, walking

heel to toe, or running, whereas a spastic gait will not change significantly according to task.
- Treatable causes of dystonia that you cannot afford to miss: Wilson disease, dopa-responsive dystonia, tardive dystonia.

Further Readings

Albanese A, Asmus F, Bhatia KP, Elia AE, Elibol B, Filippini G, et al. EFNS guidelines on diagnosis and treatment of primary dystonias. *Eur J Neurol* 2011; **18**: 5–18.

Albanese A, Bhatia K, Bressman SB, et al. Phenomenology and classification of dystonia: a consensus update. *Mov Disord* 2013; **28**: 863–873.

Balint B, Bhatia K. Dystonia: an update on phenomenology, classification, pathogenesis and treatment. *Curr Opin Neurol* 2014; **27**(4): 468–476.

Evatt ML, Freeman A, Factor S. Adult-onset dystonia. *Handb Clin Neurol* 2011; **100**: 481–511.

Fahn S, Bressman SB, Marsden CD. Classification of dystonia. *Adv Neurol* 1998; **78**: 1–10.

Fahn S. Concept and classification of dystonia. *Adv Neurol* 1988; **50**: 1–8. [PubMed: 3041755]

Fung, VSC, Jinnah HA, Bhatia K, Vidailhet M. Assessment of patients with isolated or combined dystonia: an update on dystonia syndromes. *Mov Disord* 2013; **28**(7): 889–898.

Lohmann K, Klein C. Genetics of dystonia: what's known? what's new? what's next? *Mov Disord* 2013; **28**(7): 899–905.

Phukan J, Albanese A, Gasser T, Warner T. Primary dystonia and dystonia-plus syndromes: clinical characteristics, diagnosis, and pathogenesis. *Lancet Neurol* 2011; **10**: 1074–1085.

Schneider SA, Bhatia KP. Secondary dystonia: clinical clues and syndromic associations. *Eur J Neurol* 2010; **17**(suppl 1): 52–57.

Tadic V. Dopa-responsive dystonia revisited. 2012 *Archives of Neurology*. Bethesda, MD: NCBI; 2012.

Warner TT, Bressman SB. Overview of the genetic forms of dystonia. In: Warner T, Bressman S, eds. *Clinical Diagnosis and Management of Dystonia*. London: Informa Healthcare; 2007; 27–33.

8

Ataxia

Samantha Holden, MD[1] and Deborah A. Hall, MD, PhD[2]

[1]University of Colorado School of Medicine, Aurora, Colorado, USA
[2]Department of Neurological Sciences, Section of Movement Disorders, Rush University Medical Center, Chicago, Illinois, USA

Introduction

Ataxia, meaning an absence of order, is a neurological sign characterized by incoordination and clumsiness of voluntary movements. Ataxia manifests as disturbances of gait, skilled movements, muscle tone, speech and eye movements, and is usually due to cerebellar dysfunction. The cerebellum is responsible for the coordination of motor function, and organizing the successive contractions of muscles into movement. The cerebellum is connected to multiple areas of the brain and spinal cord through feed-forward and feedback loops and ensures coordinated movements by integrating motor and sensory inputs. Therefore, ataxia is not only seen with cerebellar disease but also with any dysfunction of the associated input and output tracts, including the dorsal columns and spinocerebellar tracts of the spinal cord and peripheral nerves. Understanding the anatomy of the cerebellum and its connections is helpful in conceptualizing underlying pathology. The cerebellum is somatotopically organized, with the midline structures responsible for the trunk, head and eyes, and the more lateral hemispheres controlling the limbs. Damage to the midline vermis will affect posture and gait, and damage to the hemispheres will cause incoordination of the ipsilateral extremity.

In practice, cerebellar symptoms are rarely seen in isolation. They are frequently encountered in combination with other neurological and non-neurological signs and symptoms. This is because many causes of ataxia are related to

> ### SCIENCE REVISITED
>
> **Cerebellar anatomy**
> In addition to the described vermis and cerebellar hemispheres, there is also the flocculonodular lobe, which is connected to the vestibular system and plays a role in maintenance of equilibrium and control of eye movements.
>
> There are several deep cerebellar nuclei that receive afferent fibers into the cerebellum. These nuclei include the dentate, which is the largest nucleus and receives the input from the cerebellar hemispheres, as well as the fastigial, emboliform, and globose nuclei. The fastigial nucleus receives input from the vermis, and emboliform and globose nuclei from the paravermal zone. These nuclei then project back to the cerebellar cortex from which they received input. The input and output tracts of the cerebellum can be simplified as follows: primarily efferent fibers out through the superior cerebellar peduncle, pontine fibers through the middle cerebellar peduncle, and afferent fibers in through the inferior cerebellar peduncle.

complicated systemic diseases that lead to a potentially overwhelming clinical presentation with multiple complaints and findings. The classification of ataxic syndromes is therefore inherently complex,

Table 8.1 Clinical symptoms and signs of ataxia

Ataxic symptoms	Ataxic signs
Imbalance, frequent falls	Broad-based stance and gait
Incoordination, clumsiness, dropping things	Dysmetria, dyssynergia, dysdiadochokinesia
Slurred or slow speech	Dysarthria
Dizziness, vertigo, disequilibrium	Impaired tandem and Romberg
Blurred, double or "jumping" vision	Nystagmus, abnormal pursuit and saccades
Easy fatigability, asthenia	Hypotonia
	Postural and/or action tremor

with multiple possible underlying etiologies, many with variable or overlapping features. The precise number of individual ataxias is unknown, but there are estimated to be at least 50 unique syndromes, and possibly as many as 100, each with distinct underlying causes.

In an attempt to guide differential diagnosis, the ataxias have been split into two major categories: sporadic or hereditary. The sporadic category can be further divided into idiopathic or symptomatic, meaning there is an identifiable underlying cause determined by imaging or lab tests. The prevalence of ataxia of all causes is estimated at 60/100,000 in the United States, with 50/100,000 attributed to sporadic causes and 10/100,000 to hereditary ataxias. Though relatively rare, the ability to recognize and accurately categorize the ataxias is an essential skill for the neurologist. This chapter presents the clinical findings of ataxia, as well as a practical approach to differential diagnosis and categorization of disease. It ends with an overview of the limited treatment options currently available for ataxia.

Clinical features

Although ataxic syndromes can be variable in their clinical presentation, there will be, by definition, some combination of the cardinal features of cerebellar dysfunction, including abnormal stance, gait and eye movements, impaired coordination and control of skilled movements, and speech difficulty (Table 8.1). Impaired gait is usually the chief complaint of ataxic patients. Gait and stance are wide-based, often with staggering and irregular steps. The unsteady gait of ataxia can be attributed to inconsistent foot placement, as there is loss of the automaticity of gait. Each individual step depends on the preceding step, so without the normal return to a consistent body position between steps, there is a staggering gait

pattern. This unsteadiness may be more prominent during changes in the speed or cadence of gait, such as turning or stopping suddenly while walking. If the ataxia is mild, the gait abnormality may not be obvious on casual gait, but it can be brought out by asking the patient to walk in tandem. The patient will often need to place a foot out to the side to avoid falling. More severe gait ataxia will inhibit the ability to stand with one's feet together at all, even with eyes remaining open. At the extreme end of the spectrum, patients are unable to even stand unassisted. Stance and posture are also affected, with increased postural sway when standing, or even a more regular truncal tremor, termed "titubation." There can also be exaggerated postural reactions, which can be evaluated by testing for "rebound" on examination. Downward pressure exerted by the examiner on the outstretched arms of the patient will cause an exaggerated upward movement, or rebound, with an overcorrection in the opposite direction to the applied force.

★ TIPS AND TRICKS

Sensory ataxia

In addition to pure cerebellar ataxia, there can be sensory ataxia, caused by impaired proprioception due to a peripheral neuropathy or dorsal column dysfunction. Patients with a sensory ataxia will need to carefully watch the ground and monitor their foot placement while walking. They will also report frequent falls in the dark, or falling in the shower when closing their eyes to wash their hair. They will have a positive Romberg sign on exam, and large fiber sensory loss in the lower extremities. Most hereditary ataxias with known genetic defects, such as Friedreich ataxia, cause a combination of cerebellar and sensory ataxias.

In addition to unsteady gait, ataxic patients will complain of clumsiness and incoordination of the extremities. Their movements will be inaccurate and poorly controlled, related to difficulty properly initiating, directing and terminating movements. The normal timing of movements is lacking, with imprecise movements that start too late or accelerate too slowly, stop before appropriately reaching a target (hypometria) or accelerate too much and overshoot a target (hypermetria). This can be tested with finger-to-nose or finger-chase tests for the upper extremities and heel-knee-shin maneuvers for the lower extremities. With ataxia there is absence of the normal smoothness and ease of movements, being instead broken down into individual sequential steps (dyssynergia), as well as a lack of rhythmicity in rapidly alternating movements (dysdiadochokinesia). The faster one is asked to move, the more the movements can break down, with impairment of both acceleration and deceleration of movements.

Examination of oculomotor function is important when evaluating an ataxic patient, as clues to correct diagnosis can present themselves in abnormal eye movements. In addition to testing extraocular movements in all directions, special attention should be paid to both saccadic eye movements and smooth pursuit. Ataxic patients may display fragmentation of smooth pursuit, with difficulty smoothly tracking a target across their field of vision, as well as abnormal saccades. Saccadic eye movements, referring to the ability to quickly shift one's focus between presented targets, can become dysmetric in ataxia, with overshooting or undershooting of the eye movements. In some forms of ataxia, there can also be associated oculomotor apraxia, with impaired ability to generate saccadic eye movements at all on command, as well as difficulty coordinating head and eye movements together. However, optokinetic nystagmus will be intact in patients with oculomotor apraxia.

★ TIPS AND TRICKS

Oculomotor examination
Close examination of eye movements is very important in the ataxic patient. One should test not only extraocular movements in all directions, while looking for nystagmus, but also test both horizontal and vertical saccades, as well as for optokinetic nystagmus. Voluntary saccades should be tested for speed and accuracy.

- If downbeat nystagmus is present, one should think of anti-GAD ataxia or SCA6.
- Fixation instability, with involuntary saccades taking the patient's eyes off the target, should lead one to think of Friedreich ataxia.
- Dissociated nystagmus, with paresis of the medial rectus and nystagmus of the eye attempting to adduct, can be present in abetalipoproteinemia.
- Ophthalmoplegia may be present in SCA1, 2, or 3 (but most characteristic of SCA2), as well as later stages of ataxia with oculomotor apraxia (AOA).

The dysarthria associated with cerebellar dysfunction is often unique from that caused by pure bulbar or facial weakness. Speech is often slow, slurred and clumsy, analogous to the clumsiness of limb movements. Cerebellar speech dysfunction is often referred to as scanning dysarthria, due to the robotic, syllabic pronunciation and lack of rhythm. Cerebellar speech patterns are only a motor impairment of speech, and there is no impairment in the structure or usage of language, with no aphasia or anomia.

Hypotonia may be a cerebellar sign. As opposed to the decreased tone caused by an upper motor neuron lesion, this hypotonia is difficult to detect on motor examination. Cerebellar hypotonia may be experienced by the affected patient as asthenia (subjective weakness and easy fatigability experienced by the patient), but with normal strength testing to resistance on exam. In cerebellar dysfunction, the asthenia is of central origin, not related to neuromuscular dysfunction as can be seen in other conditions. Cerebellar hypotonia is more often seen in Friedreich ataxia and the "pure" cerebellar spinocerebellar ataxias (SCAs), including SCA6, 10, and 11. It is hypothesized that cerebellar tremors, which are often postural or action tremors of the upper extremity, are related to this hypotonia, with impaired postural stability of the arm causing lapses in tone followed by corrections, leading to the oscillation of a tremor.

Table 8.2 Categorization of ataxias: sporadic ataxias, hereditary ataxias

Sporadic ataxias		Hereditary ataxias
Symptomatic	Idiopathic	
Structural lesions or malformations: tumor, stroke, superficial siderosis	Multiple system atrophy (MSA)	Autosomal dominant
Toxic/metabolic: alcohol, heavy metals, medications	Unknown etiology	Autosomal recessive
Endocrine: autoimmune thyroiditis, anti-GAD ataxia		X-Linked
Malabsorption: gluten ataxia, vitamin B12 deficiency, vitamin E deficiency		Mitochondrial
Paraneoplastic: small-cell lung, breast, ovarian, Hodgkin lymphoma		
Demyelinating disease		
Inflammatory disease: post-viral, Whipple disease, neurosyphilis, Creutzfeldt–Jakob disease		

Diagnosis

When presented with an ataxic patient, the differential diagnosis can be daunting given an ever-expanding list of genetic diseases. The first step toward diagnosis should be distinguishing between the two main categories of ataxia: hereditary or sporadic. This categorization has largely replaced the older, neuropathological criteria for ataxia, which was previously split into either spinocerebellar degeneration or olivopontocerebellar atrophy. Taking diagnosis a step further than this initial categorization can be more difficult, with a specific etiology determined in only about half of patients presenting with a hereditary ataxia and about one-third of those with a sporadic ataxia. Regardless of the odds of determining a specific diagnosis, further investigations should include detailed family history and genealogy, as well as neuroimaging and laboratory tests (Table 8.2).

One should be cautioned against ordering a "complete ataxia panel," which is a panel of genetic testing that is offered commercially, without first narrowing down the potential diagnosis and ruling out symptomatic, potentially treatable ataxias (first-line lab tests in Figure 8.1). These panels are incredibly costly and frequently not reimbursed by insurance. When considering genetic testing, the specific tests ordered should be thoughtfully chosen based on clinical findings, rather than employing a "shotgun" approach. As genetic testing technology advances and becomes more affordable, more extensive sequencing may become readily available for elusive ataxia diagnoses. Whole exome or genome sequencing are a high-yield techniques that would allow sequencing of the entire protein coding region or the entire sequence of the patient's genome for pathogenic variants, rather than testing multiple individual genes.

Until more advanced genetic sequencing technology is offered, a thorough family history and construction of a genealogic tree may help reveal a hereditary disorder and elucidate its mode of inheritance. Ataxia present in consecutive generations with evidence of male-to-male transmission suggests an autosomal dominant disorder. One should keep in mind, however, that autosomal dominant disorders may mimic autosomal recessive inheritance, or even a sporadic disorder, due to carriers who appear clinically unaffected due to anticipation or reduced penetrance.

⬡ SCIENCE REVISITED

Anticipation and trinucleotide repeats
Anticipation refers to the earlier onset, and often worsening severity, of clinical symptoms in successive generations. This is most often seen in trinucleotide repeat diseases, caused by a mutation in which regions of trinucleotide repeats in coding or noncoding regions can become pathogenic over a certain threshold of repeats. During meiosis, trinucleotide repeats are unstable and can undergo further expansion, leading to a larger number of repeats in the germ cells, and therefore in the offspring. Expansion size is indirectly related to age of onset. Several SCAs are polyglutamine diseases, due to an expanded trinucleotide repeat of CAG. SCA2 and 7 particularly demonstrate anticipation.

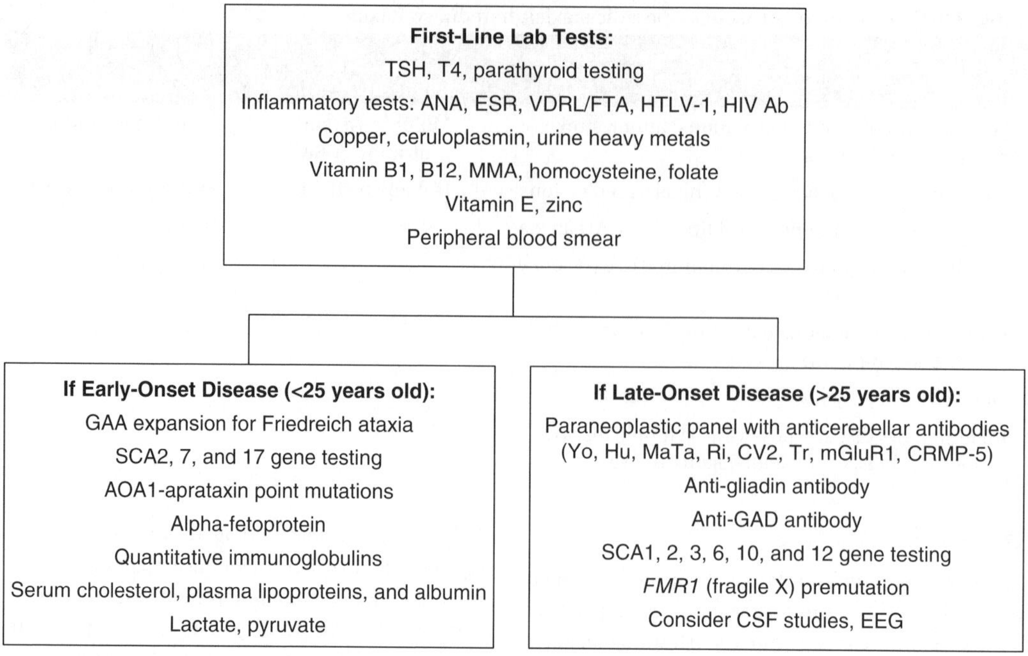

First-Line Lab Tests:

TSH, T4, parathyroid testing

Inflammatory tests: ANA, ESR, VDRL/FTA, HTLV-1, HIV Ab

Copper, ceruloplasmin, urine heavy metals

Vitamin B1, B12, MMA, homocysteine, folate

Vitamin E, zinc

Peripheral blood smear

If Early-Onset Disease (<25 years old):

GAA expansion for Friedreich ataxia

SCA2, 7, and 17 gene testing

AOA1-aprataxin point mutations

Alpha-fetoprotein

Quantitative immunoglobulins

Serum cholesterol, plasma lipoproteins, and albumin

Lactate, pyruvate

If Late-Onset Disease (>25 years old):

Paraneoplastic panel with anticerebellar antibodies
(Yo, Hu, MaTa, Ri, CV2, Tr, mGluR1, CRMP-5)

Anti-gliadin antibody

Anti-GAD antibody

SCA1, 2, 3, 6, 10, and 12 gene testing

FMR1 (fragile X) premutation

Consider CSF studies, EEG

Figure 8.1 Suggested lab tests for ataxia. TSH: thyroid stimulating hormone; ANA: antinuclear antibody; ESR: erythrocyte sedimentation rate; VDRL: Venereal Disease Research Lab; FTA: fluorescent treponemal antibody; HTLV-1: human T-cell lymphotropic virus-1; HIV: human immunodeficiency virus; MMA: methylmalonic acid; SCA: spinocerebellar ataxia; AOA: ataxia with oculomotor apraxia; GAD: glutamic acid decarboxylase.

Hereditary ataxia

Autosomal dominant

The clinical manifestations of autosomal dominant cerebellar ataxias (ADCA) are often limited to the central nervous system, as opposed to autosomal recessive diseases which usually affect multiple organ systems. ADCAs are characterized by progressive, symmetric ataxia due to involvement of the cerebellum, brainstem, and spinal cord, with a variable contribution from other neurologic symptoms (Table 8.3). ADCAs are degenerative diseases that cause steady worsening over time. This group of diseases includes the spinocerebellar ataxias (SCAs), which include an ever-increasing list of numbered syndromes. Sixty to 80% of the ADCAs are due to SCA1, 2, 3, 6, or 7 (all of which are polyglutamine diseases), with SCA3 being the common form. The common clinical presentation of a SCA is an ataxia "plus" syndrome, with some combination of obvious cerebellar dysfunction and specific associated neurological signs and symptoms, such as oculomotor

★ **TIPS AND TRICKS**

Clinical clues for SCA diagnosis

While attempting to identify a specific SCA can seem daunting, there are several distinguishing features of individual sub-types that can help narrow down diagnosis:

- Head tremor, myoclonus: SCA 2, 8, or 12
- Epilepsy: SCA 10, 13
- Neuropathy: SCA 1, 2, 3, 4, or 28
- Spasticity: SCA 1, 3, 7
- Parkinsonism: SCA 2, 3, or 17
- Dementia: SCA 13, 17
- Slow saccades: SCA 2, 3, or 7
- Early cognitive impairment: SCA17
- Staring or bulging eyes: SCA3
- MRI with pure cerebellar atrophy: SCA 5, 6, 10, 11, or 14
- MRI with brainstem atrophy: SCA 1, 2, 3, 7, or 13

Table 8.3 Autosomal dominant cerebellar ataxias[*]

	Clinical features	Oculomotor findings	Genetics
SCA1	Ataxia, dysarthria, pyramidal signs, **peripheral neuropathy**, **spasticity**, hyperreflexia, cognitive impairment	Nystagmus, slow saccades, ophthalmoparesis	CAG repeats (38–83) on 6p23, gene product is Ataxin-1
SCA2	Ataxia, dysarthria, peripheral neuropathy, hyporeflexia, **dementia**, myoclonus, parkinsonism	**Slow saccades**, ophthalmoplegia	CAG repeats (35–64) on 12q24, gene product is Ataxin-2
SCA3	Ataxia, dysarthria, spasticity, parkinsonism, lid retraction, **neuropathy**	Nystagmus, saccadic dysmetria, slow saccades, ophthalmoparesis, square-wave jerks	CAG repeats (61–84) on 14q32, gene product is Ataxin-3
SCA6	Ataxia, dysarthria, can have episodic ataxia, very slow progression, lack of family history, **later onset**	Nystagmus (**60% down-beating**), fragmented pursuit	CAG repeats (20–33) on 19p13, gene product CACNA1A
SCA7	Ataxia, dysarthria, **pigmentary retinopathy**, peripheral neuropathy, pyramidal signs, spasticity, infantile phenotypes	Fragmented pursuit, **slow saccades**	CAG repeats (37–300) on 3p14, gene product Ataxin-7
SCA8	Ataxia, dysarthria, mild sensory neuropathy, **head tremor, myoclonus**	Nystagmus, fragmented pursuit	CTG repeats (100–250) on 13q21
SCA10	Pure cerebellar syndrome, **seizures**	Nystagmus, fragmented pursuit	ATTCT Intron (9800–4500) on 12q13
SCA12	Ataxia, dysarthria, early arm tremor, late dementia, **head tremor, myoclonus**	Nystagmus, fragmented pursuit	CAG repeat (66–93) on 5q31, gene product phosphatase2A PPP2R2B
SCA14	Ataxia, dysarthria, early axial myoclonus, dystonia, peripheral neuropathy	Nystagmus, slow saccades	Missense mutations on 19q13.4, gene product is protein kinase Cg PRKCG
SCA17	Ataxia, chorea, dysarthria, **behavioral changes**, **cognitive decline, parkinsonism**	Nystagmus, fragmented pursuit, slow saccades	CAG repeats (45–63) on 6q27, gene product is TATA box-binding protein
DRPLA	Ataxia, dysarthria, chorea, seizures, dementia, myoclonus, rigidity	Nystagmus	CAG repeats (49–88) on 12p, gene product is atrophin-1
FGF14	Ataxia, dysarthria, tremor, psychiatric episodes, peripheral neuropathy	Nystagmus, fragmented pursuit	Point mutations on 13q34, gene product is fibroblast growth factor 14
EA1	Episodic ataxia, attacks lasting seconds to minutes, induced by exercise, startle or change of position, myokymia, cramping	Nystagmus between attacks	Point mutations in potassium channel gene, *KCNA1*, on 12p13
EA2	Episodic ataxia, attacks lasting minutes to hours, later permanent ataxia, vertigo, migraines	Nystagmus between attacks	Point mutations in *CACNL1A4* gene on 19p13

[*] SCA: spinocerebellar ataxia; DRPLA: dentatorubropallidoluysian atrophy; FGF14: fibroblast growth factor 14; EA: episodic ataxia. **Bolded** features and findings represent those that can be particularly helpful for narrowing clinical diagnosis, as they can be more specific for the associated condition.

findings, pyramidal or extrapyramidal features, seizures, cognitive impairment or peripheral neuropathy. The mean age of onset of the SCAs is in the third to fourth decade of life with the following caveats: SCA2, 7, 17, and 27 are commonly childhood onset and SCA6, 10, 11, and 12 are frequently seen in older adults.

Autosomal recessive

Autosomal recessive inheritance is suggested by the presence of multiple affected family members in a single generation only or by the presence of consanguinity in the family. The autosomal recessive ataxias more often present at early ages, before age 25, and manifest as multisystem diseases, affecting not only the nervous system but usually the cardiovascular, musculoskeletal, and endocrine systems as well (Table 8.4). The most frequent cause of autosomal recessive ataxia is Friedreich ataxia, which is characterized neurologically by early-onset gait ataxia, areflexia, and peripheral neuropathy related to degeneration of both cerebellar and spinal cord pathways. Extraneural manifestations of the disease include pes cavus, cardiomyopathy, diabetes mellitus, and scoliosis. Friedreich ataxia is also a trinucleotide repeat disease, but instead of a polyglutamine (CAG) repeat expansion, there is a GAA repeat expansion in the *FRDA*1 gene on chromosome 9. Unlike the autosomal dominant triplet repeat diseases, Friedreich ataxia does not demonstrate anticipation. There can be a later onset form of the disease, presenting after age 25, which is usually milder and more slowly progressive, lacking the cardiomyopathy that is the frequent cause of death in Friedreich patients.

Ataxia-telangiectasia (AT) is another autosomal recessive cerebellar ataxia that may be encountered, though it is slightly more rare than Friedreich ataxia. A clinical clue to this diagnosis is oculomotor apraxia, which is present in 96% of AT patients. Other clinical features include telangiectasia, or small dilated blood vessels near the surface of skin and mucus membranes, choreoathetosis, dystonia, immune deficiency, and predisposition to cancers. This disease has a childhood onset, with affected individuals usually wheelchair-bound by their teens, and early death before age 30. There can also be a milder phenotype, however, if there is relative preservation of the AT mutated gene product (phosphoinositol-3-kinase type enzyme).

Metabolic diseases

Metabolic diseases are usually autosomal recessive in inheritance and cause multisystem illness, typically presenting in infancy, with poor prognoses. This group of diseases includes the lipid storage disorders, urea cycle disorders, and pyruvate dehydrogenase deficiency. Although these disorders are typically seen by pediatric neurologists, it is important to be aware that several of these disorders can present in adulthood. Examples include Niemann–Pick Type C, which can present with ataxia, dementia, psychiatric symptoms, and hepatosplenomegaly, and GM-1 gangliosidosis, which can present with gait ataxia, dysarthria, and dystonia. Wilson disease and aceruloplasminemia should also be considered in this group of disorders.

X-Linked inheritance

Presence of ataxia in only male members of the family, inherited through the maternal line, implies X-linked inheritance. X-linked cerebellar ataxias are usually early-onset, slowly progressive syndromes. There can be variable phenotypes even in what are considered congenital conditions. For example, a later-onset subtype of adrenoleukodystrophy, called "adrenomyeloneuropathy," can present with ataxia, a progressive spastic paraparesis with sphincter dysfunction and adrenal failure. This disease can be diagnosed by elevated very long chain fatty acids (VLCFA) in the serum. There is also a more recently described condition, fragile X-associated tremor/ataxia syndrome (FXTAS), which is seen in older individuals, usually over age 50. This disease is characterized by a variable combination of cerebellar ataxia, tremor, parkinsonism, cognitive impairment, autonomic dysfunction, and polyneuropathy. FXTAS is another triplet repeat disease, with the underlying pathophysiology related to a premutation range expansion of the fragile X mental retardation 1 (*FMR1*) gene, with a CGG repeat between 55 and 200. Greater than 200 repeats will cause the traditionally recognized fragile X syndrome, which is a common cause of intellectual disability in boys. Patients that present with FXTAS will often have

Table 8.4 Autosomal recessive cerebellar ataxias*

	Clinical features	Oculomotor findings	Genetics
FA	Early onset gait ataxia, areflexia, dysarthria, peripheral neuropathy, pyramidal signs, scoliosis, pes cavus, cardiomyopathy, diabetes	Fixation instability, square-wave jerks, fragmented pursuit, saccadic dysmetria	GAA repeat (90–1300), *FRDA1* gene on 9q13-q21, gene product is Frataxin
AT	Ataxia, telangiectasia, choreoathetosis, dystonia, immune deficiency, predisposition to cancers	**Oculomotor apraxia,** increased latency of saccades	*ATM* gene on 11q22-q23, gene product is phosphoinositol-3-kinase type enzyme
AVED	Ataxia, dysarthria, peripheral neuropathy, head titubation, possible cardiomyopathy and retinopathy	Nystagmus, fragmented pursuit	*Alpha-TTP* gene on 8q13, gene product is alpha-tocopherol transfer protein
ABL	Ataxia, areflexia, retinal degeneration, celiac-like GI symptoms, steatorrhea, **acanthocytes on peripheral blood smear**	**Dissociated nystagmus** on lateral gaze (nystagmus of adducting eye), slow saccades	*MPT* gene on 4q22–24, gene product is large subunit of MPT
Cayman ataxia	Non-progressive gait ataxia, early-onset hypotonia, psychomotor retardation, dysarthria, tremor	Nystagmus	*ATCAY* gene on 19p13.3, gene product is caytaxin
AOA1	Ataxia, peripheral neuropathy, choreoathetosis, mild mental retardation, hypercholesterolemia, hypoalbuminemia	Oculomotor apraxia, fixation instability, fragmented pursuit, gaze-evoked nystagmus, hypometric saccades	*APTX* gene on 9p13, gene product is aprataxin
AOA2	Ataxia, choreoathetosis, peripheral neuropathy, increased alpha-fetoprotein	Oculomotor apraxia, fragmented pursuit, slow saccades	*SCAR1* gene on 9q34, gene product is senataxin
SCAN	Ataxia, sensory loss, mild hypoalbuminemia, mild hypercholesterolemia	No oculomotor findings	*TDP1* gene on 14q31, gene product tyrosyl-DNA phosphodiesterase1

* FA: Friedreich ataxia; AT: ataxia-telangiectasia; AVED: ataxia with vitamin E deficiency; ABL: abetalipoproteinemia; AOA: ataxia with oculomotor apraxia; SCAN: spinocerebellar ataxia with axonal neuropathy. **Bolded** features and findings represent those that can be particularly helpful for narrowing clinical diagnosis, as they can be more specific for the associated condition.

grandsons with intellectual disability or daughters with primary ovarian insufficiency, the latter of which is also associated with expansions in the *FMR1* gene. FXTAS can be diagnosed with a gene test for *FMR1* and all men presenting with ataxia over age 50 should be considered for screening. MRI of the brain can be supportive, with characteristic T2-hyperintensities in the middle cerebellar peduncles ("MCP sign")— (Figure 20.1b in Chapter 20 on radiology).

Mitochondrial disorders

Mitochondrial diseases can be more difficult to diagnose by genealogy alone, since mutations can occur in either mitochondrial DNA, which is inherited solely from the mother, or in the nuclear

DNA. These diseases can mimic any type of inheritance and family history is not particularly helpful. In addition, mitochondrial diseases are complicated multisystem diseases, affecting those organ systems dependent on high levels of energy production, including the brain, heart, and skeletal muscle. While ataxia is a common component of these diseases, it is usually not the presenting symptom in isolation. Examples of mitochondrial diseases with ataxia include myoclonic epilepsy with ragged red fibers (MERRF), Kearns–Sayre syndrome (KSS), and neuropathy, ataxia, and retinitis pigmentosa (NARP). MERRF presents with a variable combination of ataxia, myopathy, seizures, ophthalmoplegia, and dementia, and KSS presents with ataxia, chronic progressive external ophthalmoplegia, pigmentary retinopathy, and cardiac conduction abnormalities.

Sporadic ataxia

If a family history is not particularly helpful in narrowing down the diagnosis by mode of inheritance, the next step involves ordering neuroimaging, typically an MRI of the brain, and a thoughtfully chosen panel of laboratory tests in order to investigate symptomatic ataxias. Suggested tests are noted in Figure 8.1. In addition, it is important to keep in mind that a negative family history does not necessarily rule out a hereditary ataxia, as it could be a de novo mutation. MRI of the brain often demonstrates cerebellar atrophy, which may not be particularly specific or helpful for diagnosis, but associated patterns of atrophy in the cortex, brain stem, or spinal cord may help narrow diagnosis. A structural lesion such as a posterior fossa neoplasm or a cerebellar infarct is also easily picked up with MRI. There are several characteristic brain MRI findings that can be very useful for diagnosis if present, as listed in Table 8.5. A CT scan of the chest, abdomen, and pelvis can be considered to evaluate for an occult malignancy, should a paraneoplastic cerebellar ataxia be suspected. The above-mentioned investigations can help differentiate the various causes of sporadic ataxias, and with a simplified diagnostic algorithm as presented in Figure 8.2.

Multiple system atrophy (MSA) is a common cause of adult onset cerebellar ataxia, being responsible for about 30% of such cases. There are two sub-types of MSA, being divided into parkinsonian (MSA-P) and cerebellar (MSA-C) phenotypes. Onset is usually in the sixth decade of life, with a rapid progression and mean survival of less than 10 years after diagnosis. In addition to ataxia and parkinsonism, there is prominent autonomic dysfunction in this disease, with severe orthostatic hypotension.

Table 8.5 Characteristic MRI findings in ataxia

Ataxic syndrome	Characteristic MRI findings
Fragile-X associated tremor/ataxia syndrome (FXTAS)	Increased T2 signal in middle cerebellar peduncles (MCP sign) and in deep white matter of cerebellar hemispheres
	Mild to moderate cerebral and cerebellar atrophy
Friedreich ataxia	Atrophy of cervical cord
Ataxia with vitamin E deficiency	Mild cerebellar atrophy
Ataxia-telangiectasia (AT) Ataxia with ocular apraxia (AOA) 1 and 2 Spinocerebellar ataxia with axonal neuropathy (SCAN)	Prominent cerebellar atrophy, predominantly of the vermis
Alcoholic cerebellar degeneration	Atrophy predominantly of the anterior superior vermis and adjacent cerebellar hemispheres
Superficial siderosis	Linear T2 hypointense rim most evident along the surface of the vermis and cerebellar folia
Joubert syndrome (rare congenital ataxia)	"Molar tooth" sign at the cerebellar-midbrain junction, due to absence of the cerebellar vermis

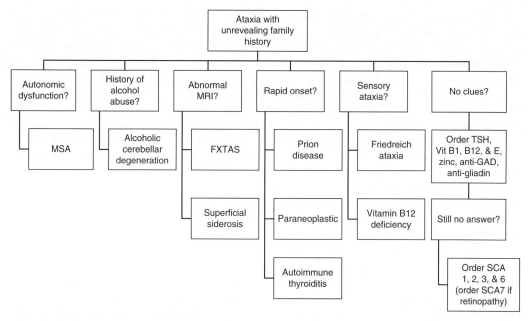

Figure 8.2 Diagnostic algorithm for sporadic ataxias.

Symptomatic ataxias due to structural lesions are often the straightforward ataxias to diagnose and usually the easiest to treat. In addition to possible strokes and tumors, a structural cause that can commonly cause ataxia is superficial siderosis. Superficial siderosis is thought to be due to repeated small subarachnoid bleeds, stemming from vascular malformations, trauma or neurosurgical procedures, and it is characterized by progressive ataxia, hearing loss, cognitive impairment, and pyramidal signs. This dysfunction is caused by the deposition of free iron and hemosiderin along the surfaces of the involved structures, namely the cerebellum, brainstem, and temporal lobes. This condition can be diagnosed by MRI and lumbar puncture.

One of the common forms of chronic cerebellar ataxia is alcoholic cerebellar degeneration, typically seen in middle-aged men with a history of chronic alcohol abuse. This presents mainly with ataxia of gait and the lower extremities, with less impairment seen in the upper extremities or with speech. Onset can be either rapid or slowly progressive, and symptoms can improve with strict abstinence from alcohol. This disease is likely related not only to the directly toxic effects of alcohol on the brain but also to thiamine deficiency, as studies have shown a reliable inverse relationship between serum vitamin B1 levels and the degree of cerebellar atrophy.

Paraneoplastic cerebellar degeneration is being increasingly recognized as a frequent cause of ataxia, with multiple cerebellar specific anti-neuronal antibodies described. The commonly associated cancers are small-cell lung, breast, and ovarian cancers, and Hodgkin lymphoma. These syndromes usually follow a sub-acute, but relentlessly progressive course, with poor response to steroids, intravenous immunoglobulin or plasma exchange, though Hodgkin lymphoma may respond. Survival ultimately depends on the underlying tumor type, if it can be discovered.

Treatment

There are few effective medications to treat ataxia, and none are FDA approved for that purpose other than acetazolamide for episodic ataxia type 2. The current mainstays of treatment are physical, occupational, and speech therapy. For gait ataxia, there is evidence that frequent and intensive gait and balance training can be effective for ataxia, with rhythmic and repetitive exercises assisting in relearning motor skills. Physical therapists should be aware that patients with cerebellar dysfunction frequently have impaired motor learning, so instructions must be explicit during training. Social workers, psychologists, psychiatrists and genetic counselors are also important members of the multidisciplinary ataxia team.

For symptomatic ataxias, treatment of the underlying cause is most effective, such as correcting nutritional deficiencies, avoiding toxins, treating underlying malignancies or immunomodulation. There have been several open-label trials for pharmacologic treatment of inherited ataxia, particularly in the SCAs, though they have been somewhat disappointing in their results. Amantadine, a NDMA receptor antagonist, is frequently used in Parkinson disease (PD) and is well tolerated in non-elderly populations. The medication may need to be used at higher doses than in PD for an effect (200–400 mg daily). Buspirone, up to 30 mg twice daily, has been shown in small case series to be effective for some patients. Both varenicline (1 mg twice daily) and riluzole (1 mg twice daily) have both been reported in isolated patients to be effective to improve gait ataxia. However, long-term use of varenicline has not been studied, and both medications are quite expensive and unlikely to be covered by insurance in the United States.

Treatment of associated symptoms that often accompany ataxia, such as tremor, dystonia, or parkinsonism, can be approached with appropriate medications for those conditions. Active research continues into disease-modifying therapies for the ataxias, focusing mainly on the polyglutamine disease. Research into the effectiveness of free radical scavengers, such as alpha-lipoic acid, mitochondrial stabilizers (like coenzyme q10 and creatine), and anti-excitotoxic agents, such as amantadine and riluzole, is underway. There have been some benefits seen in animal studies, but less dramatic improvement in human studies thus far. Other areas of research include gene therapy and stem cell therapy, as well as less invasive options like transcranial magnetic stimulation to the cerebellum.

Further Readings

Brusse E, Maat-Kievit JA, van Sweiten JC. Diagnosis and management of early- and late-onset cerebellar ataxia. *Clin Gen* 2007; **71**: 12–24.

Fahn S, Jankovic J, Hallet M, eds. *Principles and Practice of Movement Disorders*, 2nd ed. Philadelphia: Saunders, 2011.

Fogel BL, Perlman S. An approach to the patient with late-onset cerebellar ataxia. *Nat ClinPract Neurol* 2006; **2**(11): 629–635.

Ilg W, Bastian AJ, Boesch S, Burciu RG, et al. Consensus paper: management of degenerative cerebellar disorders. *Cerebellum* 2014; **13**(2): 248–268.

Klockgether T. Sporadic ataxia with adult onset: classification and diagnostic criteria. *Lancet Neurol* 2010; **9**: 94–104.

Mariotti C, Fancellu, Di Donato S. An overview of the patient with ataxia. *J Neurol* 2005; **252**: 511–518.

Perlman SL. Symptomatic and disease-modifying therapy for the progressive ataxias. *Neurologist* 2004; **10**(5): 275–289.

9

Restless Leg Syndrome

Olga Klepitskaya, MD

Department of Neurology, School of Medicine, University of Colorado, Aurora, Colorado, USA

Introduction

The earliest references to painful restlessness of the limbs dates back to ancient philosophers. The first scientific description is found in the works of a well-known seventeenth-century anatomist and physician, Sir Thomas Willis. In the following centuries, RLS was known under the term "anxietas tibiarum," which means an irritation of the lower legs. In the 1940s, Swedish neurologist, Karl Ekbom, published a series of manuscripts describing the variety of symptoms of this disorder and its negative impact on sleep and quality of life. He also noted the familial nature of this disorder and association with pregnancy, anemia, and other medical conditions. He reported that the disorder is fairly common, can be disabling, and is easily diagnosed if physicians are aware of it. He also suggested the name "restless leg syndrome." The name of the disease, however, is still a subject for debate. One reason is that although symptoms occur most commonly in the legs, they can occur in any part of the body, and the name does not reflect this distribution. Another reason is that the word "restless" does not necessarily reflect the potential severity of the symptoms. Therefore it was recently suggested that the name of the disorder should be officially changed to Willis–Ekbom syndrome.

Clinical features

Restless leg syndrome (RLS) is a chronic progressive sensorimotor disorder (Table 9.1). The diagnosis of RLS is clinical and is based on whether the patient's description of their symptoms match those outlined in the RLS diagnostic criteria. There are four essential diagnostic criteria and three supportive non-essential clinical features. Several associated non-essential symptoms have also been described.

The first essential criterion is an urge to move the legs, usually accompanied or caused by uncomfortable and unpleasant sensations in the legs. These symptoms have a certain degree of variability. For example, an urge to move can present without unpleasant sensations, or the sensations are so vague that they are difficult to describe. The most common descriptions are creeping, crawling, pulling, squeezing, itching, tingling, or restlessness. These sensations are usually bilateral, but they can be asymmetric and usually are experienced as deep "in the muscles or bones." Although legs, especially in the calf area, are most commonly affected, other parts of the body can also be involved. The symptoms can occur in the arms and even in the trunk. Of note, the feet are not as commonly affected as the calves; this can serve as a clue in a differential diagnosis with peripheral neuropathy, where sensory problems usually start in the feet (especially in the soles) and later can spread upward.

The second essential criterion is an urge to move or unpleasant sensation that begins or worsens during periods of rest or inactivity, such as laying or sitting. For example, these usually happen when the patient is in bed trying to fall asleep, watching TV, reading a book, or sitting for a prolonged period at a meeting or on an airplane. Some hospitalized

Non-Parkinsonian Movement Disorders, First Edition. Edited by Deborah A. Hall and Brandon R. Barton.
© 2017 John Wiley & Sons, Ltd. Published 2017 by John Wiley & Sons, Ltd.
Companion website: www.wiley.com/go/hall/non-parkinsonian_movement_disorders

Table 9.1 Diagnostic criteria for restless legs syndrome

Essential diagnostic criteria
1. An urge to move legs usually accompanied or caused by uncomfortable and unpleasant sensations in the legs
2. The urge to move or the unpleasant sensations begin or worsen during periods of rest or inactivity such as laying or sitting
3. The urge to move or unpleasant sensations are partially or totally relieved by movement such as walking or stretching, at least as long as activity continues
4. The urge to move or unpleasant sensations are worse in the evening or at night

Supportive nonessential clinical features
1. Positive family history of RLS
2. Positive response to dopaminergic therapy
3. Periodic limb movements of sleep (PLMS)

Associated nonessential clinical features
1. Sleep disturbances
2. Intermittent and relapsing clinical course, especially at the beginning of the disease
3. Otherwise normal physical and neurological examination

patients can develop de novo RLS or exacerbation of preexisting RLS from being immobilized or staying in bed due to acute illness. The symptoms of RLS in these situations are frequently overlooked and not treated, increasing the discomfort and suffering of already sick patients. Therefore, inpatient medical providers have to be aware of this problem, learn to recognize RLS symptoms, and treat appropriately.

The third essential criterion is that the urge to move or unpleasant sensations are partially or totally relieved by movement such as walking or stretching, at least as long as the activity continues. This usually forces patients to move, flex, and stretch their extremities. It frequently causes pacing, walking, and shaking that can be deemed socially unacceptable and affect patients' work performances. Tossing and turning at night in bed can be disturbing, not only to the patient's own sleep, but to the bed partner's sleep as well, and that in turn can negatively affect relationships.

Finally, the fourth essential criterion is that the urge to move or unpleasant sensation is worse in the evening or at night than during the day, or may only occur in the evening or night. In patients with severe symptoms, the worsening at night might not be noticeable but must be present earlier in disease. It is difficult to determine if this nighttime worsening is due to the fact that periods of inactivity (e.g., watching TV or lying in bed) are usually at night or if these circadian variations may be the predominant factor.

Supportive nonessential clinical features include a family history of RLS, good response to dopaminergic therapy, and periodic limb movements of sleep (PLMS). More than 50% of patients with RLS report a family history of RLS and even more report family history when symptoms started before the age of 45. Nearly all patents with RLS have, at least partially, an initial response to dopaminergic therapy. However, this response does not persist in all patients. The response to dopamine agonists is not as specific to RLS diagnostically as the response to carbidopa/levodopa. It has been shown that the response to the initial dose of levodopa is both sensitive (80–88%) and specific (100%) for supporting a diagnosis of RLS; however, this is not typically done as a diagnostic test in clinical practice. About 85% patients with RLS also have PLMS and some proportion have periodic limb movements during wakefulness (PLMW), in which the patient has similar movements to PLMS, but while awake. While PLMS are very nonspecific and can be associated with a variety of other disorders or can happen without any association, PLMW are more specific to RLS.

Associated nonessential features include sleep disturbances, an intermittent and relapsing clinical course (especially at the beginning of the disease), and otherwise normal physical and neurological examination. Younger patients tend to have more waxing and waning symptoms, while those older than age 50 might have a more abrupt onset, with severe and constant symptoms. Spontaneous resolution of symptoms can happen in older age. Sleep disturbance is the major health problem associated with RLS and is seen in the majority of patients. Insomnia, both with sleep onset and sleep maintenance difficulties, is a major contributor to poor quality of life in RLS patients. Patients with moderate to severe RLS sleep, on average, less than five hours per night.

Mimics of RLS

The common mimickers of RLS are akathisia, neuropathy, radiculopathy, chronic back pain, PLMW, PLMS, stereotypies, tremor, tics, painful legs and moving toes, attention deficit hyperactivity disorder (ADHD), levodopa-induced dyskinesias in Parkinson disease (PD), and metabolic conditions. Distinguishing between RLS and these disorders can be difficult and, to make things more complicated, sometimes these disorders can coexist with RLS. For example, hyperactivity in children with ADHD can be misinterpreted as a symptom of RLS. There are some clues that might be helpful in differentiation of these conditions. For example, akathisia is a motor restlessness that is usually caused by an inner sense of restlessness, rather than an unpleasant sensation in the limbs, and does not improve with movement nor worsen at nighttime. In peripheral neuropathy, pain or paresthesias are frequently experienced superficially and in the feet, while unpleasant sensations in RLS are usually experienced as deep and in the calves. Levodopa-induced dyskinesias are frequently not subjectively bothersome for PD patients, but look uncomfortable to an observer. Dyskinesia in PD can happen at any time of the day, depending on the timing of medication, and can involve any part of the body, including the face, head, neck, trunk, and extremities.

RLS is a sensorimotor disorder and the diagnosis is based on the patient's own description of their symptoms. Therefore, making this diagnosis becomes challenging in children or in individuals who are cognitively impaired. Nevertheless, a diagnosis can be made based on careful observation of patient's movements, relationship to the time of the day, response to dopaminergic therapy, and the presence of supportive features such as family history, PLMS, or sleep disturbances.

RLS is not a disorder of sleep, but rather, a disorder of wakeful restlessness. Therefore, the sleep study (polysomnography) is not essential for the diagnosis. Sleep studies, however, might be helpful to determine the presence of supportive feature of RLS such as the presence of PLMS or other sleep disorders.

Epidemiology of RLS

RLS symptoms affect 7–15% of the general adult population and almost 2% of children. However, clinically significant RLS, where symptoms are severe enough to require treatment, is less common and occurs in 1.6–2.8% of population. Both sexes and all ethnicities are affected; however, incidence is much higher in Caucasians and women. RLS is less common in persons of Indian and Asian origin.

Etiology of RLS

Primary RLS

RLS is classified as primary or secondary. Primary RLS can be sporadic or genetic. It is clear that RLS has a strong genetic predisposition, but the exact genetic inheritance is unknown and is most likely variable and multifactorial. Both autosomal dominant and recessive forms of inheritance have been described. Several genomic studies in RLS have been done. Two genome-wide association studies completed in Europe identified three gene loci associated with RLS. Notably, one of them, *MEIS1* on chromosome 2p, is thought to be partially responsible for the embryonic development of limbs.

⚝ TIPS AND TRICKS

Diagnosis of RLS

RLS is a sensorimotor disorder. Therefore the diagnosis is being made based on the patients' own reports of their symptoms, not on a physical exam or a diagnostic test, like in many other neurological disorders.

- Neurological examination is essential to rule out other neurological disorders (e.g., neuropathy, radiculopathy) that can mimic or contribute to the RLS symptoms.
- Diagnostic tests are essential to rule out secondary RLS.

⬡ SCIENCE REVISITED

Genomic studies have identified several genes associated with RLS:

- A common variant in an intron of *BTBD9* on chromosome 6p
- Homeobox gene *MEIS1* gene on chromosome 2p
- Genes encoding mitogen-activated protein kinase *MAP2K5* and transcription factor LBXCOR1 on chromosome 15q

Note: *MEIS1* gene is associated with embryonic development of limbs 1 & 2.

Secondary RLS

Secondary RLS can be diagnosed when a precipitating factor, illness, or causative agent can be identified. The most common causes of secondary RLS are iron deficiency, pregnancy, renal failure with uremia, and exposure to certain medications or substances (Table 9.2). In addition, there are disorders that demonstrate strong association with RLS, including PD, neuropathy, myelopathy, tremor, ataxia, fibromyalgia, multiple sclerosis, sleep apnea, and rheumatologic disorders.

Iron deficiency is the most common cause of secondary RLS. Many conditions that can cause iron deficiency have been implicated in precipitating RLS. Among these are blood loss, chronic proton pump inhibitors use, chronic blood donations, gastric surgery, pregnancy, and renal failure. Iron studies should be done in every patient with RLS. The most commonly tested parameters are serum iron levels and ferritin. However, serum iron levels are variable and can be impacted by a variety of dietary and lifestyle factors. Ferritin, an acute phase reactant, can have a false positive increase. Therefore, it is preferable to test the complete iron panel, including serum iron, total iron binding capacity (TIBC), iron saturation, transferrin, and ferritin. In addition, tests for vitamin B12 and folate may be beneficial because their malabsorption can occur in the same medical conditions. A kidney function test and a pregnancy test, in appropriate patients, should be performed as well.

Table 9.2 Factors known to exacerbate RLS

Factors known or likely to enhanced expressivity of RLS

Lifestyle
- Sleep
  - Irregular sleep-awake schedule
  - Sleep restriction
- Environment
  - Quite, relaxing environment
- Dietary
  - Caffeine
  - Alcohol
  - Biogenic amines
- Activity
  - Lack of
  - Overly strenuous physical activity
- Habits
  - Nicotine

Structural
- Neuropathies
  - Acquired
  - Familial
- Radiculopathies
  - Axonal
  - Demyelinating
- Myelopathies
  - Heritable
  - Acquired
  - Compressive/traumatic
- Varicose veins/ venous insufficiency
- Musculoskeletal abnormalities or injuries

Metabolic
- Iron deficiency
- Folate deficiency
- Kidney failure

Pharmacologic
- Antihistamines
  - Over-the-counter cold remedies,
  - Nasal decongestants
  - Sleeping aids
  - Antidepressants with antihistaminergic actions
    - Ex: Desyrel
    - Ex: Mirtazapine
- Antidopaminergics
  - Antiemetics
    - Metoclopramide
    - Promethazine
  - Neuroleptics
    - Typical
    - Atypical
- Antidepressants
  - Tricyclics
    - Ex: Amitriptyline
  - Tetracyclics
    - Ex: Mirtazapine, Amoxapine
  - Selective serotonin reuptake inhibitors (SSRIs)
    - Ex: Sertraline, Paroxetine, Citalopram
  - Serotonin–norepinephrine reuptake inhibitors (SNRIs)
    - Ex: Venlafaxine, Duloxetine
  - Lithium

Pathophysiology

The pathophysiology of RLS is not fully understood. Dopaminergic dysfunction and the alteration of brain iron metabolism continue to be two major concepts regarding mechanisms of RLS. Histopathological and MRI studies of the brain in RLS patients demonstrate a reduction of iron, especially in substantia nigra and putamen. Iron is intrinsically linked to dopaminergic function of the brain. It is a cofactor of tyrosine hydroxylase, an enzyme that controls the rate-limiting step of conversion from tyrosine to dopamine and is also essential for the D2 receptors' functionality. The strongest evidence of the role of dopamine in RLS pathogenesis is the dramatic and universal response of symptoms to the dopaminergic treatment and the exacerbation of symptoms after exposure to the dopamine receptors' antagonists. It has been hypothesized that a reduction in dopamine transporters and an increase of extracellular dopamine in RLS causes a relative dopamine deficiency. Opioids might also play a role in modulation of dopamine D2 receptors, and this, at least partially, can explain the beneficial effect of opioids in RLS. It has been demonstrated that the endogenous opioids beta-endorphin and met-enkephalin are decreased in the thalamus in RLS patients. In addition to the iron and dopamine hypotheses, extensive brain networks, spinal cord reflexes, and sensory systems in the peripheral nerves may be involved in the expression of RLS symptoms. For example, physiological studies have shown increased spinal excitability and decreased peripheral inhibition in RLS.

Treatment

The first step in the treatment of RLS is to identify and, if possible, eliminate any factors that can potentially cause or aggravate the symptoms (Table 9.2). Although not systematically proven, it appears that several lifestyle factors can precipitate RLS. Among them are sleep deprivation, use of caffeine and/or nicotine, and both lack of exercise and excessive strenuous exercise. Therefore, some lifestyle modification can potentially improve symptoms.

Iron deficiency should be tested for and treated if deemed appropriate. The etiology of the iron loss should also be evaluated, as it may be due to a serious medical condition. The Willis–Ekbom Disease Foundation treatment algorithm recommends iron repletion when ferritin is less than 20 mg/ml. Ferritin levels between 20 and 50 mg/ml have been associated with increased severity of RLS symptoms and augmentation. Treatment of patients with ferritin levels even less than 75 mg/ml can improve symptoms. Therefore iron supplementation is recommended on a case-by-case basis. Oral iron supplementation along with ascorbic acid, to enhance absorption, could be considered. The usefulness of IV iron formulations is controversial and was proved to be effective only in patients with end stage renal disease.

★ TIPS AND TRICKS

Iron in RLS treatment

- Every RLS patient should be tested for iron deficiency.
- The preferable test is a complete iron panel: serum iron, total iron binding capacity, percent iron saturation, transferrin, and ferritin.
- If present, the cause of iron deficiency should be further investigated.
- Iron repletion is recommended when ferritin is less than 20 mg/ml or percent iron saturation is less than 20%.
- Iron repletion is recommended for patients with severe symptoms or augmentation and low ferritin levels (20–50 mg/ml) on a case-by-case basis.
- The common iron treatment regiment is oral ferrous sulphate 325 mg, three times a day along with 100–200 mg of vitamin C to enhance absorption.
- Follow up laboratory tests are recommended every 3–6 months. If normalized, iron repletion can be stopped.
- Empirical treatment with iron is not advised because it can lead to iron overload.
- Oral iron therapy is usually well tolerated but can cause constipation and abdominal discomfort.
- Intravenous iron treatment has been demonstrated to be useful only in patients with end stage renal disease.

Many medications are known to cause or worsen RLS; therefore medication reconciliation and, if possible, discontinuation of offending medications are essential in a RLS treatment plan (Table 9.2). All classes of antidepressants can worsen RLS symptoms. Unfortunately, RLS patients can be depressed due to the severity of their symptoms and sleep disturbances and will need treatment for their depression. This makes treatment of patients with both RLS and depression challenging. Antidepressants that are both a norepinephrine and dopamine reuptake inhibitor, such as bupropion (Wellbutrin), may be less likely to exacerbate RLS symptoms. It is important to inquire about current and past medications, including asking if any medications were recently stopped. Rapid decrease in doses or sudden discontinuation of dopaminergic medications and opioids can provoke RLS symptoms. For example, in PD patients, it is occasionally necessary to decrease or discontinue dopamine agonists that are being used to treat motor symptoms, either due to side effects or other reasons. This, in turn, can bring out RLS symptoms in these patients. Therefore, a decrease in dose should be done very gradually, and if needed, smaller doses of dopamine agonists at night should be reinstituted or other RLS treatment should be considered.

The first-line pharmacologic treatment of RLS is dopamine agonist drugs (Table 9.3). These medications have been extensively studied in clinical trials, have shown high efficacy, and have been approved by US FDA for this indication, including pramipexole (Mirapex), ropinirole (Requip), and the rotigotine transdermal patch (Neupro). They are not as effective if taken after symptoms have already started, so it is recommended to take these medications about 90 to 120 minutes prior to the typical time of symptom onset. Dopamine agonists relieve symptoms in 70–90% of the patients. Doses needed to control symptoms are lower than those typically needed in PD. In the smaller dosages, they are less likely to cause the side effects that are typical for this class of medication. Nevertheless, even in these doses, side effects can be seen, and patients should be advised of the possibility of excessive daytime sleepiness, impulse control disorders, nausea, or swelling of the legs.

The most troubling side effects of dopaminergic treatment are rebound and augmentation. Rebound is a reoccurrence of RLS symptoms occurring in conjunction with decreasing half-life of the medication, usually in the early morning hours. Augmentation is characterized by the shift of RLS symptoms to an earlier time of the day, shorter latency of symptom onset, spreading of the urge to move to other limbs or parts of the body, shorter duration of the benefit of medication, and paradoxical reaction to medication (increased intensity with increased dose and decreased intensity with decreased dose). Augmentation is a difficult to manage complication of the treatment of RLS. It can occur during treatment with either dopamine agonists or levodopa, but is much more common with levodopa. Levodopa has the highest rate of augmentation, occurring in close to 70% of patients. Therefore levodopa is not recommended for everyday treatment, but it can be used for patients with sporadic symptoms or as a "rescue" medication for anticipated period of inactivity, such as a prolonged airplane or a car ride. The longer acting dopamine agonists may show a lower rate of augmentation and a high efficacy of symptoms control in some patients.

☆ TIPS AND TRICKS

Management of augmentation

- Avoid chronic treatment with levodopa.
- Use longer acting dopamine agonists.
- Recommend earlier doses of dopamine agonists if mild augmentation occurs.
- Reevaluate iron stores and start iron replacement treatment in cases of low ferritin levels.
- For severe or recurrent augmentation, decrease doses or discontinue dopamine agonists and initiate different pharmacological therapy.

Gabapentin and its derivatives have also been well studied and have demonstrated efficacy comparable with dopamine agonists. In fact, pregabalin (Lyrica) showed equal or superior efficacy compared to pramipexole, without causing typical dopamine agonists side effects. These medications can be especially beneficial in patients with coexisting neuropathic pain or other pain syndromes. A longer acting gabapentin derivative, gabapentin enacarbil extended-release (Horizant), was recently been approved by the US FDA for RLS treatment.

Table 9.3 Pharmacologic treatments for RLS

Medications	Recommended daily dose	Recommended use and benefits	Potential side effects
Dopaminergic treatment			
Dopamine agonists		First line of treatment	• Excessive daytime sleepiness
Pramipexole*	0.25–0.75 mg		• Impulse control disorders
Ropinirole*	0.25–4.0 mg		• Pedal edema
Rotigotine*	1–3 mg		• Nausea
			• Rebound
			• Augmentation
Cabergoline†	0.5–2.0 mg		• Cardiac valve defects
Levodopa	100–200 mg	• Second line of treatment	• Highest incidence of augmentation
		• Recommended for intermittent use and as a rescue medication	
Gabapentin and its derivatives		• Second line of treatment	• Somnolence,
Gabapentin enacabril*	600 mg	• Beneficial for patient with other pain issues.	• Cognitive difficulties
Gabapentin	800–3000 mg	• Low augmentation potential.	
Pregabalin	75–350 mg		
Opiods and opiod receptor agonists		• Second line of treatment	• Sleep apnea
Oxycodone	5–30 mg	• Beneficial for patient with other pain syndromes.	• Somnolence
Propoxyphene napsylate	100–200 mg	• Low augmentation potential.	• Addiction & tolerance: not common in RLS patients without prior history
Propoxyphene hydrochloride	65–130 mg	• Intermittent use for severe RLS is preferable.	
Codeine	30–60 mg	• Chronic use with long acting formulations with caution	
Tramadol	50–100 mg	• Preferable pharmacological treatment in pregnancy	
Methadone	10–40 mg		

(Continued)

Table 9.3 (*Cont'd*)

Medications	Recommended daily dose	Recommended use and benefits	Potential side effects
Benzodiazepines		• Second line of treatment	• Sleep apnea
Triazolam	0.125–0.5 mg	• Beneficial for patients with insomnia	• Somnolence
Clonazepam	0.25–1.0 mg	of other etiologies	• Addiction & tolerance: not common
Zolpidem	5–10 mg		in RLS patients without prior history
Temazepam	15–30 mg		• Unsteadiness
			• Cognitive difficulties, especially in
			the elderly
Others		Third line of treatment	
Amantadine	100–300 mg		
Carbamazepine	200–400 mg		
Valproic acid	600 mg		
Clonidine	0.1–0.5 mg		
Transdermal lisuride	3–6 mg every other day		

* Approved by FDA for treatment of RLS.
† Not available in US, available in Europe.

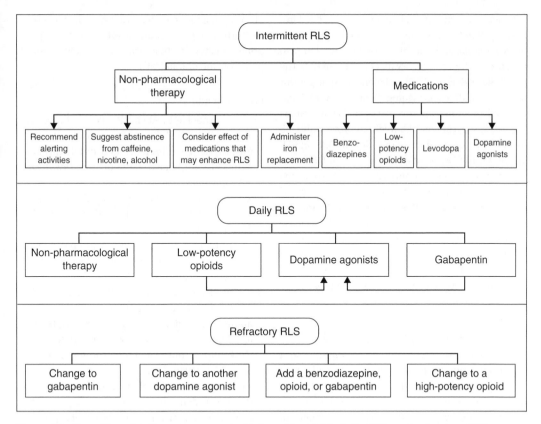

Figure 9.1 Algorithms for the management of intermittent RLS, daily RLS, and refractory RLS.
Source: Adapted from Silber (2004).

Opioids and opioid agonists were shown to be effective for RLS. Concerns regarding long-term opioid use, such as addiction, tolerance, and sleep apnea, limit their utility. Nevertheless, intermittent use of low-potency opioids may be beneficial, especially for treatment of severe RLS. When more regular treatment with opioids is needed, long-acting options such as methadone should be considered.

Benzodiazepines are also helpful, especially in patients who have severe sleep disturbances. These medications improve sleep and decrease leg discomfort and the urge to move. Clonazepam has been studied the most and demonstrated efficacy and safety, even in older patients. However, due to a long duration of action, it can result in side effects of morning drowsiness, cognitive impairment, and unsteadiness. The side effects of addiction and tolerance rarely occur in RLS patients, without a previous history of addiction. Just as with opioid treatment, sleep apnea is common and must be monitored.

Other medications and medication groups (or their combinations) might be useful for treatment of RLS, but evidence is lacking (Table 9.3). In 2008, an expert task force of the Movement Disorders Society published a systematic review with evidence-based recommendation on treatment of RLS. The algorithm for management of mild, moderate, and refractory RLS has been proposed to guide treatments (Figure 9.1).

Treatment of RLS in pregnancy is a challenge. Most medications used to treat RLS are not recommended for pregnant women. Non-pharmacological management should be tried first and iron deficiency should be treated. Some evidence suggests that folate, magnesium, and B12 might be helpful in pregnancy. If pharmacological treatments are necessary, opioids can be tried with caution. Although treatment with dopamine agonists is not recommended, there are several reports of successful use of dopamine agonists for treatment of PD in pregnant women.

Other less conventional treatments of RLS have been explored. For instance, botulinum toxin injections in the affected limbs were used in the attempt to interrupt peripheral sensory mechanisms of RLS. The possibility of deep brain stimulation (DBS) surgery for treatment of RLS is intriguing. Similarity of RLS and PD, and profound improvements of PD symptoms with DBS, suggest that RLS might improve with DBS as well. The observations of the effect of DBS on RLS symptoms in PD patients who underwent DBS were non-conclusive: both improvement and worsening were described. Exercise has also been implemented for treatment of RLS with some success. The mechanism of exercise's effects is likely mediated by increase of endogenous opioids. Melatonin has been postulated to improve RLS by normalizing circadian rhythms, but it failed to show efficacy in a clinical trial, and instead showed worsening of the symptoms.

Prognosis

The course of RLS is variable; spontaneous remissions and relapses are common. If symptoms start during an early age, the progression is usually slow. In many cases, however, RLS symptoms worsen over the years and eventually can become severe.

The negative impact of RLS on patients' quality of life (QoL) cannot be underestimated. RLS is associated with serious disruption of sleep. This, in turn, causes chronic sleep deprivation, impairment in cognitive function, depression, decrease in work performance, and many other problems. Studies on QoL in RLS patients demonstrated substantial impairment in all domains, including greater bodily discomfort as well as impairment in physical and mental functioning. Scores from the QoL questionnaire were significantly lower in the RLS group as compared to an age and sex-adjusted general population group. In fact, the impairments of QoL in the RLS group were the same as (or even worse than) the impairments of the group of patients suffering from other common chronic medical conditions, such as type 2 diabetes mellitus. In addition, it has been shown that RLS patients have worse job performance by 13.5% compared to non-RLS patients. Strong correlation between severity of symptoms and loss of work productivity was observed. All of this underscores the serious, and potentially disabling, nature of RLS; the importance of early recognition of the symptoms; the creation of the correct diagnosis; and the initiation of an appropriate treatment that can potentially improve patients' QoL dramatically.

Further Readings

Abetz L, Arbuckle R, Allen RP, Mavraki E, Kirsch J. The reliability, validity and responsiveness of the Restless Legs Syndrome Quality of Life questionnaire (RLSQoL) in a trial population. *Health Qual Life Outcomes* 2005; **3**:79.

Allen RP, Earley CJ. Augmentation of the restless legs syndrome with carbidopa/levodopa. *Sleep* 1996; **19**: 205–213.

Allen RP, Earley CJ. Restless legs syndrome: a review of clinical and pathophysiologic features. *J Clin Neurophysiol* 2001; **18**: 128–147.

Allen RP, Picchietti D, Hening WA, et al. Restless legs syndrome: diagnostic criteria, special considerations, and epidemiology. A report from the restless legs syndrome diagnosis and epidemiology workshop at the National Institutes of Health. *Sleep Med* 2003; **4**: 101–119.

Allen RP, Bharmal M, Calloway M. Prevalence and disease burden of primary restless legs syndrome: results of a general population survey in the United States. *Mov Disord* 2011; **26**: 114–120.

Aukerman MM, Aukerman D, Bayard M, Tudiver F, Thorp L, Bailey B. Exercise and restless legs syndrome: a randomized controlled trial. *J Am Board Fam Med* 2006; **19**: 487–493.

Happe S, Trenkwalder C. Role of dopamine receptor agonists in the treatment of restless legs syndrome. *CNS Drugs* 2004; **18**: 27–36.

Ondo WG, Jankovic J, Simpson R, Jimenez-Shahed J. Globus pallidus deep brain stimulation for refractory idiopathic restless legs syndrome. *Sleep Med* 2012; **13**: 1202–1204.

Rye DB, Trotti LM. Restless legs syndrome and periodic leg movements of sleep. *Neurol Clin* 2012; **30**: 1137–1166.

Silber MH, Ehrenberg BL, Allen RP, et al. An algorithm for the management of restless legs syndrome. *Mayo Clin Proc* 2004; **79**: 916–922.

Trenkwalder C, Hening WA, Montagna P, et al. Treatment of restless legs syndrome: an evidence-based review and implications for clinical practice. *Mov Disord* 2008; **23**: 2267–2302.

10

Hemifacial Spasm and Other Facial Movement Disorders

Tao Xie, MD, PhD[1], Ifeoma Nwaneri, MD[2] and Un Jung Kang, MD[3]

[1]Department of Neurology, University of Chicago Medical Center, Chicago, Illinois, USA
[2]Reston Hospital Center, Springfield, VA
[3]Department of Neurology, Columbia University Medical Center, New York, USA

Hemifacial spasm

Definition/clinical features

Hemifacial spasm (HFS) is characterized by involuntary and irregular clonic or tonic contraction of facial muscles innervated by the ipsilateral facial nerve. In the US Caucasian population, the average prevalence of HFS is 7.4 per 100,000 in men and 14.5 per 100,000 in women, with the highest incidence in the 40 to 79 age group. The prevalence in Asian populations appears to be higher than that in the Caucasian population for reasons that are not well understood.

The onset of HFS is usually insidious, beginning with involuntary twitching of the unilateral lower eyelid orbicularis oculi muscle, which gradually progresses to involve other ipsilateral facial muscles, including the frontalis, corrugator, procerus, levator labii superioris, superioris alacque nasi, nasalis, depressor septi nasi, zygomaticus major and minor, orbicularis oris, depressor auguli oris, mentalis, depressor labii inferioris, levator anguli oris, buccinator, rizorius, and platysma. The spasms are usually very brief, but can occur in runs and are often brought on when the patient voluntarily and forcefully contracts the facial muscles (Video 10.1). Facial spasms may persist during sleep, and are frequently exacerbated by stress, fatigue, and anxiety. HFS is usually unilateral, but bilateral HFS has also been reported, accounting for about 3% of HFS cases. Bilateral HFS usually starts on one side and progresses to involve the other side in several months to years, with the latter being less severely involved and the bilateral contractions being asynchronous and asymmetrical.

Although most cases of HFS are sporadic, familial cases have been described, suggesting an underlying genetic component in some cases. Familial cases appear to have an autosomal dominant pattern of inheritance with low penetrance and clinical features overlapping with idiopathic cases of HFS, except for a younger age at onset.

☼ SCIENCE REVISITED

Etiology and mechanism of HFS

The most prevalent accepted etiology of HFS is compression of the facial nerve at the root exit zone by a vascular abnormality in the posterior fossa, which accounts for 95% of HFS cases. Biopsy of the compressed nerve typically shows demyelination. In a study of 115 patients undergoing microvascular decompression surgery, the anterior inferior cerebellar artery was mostly involved (43%), followed by the posterior inferior cerebellar artery (31%), vertebral artery (23%), and a large vein (3%). Tumor at the cerebellar pontine angle probably accounts for 4% of HFS cases. Other reported causes of HFS include Bell palsy, peripheral facial nerve injury, stroke, demyelinating disease, headache, and familial inheritance, as listed in Table 10.1.

Non-Parkinsonian Movement Disorders, First Edition. Edited by Deborah A. Hall and Brandon R. Barton.
© 2017 John Wiley & Sons, Ltd. Published 2017 by John Wiley & Sons, Ltd.
Companion website: www.wiley.com/go/hall/non-parkinsonian_movement_disorders

Pathophysiology

The mechanism of HFS has not been fully elucidated, but there are two leading hypotheses to describe the proposed mechanism of HFS: the nerve origin hypothesis and the facial nucleus hypothesis. According to the nerve origin hypothesis, the region of the compressed and demyelinated nerve produces abnormal discharges that precipitate spasms. The demyelinated nerve can produce spontaneous discharges, referred to as ectopic discharges. Additionally, there can be lateral transmission of activity between demyelinated nerve axons, which is referred to as ephaptic transmission. Ephaptic transmission is believed to account for subsequent involvement of the rest of the facial muscles. Rapid amelioration of symptoms following decompression surgery strongly argues for the nerve origin hypothesis. The facial nucleus hypothesis proposes that peripheral facial nerve lesions lead to hyperexcitability of the facial nucleus and the discharges arise from this nucleus. Studies demonstrating hyperexcitability of the blink reflex in HFS argues in favor of facial nucleus involvement.

Differential diagnosis

A comprehensive history and neurologic exam must be performed to diagnose HFS and to evaluate for other possible etiologies that may mimic HFS, including blepharospasm, facial tics, tardive dyskinesia, dopaminergic medication related dyskinesia, oromandibular dystonia, masticatory spasm, facial myokymia, facial myoclonus, facial myorhythmia, facial dystonia, aberrant synkinesia, and psychogenic facial movements, as are summarized in Table 10.2. Spontaneous dyskinesias in the elderly and dyskinesias seen in edentulous individuals or those with poorly fitting dentures should also be considered in the differential diagnosis. Although brain MRI and MRA imaging are normally used to investigate patients with HFS, identifying vascular compression may not always be pathognomonic for a direct cause because this finding can also be detected on the asymptomatic side and in control subjects, suggesting vascular compression alone may not be sufficient to cause HFS.

Treatment

Treatment of HFS includes oral medications, intramuscular botulinum toxin injection, and surgical management. Oral medications such as antiepileptics, anticholinergics, benzodiazepines, muscle relaxants, and tetrabenazine are infrequently prescribed for HFS due to their poor effectiveness and potential side effects. Botulinum toxin injections have become the major treatment of choice for HFS given demonstrated effectiveness and minimal side effects. Treatment success is achieved in 76–100% of patients; however, the beneficial effects are temporary and repeat injections are typically needed every three to four months on average. Patients generally tolerate this procedure well, and rarely develop tolerance to the treatment. Transient side effects such as facial weakness, ecchymosis, diplopia, ptosis, lid edema, dry eye, and lacrimation are minimal in experienced hands. (Further information about botulinum toxins is included in Chapter 7 on dystonia.)

Surgical treatment of HFS is an option in patients who are unresponsive to or develop tolerance to botulinum toxin injections, who cannot tolerate life-long facial injections, or who have concerns about facial weakness, atrophy, or other side effects from repeated injections. The main surgical procedure used to treat HFS is microvascular decompression (MVD) of the facial nerve at the cerebellar pontine angle via a lateral sub-occipital approach. The rationale for MVD is that a vast majority of HFS cases are caused by vascular compression of the facial nerve at the root exit zone from the brainstem. The goal of MVD is to physically separate the compressive aberrant artery from the facial nerve. This procedure can be curative in about 90% of patients, but it is associated with some risk of complications.

Other surgical options such as sectioning of the peripheral nerve trunk or its branches, unilateral removal of the orbicularis oculi and corrugator superciliaris muscles, injection of alcohol or phenol into the facial nerve, and percutaneous puncture of the facial nerve at the stylomastoid foramen have all been used with varying success in the past, but these procedures are rarely used today.

EVIDENCE AT A GLANCE

Effectiveness and complications of microvascular decompression

A thorough review by Miller and Miller in 2008, on the safety and effectiveness of MVD for the treatment of HFS based on 5685 patients from studies published in the English language from

Table 10.1 Etiologies of HFS

Vascular abnormality	Mass lesion	Bony lesion or structural abnormality	Demyelinating	Stroke	Headache	Infection and inflammation	Facial nerve injury	Familial
AV malformation	Parotid tumor	Paget's disease			Migraine	Otitis media		
AV fistula	CP angle lipoma	Marfan's syndrome			Cluster	Neurocysticercosis		
Fusiform aneurysm	Acoustic neuroma	Chiari malformation				Tuberculous meningitis		
Venous angioma	Arachnoid cyst	Focal bone hyperostosis				Bell's palsy		
ECA compression	Meningioma							
Vertebrobasilar dolichoectasia	Schwannoma							
	Hemangioma							
	Glomus jugulare tumor							
	Astrocytoma							
	Ependymal cyst							
	Pontine glioma							
	Epidermoid cyst							
	Cerebellar gangliocytoma							

Source: Yaltho 2011. Adapted with permission of John Wiley & Sons, Ltd.
HFS, hemifacial spasm; AV, arteriovenous; ECA, external carotid artery; CP, cerebellar pontine.

2000 to 2011. Primarily, they found that complete resolution of symptoms following MVD occurred in 91.1% of patients over a median 2.9-year follow-up period, with HFS symptoms recurring only in 2.4% of patients and 1.2% needing to undergo repeat MVD. Transient complications included facial palsy (9.5%), hearing deficit (3.2%), and cerebrospinal fluid leak (1.4%). Permanent complications included hearing deficit (2.3%), facial palsy (0.9%), stroke (0.1%), and death (0.1%). In another study by Illingworth and Jakubowski, in 1996, 72/78 (92.3%) patients remained free of any spasms at a mean follow-up period of 8 years, and 8 were left with permanent postoperative deficits with the common complication being unilateral sensorineural deafness. A causative vessel was found at the root exit zone of the facial nerve in 81/83 (97.6%) patients. Overall, MVD successfully relieves HFS in more than 90% of patients with low rates of symptom recurrence and rare permanent complications.

Blepharospasm

Definition/clinical features

Blepharospasm is a focal dystonia characterized by excessive involuntary contraction of the orbicularis oculi muscles (pretarsal, preseptal, and periorbital muscles) and adjacent upper facial muscles (e.g., procerus, depressor supercilii, corrugator muscles), leading to repetitive blinking or sustained eyelid closure (Video 10.2). Involuntary contractions usually occur on both sides synchronously but can differ in prominence. The persistent involuntary spasms of eyelid closure can be severe enough to cause functional blindness. On average, blepharospasm begins at the age of 55 and has a prevalence of 17 per 100,000 people. Women are more often affected than men (1.8:1). Provoking factors of spasms include reading, driving, stress, fatigue, and exposure to bright light. Alleviating factors include relaxation, walking, talking, and sleep. Some patients develop techniques using other muscles innervated by the facial nerve or acts of mental concentration to decrease the frequency and intensity of the spasms. Other tricks used to decrease the frequency and intensity of spasms include humming, singing, whistling, yawning, coughing, mouth opening, nose picking, chewing, eating, rubbing the eyelids, covering one eye, solving puzzles, and applying pressure on particular parts of the face.

Blepharospasm may occur in isolation with no associated etiology, which is termed primary, benign, essential, or idiopathic blepharospasm. Blepharospasm can also occur in association with other disease entities, such as Parkinson disease and atypical parkinsonian disorders like progressive supranuclear palsy. It can occur in conjunction with dystonic movements of lower facial, oral, jaw, or cervical muscles, as seen in Meige syndrome. Meige syndrome is manifested by segmental dystonia consisting of blepharospasm and oromandibular dystonia, with possible cervical involvement or more widespread dystonia. In the idiopathic form of Meige syndrome, symptoms usually start in the fifth or sixth decade of life with a twofold higher incidence in women. Blepharospasm is typically the most frequent initial complaint. Apart from the primary form, Meige syndrome can also been seen as a tardive movement disorder after neuroleptic treatment.

> **⚙ SCIENCE REVISITED**
>
> The exact cause of essential blepharospasm is unknown. Unless there are clinical signs/symptoms pointing to a symptomatic cause, adults presenting with blepharospasm usually do not require extensive etiological investigations because no specific abnormality or lesion has been identified on brain imaging or autopsy of most patients with blepharospasm. Prior head trauma with loss of consciousness, family history of dystonia, and prior eye disease may increase the risk of developing blepharospasm. Older age at onset, female gender, and prior head/face trauma are risk factors for the spread of dystonia to other muscles. Dopaminergic medications, nasal decongestants containing antihistamine and sympathomimetics, and neuroleptics have been reported to cause blepharospasm.

Pathophysiology

The protractor muscles (corrugator, procerus, depressor supercilii, and orbicularis oculi muscles) are responsible for eyelid closure and the retractor muscles (levator palpebrae, Müller's, and frontalis muscles) open the upper eyelids. Electrophysiological studies of patients with blepharospasm have identified abnormalities in the R2 component of the blink reflex, indicating increased excitation of brainstem somatosensory pathways.

Differential diagnosis

As with HFS, a comprehensive history, ophthalmologic and neurologic exams must be performed to diagnose blepharospasm and to evaluate for other possible etiologies that may mimic this condition. Reflex irritation of the eyes is a common cause of blepharospasm, which can occur in the setting of ocular conditions such as keratitis sicca, spastic entropion, eyelash abnormalities, blepharitis, anterior uveitis and posterior subscapular cataracts. Apraxia of eyelid opening (AEO) is another important diagnostic consideration. AEO is a non-paralytic motor abnormality characterized by difficulty in initiating lid elevation in the absence of visible contraction of the orbicularis oculi muscles. It is attributed to the absence of contraction or even inhibition of the levator palpebrae muscle. Descending control of the blink circuits is presumably impaired due to dysfunction of the cortical-striatal–thalamic–cortical circuits. AEO can also be seen in patients with Parkinson disease and atypical parkinsonian disorders, such as progressive supranuclear palsy. The prevalence of AEO concomitant with blepharospam varies from 7 to 75% in the literature, and 37% as noted by Yoon et al.

Orbicularis myokymia, a condition characterized by localized fascicular contractions within the orbicularis oculi muscles, can also mimic blepharospasm, although it is usually unilateral and commonly manifests after physical exertion, caffeine consumption, emotional stress or fatigue. Orbicularis myokymia can also be seen in brainstem lesions and multiple sclerosis.

Other conditions that can resemble blepharospasm include facial tics, tardive dyskinesia, dopaminergic medication-related dyskinesia, oromandibular dystonia, masticatory spasm, facial myokymia, facial myoclonus, facial myorhythmia, facial dystonia, aberrant synkinesia, and psychogenic facial movements, as previously discussed in detail in the differential diagnosis of HFS (Table 10.2).

Treatment

Due to the lack of understanding of the etiology and pathophysiology of essential blepharospasm, there is no cure. The main objective in the treatment of blepharospasm is to decrease or abolish the unwanted, repeated forced closure of the eyelids. Treatment is largely symptomatic and includes oral medication therapy, intramuscular botulinum toxin injection, and surgical management. Available oral medication treatments include trihexyphenidyl, baclofen, clonazepam, and tetrabenazine.

The generally poor response to medications and/or the adverse effects of medications make botulinum toxin injection therapy the major treatment of choice in clinical practice. Treatment success is achieved in 72–98% of patients; however, the beneficial effects are temporary and repeat injections are typically needed every three to four months, on average. Patients generally tolerate this procedure well, and rarely develop tolerance to the treatment. Side effects are minimal in experienced hands. In those patients who do not benefit from medications and botulinum toxin injections, surgical options are available. Deep brain stimulation has been tried in the treatment of blepharospasm, showing some success in patients with Meige syndrome. Orbital myectomy is rarely performed today.

EVIDENCE AT A GLANCE

The effectiveness and complications in the use of botulinum toxin for blepharospasm

The effectiveness of botulinum toxin in treating blepharospasm was demonstrated in double-blind, placebo controlled trials by Fahn et al in 1985 and Jankovic and Orman in 1987. Average latency from the time of injection to the onset of symptomatic improvement was 4.2 days; average duration of maximum benefit was 12.4 weeks, but the total benefit lasted an average of 15.7 weeks, with about a 72–98% improvement in severity. While about 40% of all those treated with botulinum toxin had

Table 10.2 Differential Diagnosis of HFS

Diseases	Nature of contraction	Site of involvement	Other distinguishing features
HFS	Mostly unilateral but it can be bilateral. If bilateral, spasms are asymmetric and asynchronous, and there is a long latency of symptom onset from one side to the other	Symptoms usually start in the lower eyelid orbicularis oculi muscle and gradually progress to involve other facial muscles with time	Positive "Babinski sign" (distinct from the extensor toe response) with elevation of the eyebrow on eye closure distinguishes HFS from unilateral blepharospasm
Blepharospasm	Symmetric and synchronous	Bilateral orbicularis oculi, depressor supercilii, corrugator, and procerus muscles. Other facial muscles are frequently involved	Sensory trick Photophobia, dry eye
Tics	Suppressible and semi-voluntary or involuntary	Commonly associated with motor tics elsewhere in the body, including vocal or phonic tics	Premonitory sensations and tension prior to the tic, which is released after the tic movement
Oromandibular dystonia	Bilateral sustained or repetitive muscle contraction	Mouth, jaw, tongue, pharynx, and other muscles not innervated by the facial nerve	Sensory trick
Tardive dyskinesia	Choreic or dystonic movements	Orobuccal lingual area, and other facial areas or body parts	History of neuroleptic or select antiemetic use in the past
Levodopa dyskinesia	Choreic or dystonic movements	Orobuccal lingual area, and other facial areas or body parts	History of levodopa use in the past
Masticatory spasms	Usually unilateral contraction of muscles innervated by the motor trigeminal nerve resulting in painful jaw closure	Masseter, temporalis, and pterygoid muscles	

Facial myokymia	Contraction of small muscles or fascicles causes undulating rippling movements beneath the skin	Facial muscles	Characteristic EMG finding: doublets, triplets or multiplets in single motor unit bursts
Facial myoclonus	More rhythmic and continuous	Facial muscles	
Facial myorhythmia	Coarse 1–3 Hz rhythmical, tremor-like involuntary movements	Mostly oculomasticatory myorhythmia	Highly characteristic of Whipple's disease
Facial dystonia	Patterned, sustained contractions	Forehead, eyelids, and lower face	
Synkinesia		Facial muscles	Often accompanied or followed by facial movements in HFS, while it follows voluntary contraction of the facial muscles in Bell's palsy
Psychogenic facial movements	Acute onset, with inconsistent and incongruous features	Any part of the face or other body parts	Movements vary and can be reduced or abolished with distraction, suggestion or psychotherapy

Source: Tan 2002. Adapted with permission of John Wiley and Sons, Ltd.

side effects of dry eyes, ptosis, blurred vision, diplopia, lid edema, or local hematoma formation, the complications were generally minimal and usually improved spontaneously in less than 2 weeks. Only 2% of these reported complications affected patient function. Even after frequent botulinum toxin treatments, there is no apparent decline in benefit and the frequency of complications actually decreases, which may be due to the injector's enhanced experience and injection techniques.

Using botulinum toxin for blepharospasm
An understanding of muscular anatomy is critical to ensure optimal results. Targeting the pretarsal rather than the preseptal portion of the orbicularis oculi muscle yields the best results, with longer effective treatment duration and fewer side effects, as reported by Cakmur et al. and supported by our clinical experience. Injection close to the upper eyelid midline levator palpebrae muscle should be avoided as this will likely lead to ptosis. Injection into the medial two thirds of the lower eyelid should also be avoided to prevent diplopia from inferior oblique muscle weakness. Common reasons for the lack of efficacy include under-dosing, improper injection technique, presence of eyelid opening apraxia, and resistance to botulinum toxin from antibody formation, especially in patients with a history of exposure to large doses and frequent injections. However, the likelihood of treatment failure due to the presence of blocking antibody is very low. Switching to alternative botulinum toxin formulations (e.g., from botulinum-A toxin to B, and vice versa) can be tried and may show some benefit in refractory patients.

Facial tics and Tourette syndrome

Tics are recurrent, non-rhythmic motor movements (motor tics) or sounds (vocal or phonic tics). Both motor and phonic tics are often preceded by premonitory sensations, which are very helpful in differentiating tics from other hyperkinesias. The premonitory phenomenon can be bodily discomforts in the region of the tics or mental urges, which can be released by the tics movements. For most people, there is a tension that builds up just prior to a tic, and is ultimately released once the tic occurs. Some people are not aware of this premonitory urge, especially the pediatric population. Most tics are semi-voluntary (also called unvoluntary). Tics can be completely suppressed for a brief period of time in public or school and released when the patients come home. Tic frequency may increase during stress, fatigue, boredom, or emotional situations, and may decrease while relaxing or focusing on a task. Facial tics are often just part of tics that involve other parts of the body.

Tourette syndrome (TS) is a neurological disorder of both motor and vocal/phonic tics usually starting during childhood and often accompanied by a variety of neurobehavioral comorbidities such as attention deficit hyperactivity disorder (ADHD), obsessive-compulsive disorder (OCD), affective disorders and poor impulse control. The average age at onset of tics is 6 years old, and the tics become more severe around age 10. By 18 years of age, about 50% of patients are tic-free. Although TS is usually considered a childhood disease, symptoms may also occur in adults, which mostly represents a recurrence of symptoms but can also be a new onset of symptoms. Causes of tics are seen in Table 10.3, and can more often be secondary when onset is during adulthood. Facial, neck, and trunk tics dominate in adult TS, with fewer phonic tics than that of children. (See Chapter 5 on tics and Tourette syndrome for more detail.)

Differential diagnosis

Facial tics should be differentiated from other non-tic facial movements such as HFS, blepharospasm, and various other facial movements as aforementioned in this chapter, particularly those listed in Table 10.2. Performing a comprehensive history and neurologic exam is essential to help distinguish between these types of facial movements.

Treatment

The treatment plan should take into consideration the motor symptoms and the neuropsychiatric comorbidities. Counseling and behavioral modifications may be sufficient for those with mild symptoms. For those with more severe symptoms that disrupt quality of life, or academic or professional

Table 10.3 Causes of Tics

A. Primary

1. Tourette Syndrome
2. Transient motor or phonic tics (<1 year)
3. Chronic motor or phonic tics (>1 year)

B. Secondary

1. Inherited
   a. Huntington disease
   b. Primary dystonia
   c. Neuroacanthocytosis
   d. Neurodegeneration with brain iron accumulation
   e. Tuberous sclerosis
   f. Wilson disease
2. Infections: encephalitis, Creutzfeldt-Jakob disease, neurosyphilis, Sydenham disease
3. Drugs: amphetamines and other CNS stimulants, cocaine, carbamazepine, phenytoin, phenobarbital, lamotrigine, antipsychotics, and other dopamine receptor-blocking drugs (tardive tics, tardive tourettism)
4. Toxins: carbon monoxide
5. Developmental: static encephalopathy, mental retardation syndromes, chromosomal abnormalities, autistic spectrum disorders (Asperger syndrome)
6. Chromosomal disorders: Down syndrome, Kleinfelter syndrome, XYY karyotype, fragile X syndrome, triple X and 9p mosaicism, partial trisomy 16, 9p monosomy, paracentric inversion, 15q13;q22.3, Beckwith-Wiedemann syndrome
7. Head and peripheral trauma
8. Other: stroke, neurocutaneous syndromes, schizophrenia, neurodegenerative diseases

C. Related manifestations and disorders

1. Stereotypies/habits/mannerisms/rituals
2. Self-injurious behaviors
3. Motor restlessness
4. Akathisia
5. Compulsions
6. Excessive startle
7. Jumping Frenchman, "ragin' Cajuns" of Louisiana, latah of the Malays, and myriachit of Siberia

Source: Jankovic 2011. Reproduced with permission of John Wiley & Sons, Ltd.

performance, medications are indicated. In general, principles of medication management include initiation at low doses with up-titration to the lowest effective dose and giving each medication an adequate trial. Although the classic neuroleptics (e.g., haloperidol and pimozide) are effective in treating facial tics, they can cause sedation, weight gain, hepatic and cardiac side effects, parkinsonism, and tardive dyskinesia. The atypical neuroleptics, such as risperidone, tiapride or aripiprazole, are also effective in treating tics with low risk of adverse reactions, as reviewed by Roessner et al. Overall, medications such as guanfacine and clonidine are often recommended to be considered first. It is worth noting that tetrabenazine, a dopamine depletor, is emerging as an important effective medication for tics. Tardive dyskinesia is extremely rare with tetrabenazine. Possible side effects of the tetrabenazine include drowsiness, depression, parkinsonism, and akathisia. Botulinum toxin at the site of bothersome tics, such as eyelids, has proved effective. Deep brain stimulation has been used well in treating severe medication refractory TS, based on the limited efficacy data. Management of tics also involves the treatment of neurobehavioral comorbidities, such as ADHD, OCD, and impulsive control disorder. (For more detail on the treatment of tics, see Chapter 5 on tics and Tourette syndrome.)

Further Readings

Cakmur R, Ozturk V, Uzunel F, Donmez B, Idiman F. Comparison of preseptal and pretarsal injections of botulinum toxin in the treatment of blepharospasm and hemifacial spasm. *J Neurol* 2002; **249**: 64–68.

Campos-Benitez M, Kaufmann AM. Neurovascular compression findings in hemifacial spasm. *J Neurosurg* 2008; **109**: 416–420.

Fahn S, Jankovic J. Restless legs syndrome and peripheral movement disorders. In: Fahn S, Jankovic, eds., *Principles and Practice of Movement Disorders*. Philadelphia: Churchill Livingstone, Elsevier, 2007: 580–581.

Grandas F, Elston J, Quinn N, Marsden CD. Blepharospasm: a review of 264 patients. *J Neurol Neurosurg Psychiatry* 1988; **51**: 767–772.

Illingworth RD, Jakubowski DGP. Hemifacial spasm: a prospective long term followup of 83 cases treated by microvascular decompression at two neurosurgical centers in the United Kingdom. *J Neurol Neurosurg Psychiatry* 1990; **60**: 72–77.

Jost WH, Kohl A. Botulinum toxin: evidence-based medicine criteria in blepharospasm and hemifacial spasm. *J Neurol* 2001; **248**(suppl 1): 21–24.

Kenney C, Jankovic J. Botulinum toxin in the treatment of blepharospasm and hemifacial spasm. *J Neural Transm* 2008; **115**: 585–591.

Limotai N, Go C, Oyama G, Hwynn N, Zesiewicz T, Foote K, Bhidayasiri R, Malaty I, Zeilman P, Rodriguez R, Okun MS. Mixed results for GPi-DBS in the treatment of cranio-facial and cranio-cervical dystonia symptoms. *J Neurol* 2011; **258**: 2069–2074.

Miller LE, Miller VM. Safety and effectiveness of microvascular decompression for treatment of hemifacial spasm: a systematic review. *Brit J Neurosurg* 2011; doi 10.3109/02688697.2011.641613.

Nutt JG, Muenter MD, Aronson A, Kurland LT, Melton J. Epidemiology of focal and generalized dystonia in Rochester, Minnesota. *Move Disord* 1988; **3**: 188–194.

Patel BCK. Surgical management of essential blepharospasm. *Otolaryngol Clin N Am* 2005; **38**: 1075–1098.

Roessner V, Schoenefeld K, Buse J, Bender S, Ehrlich S. Pharmacological treatment of tic disorders and Tourette syndrome. *Neuropharmacology* 2013; **68**: 143–149.

Tan EK, Chan LL. Clinico-radiologic correlation in unilateral and bilateral hemifacial spasm. *J Neurol Sci* 2004; **222**: 59–64.

Tan EK, Jankovic J. Bilateral hemifacial spasm: a report of five cases and a literature review. *Mov Disord* 1999; **14**: 345–349.

Tan NC, Chan LL, Tan EK. Hemifacial spasm and involuntary facial movements. *Q J Med* 2002; **95**: 493–500.

Yaltho TC, Jankovic J. The many faces of hemifacial spasm: differential diagnosis of unilateral facial spasms. *Mov Disord* 2011; **26**: 1582–1592.

Yoon WT, Chung EJ, Lee SH, Kim BJ, Lee WY. Clinical analysis of blepharospasm and apraxia of eyelid opening in patients with parkinsonism. *J Clin Neurol* 2005; **1**: 159–165.

11

Periodic Limb Movements of Sleep and REM Sleep Behavior Disorder

Aleksandar Videnovic, MD

Department of Neurology, Massachusetts General Hospital, Harvard Medical School, Boston, Massachusetts, USA

Introduction

Periodic limb movements of sleep (PLMS) are repetitive stereotyped movements of the lower extremities during sleep. The upper extremities can also be involved, much less frequently. PLMS were initially described as "nocturnal myoclonus" by Symonds in 1953. The first polysomnographic characterization of PLMS was done by Lugaresi and colleagues in 1972.

Epidemiology

Reported prevalence of PLMS in the general population varies between 5–11%. In a large population-based study of almost 19,000 participants, the prevalence of PLMS was 3.9%. The prevalence of PLMS increases with age. While PLMS occur rarely in individuals below age 30, up to half of people older than 65 years may have PLMS. PLMS are rare in the pediatric population, affecting 1.2% of children without a co-morbid disorder. Children with attention deficit/hyperactivity disorder and low ferritin levels have an increased incidence of PLMS. Men and women are equally affected by PLMS.

> ### ⚜ SCIENCE REVISITED
>
> The pathophysiology of PLMS has not been fully elucidated. There is increasing evidence from clinical, pharmacological, and radiologic investigations that points to reduced cerebral dopaminergic activity in patients with PLMS, likely at the level of postsynaptic dopamine receptors. A dysfunction of the opiate system has been associated with PLMS as well. It has been suggested that the role of the opiate system in the pathogenesis of PLMS may be primarily mediated by dopaminergic mechanisms.

Clinical features

PLMS typically manifests as dorsiflexion of the big toe and ankle with occasional flexion of the knee and hip, lasting between 0.5 and 5 seconds. The frequency of movement is approximately every 20 to 40 seconds. PLMS are longer and more frequent during NREM sleep compared with REM sleep. In general, PLMS are more numerous during the first half of night. There is a substantial night-to-night variability in the occurrence of PLMS. The frequency of PLMS is expressed as the PLMS index, defined as the number of PLMS per hour of total sleep time. A PLMS index greater than 5 per hour is considered abnormal. Another measurement is the PLMS-arousal index, calculated as the number of PLMS followed by an arousal per hour of total sleep time, and used to estimate sleep disturbance related to PLMS. Studies that examine relationships between subjective sleep complaints and frequency of PLMS reveal conflicting

Non-Parkinsonian Movement Disorders, First Edition. Edited by Deborah A. Hall and Brandon R. Barton.
© 2017 John Wiley & Sons, Ltd. Published 2017 by John Wiley & Sons, Ltd.
Companion website: www.wiley.com/go/hall/non-parkinsonian_movement_disorders

results. It is likely that the arousals associated with PLMS, rather than PLMS itself, are clinically significant when it comes to the impact of PLMS on sleep and alertness. Periodic limb movements may also occur during wakefulness. These movements are referred to as periodic limb movement in wake (PLMW). PLMW are more specific for restless legs syndrome (RLS) than PLMS.

PLMS can be classified as idiopathic or associated with several disorders such as periodic limb movement disorders (PLMD), RLS, non-sleep medical disorders, or various medications. PLMS are frequently an incidental finding on a polysomnogram (PSG). It is important to point out that while PLMS co-exist frequently with other sleep disorders causing sleep fragmentation and daytime sleepiness, they are not always associated with sleep disruption.

PLMD is a sleep disorder characterized by episodes of PLMS associated with insomnia or daytime sleepiness that cannot be explained by another primary sleep disorder. In addition to causing non-restorative sleep in affected individuals, PLMS can negatively affect sleep of the patient's bed partners, who frequently report being kicked at night. The association between PLMS and RLS is particularly strong. Up to 95% of patients with RLS have PLMS. Some studies report strong correlations between the PLMS index and severity of RLS, while others do not. PLMS are commonly seen in patients affected by sleep disordered breathing, such as obstructive sleep apnea. Treatment of obstructive sleep apnea may result in a reduction of PLMS. REM sleep behavior disorder (RBD) is frequently associated with PLMS. It is estimated that up to 70% of patients with RBD have an abnormal PLMS index. Association between narcolepsy and PLMS has been reported as well.

In addition to other sleep disorders, PLMS are frequently seen in several non-sleep disorders. Literature addressing the prevalence of PLMS in non-sleep disorders is quite scarce. Patients with hypertension, advanced renal disease, chronic lung disease, sleep apnea, rheumatologic diseases, and alcohol abuse commonly have PLMS. Emerging recent literature suggests an association between PLMS and increased risk for cardiovascular disease on the basis of a significant increase in heart rate and systolic blood pressure during PLMS. Neurological disorders associated with PLMS include Parkinson disease, amyotrophic lateral sclerosis, stiff-person syndrome, myelopathies, and several forms of neuropathy. Several classes of medications have been associated with an increase in PLMS. Antidepressants and lithium carbonate, as well as a withdrawal from benzodiazepines and anticonvulsants, can cause and/or exacerbate PLMS. Among antidepressants, selective serotonin reuptake inhibitors, venlafaxine, and tricyclic antidepressants are commonly associated with PLMS.

> ### ⚓ CAUTION
> Several classes of medications can provoke and/or exacerbate PLMS. These include psychoactive substances like lithium, tricyclic antidepressants, selective serotonin reuptake inhibitors, and venlafaxine. Similarly, withdrawal of benzodiazepines, barbiturates, and anticonvulsants may exacerbate PLMS.

Differential diagnosis

Several conditions should be considered in the differential diagnosis of PLMS. These include hypnic myoclonus (an involuntary twitch during transition to sleep), fragmentary myoclonus (a series of very brief muscle contractions usually involving fingers, toes and corners of the mouth), myoclonic epilepsy, and segmental myoclonus. In addition to these conditions, several limb movements with EMG burst may be confused for PLMS. These include REM twitches, hypnagogic foot tremors (a rhythmic movement of feet/toes that occurs at the transition between wake and sleep or during light NREM sleep), and alternating leg muscle activation (ALMA), which is characterized by quick alternating pattern of bilateral anterior tibialis activation. REM-related muscle twitches occur during REM sleep, as opposed to PLMS, which emerge in non-REM sleep. Foot tremors and ALMA are shorter lasting and do not exhibit a typical periodicity of PLMS.

Diagnosis

The diagnosis of PLMS is based on clinical interview and PSG. According to the American Academy of Sleep Medicine Scoring Manual, PSG features of PLMS include leg movement of 0.5–10 seconds in duration, with amplitude that is at least 8 μV higher than the baseline EMG activity recorded from the anterior tibialis muscles (Figure 11.1). To qualify as a

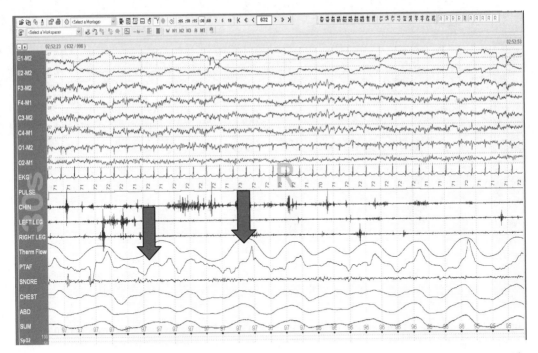

Figure 11.1 Excessive electromyographic activity in the chin and limbs during REM sleep in a patient with RBD (gray arrows illustrate two episodes of movement). (*See insert for color representation of the figure.*)

periodic sequence of movements, there must be a minimum of 4 repetitive limb movements appearing every 5–90 seconds. Limb movements are not scored if they occur 0.5 seconds before or after an apnea or hypopnea. Similarly, an arousal and limb movement should be considered associated with each other when there is a less of 0.5 seconds between a movement and arousal.

The diagnosis of PLMD is based PSG evidence of PLMS and a detailed sleep history that excludes other causes of sleep disturbance. PLMW are observed during the awake portion of the PSG or during the "suggested immobilization test" (SIT). During a SIT, an individual is sitting up with legs outstretched and instructed to stay awake and does not move legs for 1 hour. Leg movements are measured using EMG from the anterior tibialis muscles. PLMW of ≥ 40/h are suggestive of RLS.

Treatment

Treatment of PLMS/PLMD should be considered only after other co-morbid sleep and medical disorders have been appropriately diagnosed and treated. The common pharmacological compounds used in the treatment of PLMS/PLMD are dopaminergic drugs, benzodiazepines and opioids. This approach has emerged from the success of L-dopa and dopamine agonists in treating symptoms of RLS. Only a few open-label clinical studies have examined the efficacy of dopaminergic and non-dopaminergic pharmacological agents for PLMD. These studies included L-dopa, ropinirole, clonazepam, melatonin, gabapentin, valproic acid, and opioids. While opioids such as methadone, morphine, codeine, and oxycodone successfully alleviate PLMS, their use remains limited due to the risk for abuse and addiction. Further clinical investigations employing controlled, blinded, randomized research methods are needed to understand the optimal treatment choices for PLMS/PLMD and associated symptoms of poor sleep and daytime alertness.

REM sleep behavior disorder (RBD)

Rapid eye movement (REM) sleep behavior disorder (RBD) is a parasomnia initially reported by Schenck and colleagues in 1986. The clinical hallmarks of rapid eye movement (REM) sleep behavior disorder

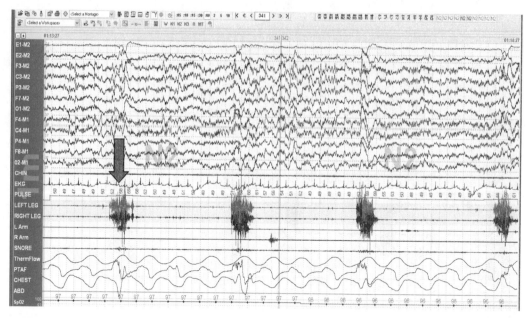

Figure 11.2 Sequence of four periodic limb movements of sleep from a polysomnography recording (gray arrow illustrates the first limb movement). (*See insert for color representation of the figure.*)

(RBD) are motor behaviors and vocalizations that surround very vivid and usually aggressive, action filled dreams during REM sleep. Individuals attempt to react to these dreams ("act them out"), which eventually results in awakenings, sleep interruption, and frequent injuries. The pathophysiological mechanism that drives movements and behaviors associated with RBD is a loss of muscle atonia during REM sleep. This loss of normal muscle atonia during REM sleep represents the neurophysiologic signature of RBD (Figure 11.2).

Epidemiology

The prevalence data for RBD in the general population are sparse. The commonly quoted study reported RBD prevalence of 0.5% in the general population. Due to the methodological constraints of the study, this number may not reflect accurately the true frequency of RBD. RBD usually emerges around the age of 50. There is a strong male predominance in RBD.

Clinical features

A broad spectrum of behaviors associated with dream enactment in RBD has been reported. Behaviors include kicking, punching, flailing, grabbing, jumping

out of bed, and sitting up in bed. Vocalizations associated with RBD are quite variable as well and may include whispering, screaming, shouting, laughing, talking, mumbling, and singing. On some occasions, patients modify their voices to reflect the dream content. Commonly, dreams display negative emotions and violent content, and depict events of being attacked, chased by someone, or robbed. Pleasant dreams have been reported in minority of cases. A paradoxical improvement in movements and vocalizations associated with RBD dream enactment behaviors have been recently reported in patients affected by parkinsonism. Among Parkinson disease (PD) patients with co-existent RBD, the quality of movement and strength of voice seems to improve during RBD compared with wakefulness. While the mechanisms behind this clinical observation remain unknown, this phenomenon suggests a modified role of the extrapyramidal system in the control of movements during REM sleep.

Frequency, complexity, and severity of behaviors in RBD vary significantly across different nights, and may vary throughout a single night. Abnormal behaviors can emerge infrequently or manifest several times within one night. Similarly, the severity of injures is quite variable. Some patients sustain minor bruising and lacerations, while others suffer from fractures and large hematomas. Most aggressive behaviors are exhibited by older men. According to a recent comprehensive review of RBD, a total of 41 cases of RBD associated with potentially lethal behaviors have been reported in the literature.

SCIENCE REVISITED

The main anatomical structures involved in the regulation of REM sleep are located in the pontine tegmentum and medial medulla. These include pedunculopontine (PPN) and laterodorsal (LTD) nuclei, locus coeruleus (LC), peri-locus coeruleus area, and medullary magnocellularis and gigantocellularis nuclei. It has been proposed that two independent neuroanatomical pathways are involved in RBD. A "direct" pathway leading to REM sleep atonia involves sublaterodorsal nucleus (or its analogous nucleus in humans) and its projections to spinal interneurons. The "indirect" contributing pathway conducts inputs from magnocellular reticular formation to spinal interneurons. The location and connections of "locomotor generators" that are responsible for complex behaviors in RBD have not been fully elucidated.

Differential diagnosis

Several conditions can mimic RBD and need to be distinguished from RBD. These conditions include non-REM parasomnias, sleep disordered breathing, seizures, periodic limb movements during sleep, and normal dream-enactment behaviors. Sleep walking, sleep terrors, and confusional arousals occur in non-REM sleep and are associated with confusion and amnesia. Arousals associated with oxygen desaturations during episodes of sleep disordered breathing may be accompanied with short lasting movements and vocalizations that resemble behaviors of RBD. PSG is critical in distinguishing these disorders from RBD.

CAUTION

Not everything that sounds and appears like RBD is RBD. A spectrum of similar conditions needs to be considered throughout the diagnostic process.

Diagnosis

The International Classification of Sleep Disorders (ICDS-2) established the diagnostic criteria for RBD. The diagnosis of RBD is based on a history of abnormal behaviors while asleep and excessive muscle activity during REM sleep on PSG.

Getting collateral historic information from the bed partner remains a critical step in diagnosing RBD, since patients frequently do not have recollections of their dreams and are unaware of their abnormal sleep behaviors. Minor movements and soft vocalizations may frequently be overlooked by bed partners of individuals affected by RBD. Several questionnaires have been developed as screening tools for RBD. These include the RBD Questionnaire–Hong Kong (RBD-HK), the Mayo Sleep Questionnaire, and the REM Sleep Behavior Disorders Screening Questionnaire. Among these, only the RBD-HK measures both the frequency and severity of RBD symptoms. While these instruments may capture symptoms suggestive of RBD, an overnight PSG is needed to establish the diagnosis of definitive RBD. PSG is needed to evaluate for the loss of muscle atonia during REM sleep as well as to identify sleep abnormalities and behaviors that may mimic RBD. It is, however, important to note that the cutoff for abnormal muscle activity in REM sleep is not yet determined. Furthermore, there is no consensus in regard to the methodology used to measure excessive muscle activity throughout REM sleep. Several visual and computerized ascertainment methods of excessive muscle activation in REM sleep have been developed and utilized primarily for research purposes. An additional challenge in assessing REM-related muscle activation is the dilemma of which muscles should be studied. The highest rate of phasic EMG activity during REM sleep in individuals with RBD was found with simultaneous recordings of the mentalis, flexor digitorum superficialis, and extensor digitorum brevis muscles.

TIPS AND TRICKS

Individuals with RBD may not be aware of their dream enactment behaviors and may not recall dreams. Interviewing their bed partners is therefore a critical step in order to establish the diagnosis as well as to establish frequency and severity of the disorder.

RBD and neurodegenerative disorders

A large body of evidence that links RBD with several neurodegenerative disorders has emerged over the past decade. RBD frequently predates the characteristic clinical motor or cognitive presentation of these disorders. Commonly, RBD has been associated with synucleinopathies, a group of neurodegenerative disorders characterized by accumulation of alpha synuclein. The common synucleinopathies are PD, dementia with Lewy bodies (DLB), and multiple system atrophy (MSA). RBD is especially common in this group of disorders, affecting 15–60% of patients with PD and 80–100% of patients with DLB and MSA. RBD can emerge decades prior to the onset of the diagnostic motor features of a neurodegenerative disorder. Longitudinal studies of individuals affected by idiopathic RBD revealed development of a synucleinopathy in 50–80% of cases. The estimated risk of a neurodegenerative disorder in the individual affected by RBD is approximately 18% at 5 years, 41% at 10 years, and 52% at 12 years. The link between RBD and synuclein pathology remains a scientific mystery. In contrast to synucleinopathies, RBD is exceedingly rare in tauopathies, such as Alzheimer disease (AD) and progressive supranuclear palsy (PSP).

RBD is considered one of the main prodromal markers of a synucleinopathy. It is therefore not surprising that patients with RBD have subtle abnormalities in many domains that are affected in PD and other synuclein disorders. These include alterations in olfaction, color vision, cognition, and autonomic function. Brain imaging studies in individuals with RBD revealed decreased levels of dopamine transporters in the basal ganglia that progressively decrease over time as motor signs of parkinsonism gradually emerge.

PD patients with co-existent RBD are somewhat different phenotypically from those PD patients without RBD. They are more likely to have an akinetic-rigid phenotype as opposed to tremor-predominant disease and are prone to more frequent falls and gait impairment. RBD has been associated with longer duration of PD symptoms, a higher dose of dopaminergic medications, and presence of autonomic dysfunction. Age, disease severity, and daytime sleepiness do not seem to be strongly associated with RBD in PD. In DLB, RBD has been associated with a shorter duration of dementia and earlier onset of parkinsonism and visual hallucinations.

A large proportion of patients with neurodegenerative disorders is unaware of their RBD-related symptoms and does not recall unpleasant, frightening dreams. The sensitivity of clinical interviews in diagnosis RBD may be low as 33%. It is therefore very important to interview bed partners and perform video PSG in order to properly assess for RBD as well as exclude other conditions that may mimic RBD.

> ### ⚗ SCIENCE REVISITED
>
> RBD may be one of the earliest markers of a neurodegenerative disease such as Parkinson disease and dementia with Lewy bodies. This makes the RBD population very attractive for clinical trials of potential neurodegenerative disease modifying agents, once they become available.

Treatment

Assuring safety of the sleep environment is one of the main aspects in treating RBD. Removing potentially harmful objects from the bedroom, rearranging furniture, placing a mattress on the floor, installing padded bed railings, and padding the bedroom floor are some of the measures directed toward minimizing injuries associated with RBD. The most commonly used medications in the treatment of RBD are clonazepam and melatonin. The evidence for the effectiveness of these two agents emerged from small, open-label studies and case series. Clonazepam decreases phasic, and melatonin decreases tonic electromyographic activity during REM sleep. Melatonin (3–15 mg at bedtime) is well tolerated and was effective in a recent small double-blind clinical study. Clonazepam (0.5–2 mg at bedtime) is effective in suppressing dream enactment behaviors and unpleasant dream recall. Side effects may include sleepiness, dizziness, and urinary incontinence at night. This medication should be avoided in RBD patients with co-existent sleep disordered breathing and dementia. The co-administration of melatonin and clonazepam may be effective in patients who respond sub-optimally to either agent alone. Rivastigmine, donepezil, zopiclone, and pramipexole have also been reported to be effective in several small open-label studies.

⚠ CAUTION

Motor behaviors associated with RBD may result in serious injuries. Patients may not recognize a potential for injuries at the time of the diagnosis. Education about the RBD and implementation of safety measures within the sleep environment is therefore the most important initial therapeutic intervention.

Further Readings

AASM. *The International Classification of Sleep Disorders*, 2nd ed. Westchester, IL: American Academy of Sleep Medicine, 2005.

Arnulf I. REM sleep behavior disorder: motor manifestations and pathophysiology. *Mov Disord* 2012; **27**: 677–689.

Boeve BF, Silber MH, Saper CB, et al. Pathophysiology of REM sleep behaviour disorder and relevance to neurodegenerative disease. *Brain* 2007; **130**: 2770–2788.

De Cock VC, Vidailhet M, Leu S, et al. Restoration of normal motor control in Parkinson's disease during REM sleep. *Brain* 2007; **130**: 450–456.

Eisensehr I, Linke R, Tatsch K, et al. Increased muscle activity during rapid eye movement sleep correlates with decrease of striatal presynaptic dopamine transporters. IPT and IBZM SPECT imaging in subclinical and clinically manifest idiopathic REM sleep behavior disorder, Parkinson's disease, and controls. *Sleep* 2003; **26**: 507–512.

Frauscher B, Iranzo A, Hogl B, et al. Quantification of electromyographic activity during REM sleep in multiple muscles in REM sleep behavior disorder. *Sleep* 2008; **31**: 724–731.

Iranzo A, Santamaria J, Tolosa E. The clinical and pathophysiological relevance of REM sleep behavior disorder in neurodegenerative diseases. *Sleep Med Rev* 2009.

Karatas M. Restless legs syndrome and periodic limb movements during sleep: diagnosis and treatment. *Neurologist* 2007; **13**: 294–301.

Lugaresi E, Coccagna G, Mantovani M, Lebrun R. Some periodic phenomena arising during drowsiness and sleep in man. *Electroencephalogr Clin Neurophysiol* 1972; **32**: 701–705.

Ohayon MM, Caulet M, Priest RG. Violent behavior during sleep. *J Clin Psychiatry* 1997; **58**: 369–376; quiz 377.

Ohayon MM, Roth T. Prevalence of restless legs syndrome and periodic limb movement disorder in the general population. *J Psychosom Res* 2002; **53**: 547–554.

Postuma RB, Gagnon JF, Vendette M, Fantini ML, Massicotte-Marquez J, Montplaisir J. Quantifying the risk of neurodegenerative disease in idiopathic REM sleep behavior disorder. *Neurology* 2009; **72**: 1296–1300.

Salas RE, Rasquinha R, Gamaldo CE. All the wrong moves: a clinical review of restless legs syndrome, periodic limb movements of sleep and wake, and periodic limb movement disorder. *Clin Chest Med* 2010; **31**: 383–395.

Schenck CH, Bundlie SR, Ettinger MG, Mahowald MW. Chronic behavioral disorders of human REM sleep: a new category of parasomnia. *Sleep* 1986; **9**: 293–308.

Symonds CP. Nocturnal myoclonus. *J Neurol Neurosurg Psychiatry* 1953; **16**: 166–171.

12

Stereotypies

Michael Rotstein, MD

Tel Aviv Sourasky Medical Center, Tel Aviv, Israel

Introduction

All humans of all ages and cultures engage in repetitive behavior at one time or another, usually related to specific situations and states of variable arousal. Foot tapping, nail biting, arm waving, hand flapping, and other repetitive movements and behaviors might be seen frequently with spectators at a baseball game culminating to its peak, while the player at bat may engage in his own series of idiosyncratic repetitive movements prior to taking his position over the plate. Young children are more likely to display ritualistic and repetitive behaviors and movements that appear to be part of their normal repertoire.

Definitions

Patterned repetitive movements have been classified as stereotypies, habits, compulsions, and mannerisms, and overlapping definitions are common. Whatever the definition, repetitive movements might come to attention when patterns become unusually noticeable, are peculiar in appearance, or cause interference with daily activities.

The definition of stereotypies continues to change. Since it was first termed in Meige and Feindel's book on tics in 1907, various definitions and inclusion critieria have been described. A commonly used definition of stereotypies is "involuntary or unvoluntary, coordinated, patterned, repetitive, rhythmic, seemingly purposeless movements or utterances." A more recent definition is "a non–goal-directed movement pattern that is repeated continuously for a period of time in the same form and on multiple occasions, and which is typically distractible." In essence, stereotypies are patterned, repetitive, non-purposeful movements occurring during predicted situations, experienced by the individual as a non-intrusive, positive phenomenon that may serve a specific purpose.

> ### ⚙ SCIENCE REVISITED
>
> The pathophysiologic mechanisms of stereotypies are unknown. As stereotypies are associated with developmental abnormalities including autism and mental retardation, a neurological basis for the phenomenon is suspected, with some investigators suggesting dysfunction of cortico–striatal–thalamo–cortical circuitry. Imaging findings are unrevealing in normally developed children. As stereotypies are noted with socially isolated animals, some emphasize social isolation as a key to appearance of chronic stereotypic behavior, thus viewing autism and mental retardation as a form of sensory deprivation and stereotypies being a way of the individual to increase self-stimulation. Familial aggregation of stereotypies may bring about genetic studies in the future.

Non-Parkinsonian Movement Disorders, First Edition. Edited by Deborah A. Hall and Brandon R. Barton.
© 2017 John Wiley & Sons, Ltd. Published 2017 by John Wiley & Sons, Ltd.
Companion website: www.wiley.com/go/hall/non-parkinsonian_movement_disorders

Clinical presentation

Stereotypies in children

Stereotypies appear before the age of two years in most children, and may present as early as 4–6 months old, and rarely start after three years old. They may occur many times daily and tend to continue in a rather fixed pattern of frequency and appearance for months and sometimes a few years. Episodes are characterized as paroxysmal events occurring for a few seconds; however, extended periods of movement may occur, often with stereotypies occurring at times of boredom or imaginative activity. The episodes may be quite similar to each other in appearance, length, and the situation in which they may appear. A normally developed child may exhibit one stereotypic movement over extended periods of time. However, the characteristics of the stereotypic movement may change over the years from infancy to early or late childhood. For example, an infant presenting with distal upper and lower extremity twirling may progress over time to have a typical bilateral arm movement, or initial high amplitude hand flapping may give way over time to a less pronounced finger posturing.

EVIDENCE AT A GLANCE 1

Two large parent questionnaire based studies tested the prevalence of stereotypic behavior in normally developed children. "Repetitive behaviors" were reported by 1492 parents in 41%, 56%, 62%, 55%, 57%, and 49% of children aged <12 mo, 12–23, 24–35, 36–47, 48–59, and 60–72 mo, respectively. On repetitive behaviors occurring at least once daily, 679 parents reported spinning (59.6%), pacing to and fro (39.5%), repetitive hand and/or finger movements (31.3%), and body rocking (20.1%) in normally developed two-year-olds.

Though not triggered specifically by a single event, stereotypies may occur in specific stimulating situations such as while a child is joyous, excited, or in anticipation (e.g., receiving a gift or watching a thrown bowling ball going down the aisle), while bored, daydreaming, or engrossed in a specific activity (e.g., in front of a TV or computer screen) as well as when fatigued or anxious. Stereotypies are commonly seen by parents during meals, TV watching, play, prior to sleep, or while sitting in a car. Teachers may describe movements in the classroom, sometimes during episodes of lapsed attention.

The common appearance of stereotypic movement includes any combination of bilateral finger, hand, and/or arm movement or posturing, called complex motor stereotypies by some experts. This may include wiggling or twirling of the fingers ("piano playing"), high amplitude hand or arm flapping, or various posturing of the arms, hands, or fingers in a flexion or extension position. The arms may be elevated at the sides of the body creating a "flying" appearance during hand flapping or finger twirling or may be positioned in a neutral down going position. The hands are sometimes placed in the midline, posturing and wiggling together, giving the appearance of "hand washing." Limb movements are occasionally accompanied by lower facial grimacing, such as mouth opening, tongue movement, or platysma involvement. Some cases are accompanied by additional body movements during hand motion such as jumping, crouching, or truncal posturing. Episodes of upper limb movement usually last for several seconds; however, extended episodes lasting more than a minute are rare.

Another common movement is head nodding. Nodding is a continuous to-and-fro movement that may continue for extended periods of time. The movement may be a side-to-side tilt or turn of the head, or a back-and-forth movement. Nodding is usually not accompanied with additional hand, arm, or mouth movement; however, sometimes one notices ocular deviation during episodes. In contrast to paroxysmal upper limb movement, head nodding may appear most during times of boredom or when fatigued and less so with stimulating situations.

Stereotypies may be quite predictable. Parents may know how and when to bring about an episode. During history taking in the office, they may ask the physician to note the child while sitting bored on the chair, or might try and interest the child in a book or toy they know may "bring out" the movement. Likewise, parents are readily able to obtain home videos of the child during the episodes, as their occurrence in specific settings is predictable.

An important part of stereotypic behavior is the subjectively positive, non-intrusive experience described by the child. When asked directly, children usually are aware of the stereotypic behavior, enjoy their stereotypies, and may give insight to their own perception of the behavior. Occasionally, the child may disclose the movements to be part of an imaginative game. Some children describe fighting imaginative dragons, swordplay, or acting out a favorite movie or video game as part of their own experience.

Stereotypies in infants

Infants present with numerous stereotypies. A common stereotypic behavior is body rocking. This is also a to-and-fro movement of body parts occurring in various positions. An infant may stand on hands and knees, rocking back and forth on all fours, not unlike head nodding in an older child. Sometimes rocking is confined to a body part, such as a child lying supine and rocking his legs, flexed at the knees, from side to side. Likewise, the supine infant may rock his head from side to side in a slow, high amplitude continuous motion. Body rocking may be accompanied with head banging, in which the to-and-fro motion of the body is performed against a surface such as the siding of the infant's bed. Distal limb twirling occurs with the infant in a supine position or while in an infant seat. Hands and feet are twirled, usually in a symmetric hand and/or leg movement. These infantile stereotypies may last for minutes, and occur during "down times" such as sitting in the car or before falling asleep. They are readily suppressible with distraction.

Infantile gratification behavior, also termed infantile masturbation, is a characteristic repetitive movement of the lower extremities and pelvis occurring mostly in young girls, usually after the age of 3 months and before 3 years. The movement includes placing pressure on the perineum by body and lower extremity posturing and back-and-forth motion of the pelvis and lower extremities. There is usually an accompanying vocalization such as mild grunting as well as facial flushing or diaphoresis. As all stereotypies, these episodes may last for minutes to hours if not distracted. This specific movement pattern may cause parental concern, and parents should be reassured regarding this self-limiting, benign, non-sexual activity.

There have been other movement patterns and behaviors such as thumb sucking, nail biting, and hair twirling that are incorporated under the broad term of stereotypic behavior. These movements tend to present as continuous non-paroxysmal habitual behaviors appearing from infancy at times of boredom, stress, or need for self-relaxation. These habits seem to be rather different in that the movement patterns are not a non-purposeful non-goal-oriented movement, and their inclusion as stereotypies should be further delineated.

Stereotypies in autistic children

Autism spectrum disorder (ASD) is a neurodevelopmental disability consisting of a wide range of impairment in social interaction and communication accompanied by restricted and stereotyped behavior, interests, or activities. It is common to diagnose children with ASD prior to the age of 3 years. ASD has been diagnosed with continued increasing frequency over the past two decades, and current prevalence of ASD is estimated as high as 1:50 children aged 6–17, based on parental reports.

The appearance of stereotypies is part of the requirements for the diagnosis of ASD, and is a common occurrence in both children and adults with ASD. Some neurodevelopmental autistic syndromes have stereotypies as a hallmark of the movement abnormality. A classic example of this are the hand washing midline movements seen in girls with Rett syndrome (in which mutations in the methyl CpG binding protein 2 gene cause autism, dementia, and other motor difficulties).

Many parents noting stereotypic movements in their child have concerns whether this occurrence may implicate ASD in the child. When assessing stereotypies in a young child, a full developmental history should be elicited and red flags should be addressed.

☠ CAUTION

When assessing a child with stereotypies, beware of the possibility of secondary stereotypies, such as developmental disability or sensory deprivation. One or more findings in a child at any age in addition to stereotypic behavior should prompt further neurodevelopmental or metabolic/genetic workup. A consultation with a child development specialist might be in order.

- An abnormal neurological examination
- Dysmorphic facial or body features
- An abnormal hearing exam
- An abnormal visual exam
- Head circumference below the 5th percentile or a decline in head circumference percentiles over time
- Failure to achieve gross motor, fine motor, language, or social/adaptive developmental milestones
- Occurrence of red flags for autism (see Tips and Tricks below)

✶ TIPS AND TRICKS

Red flags for autism/pervasive developmental disorder
As modified from the DSM-IV criteria for autistic disorder, features of autistic children may include in addition to stereotypies:

Impaired social interaction:
- Decreased eye contact, use of facial expression, body posture, or hand gestures to communicate needs
- Decreased need or ability to interact with children in an age appropriate manner
- Decreased need to share interests with other people, such as showing, bringing, or pointing out objects of interest to other people
- Not actively participating in simple social play or games
- Preferring solitary activities, involving others in activities only as tools or "mechanical" aids
- Impaired communication with others

Delayed development of spoken language:
- Impaired ability to initiate or sustain a conversation with others
- Repetitive use of language or strange "idiosyncratic" language
- Impaired "make-believe" play or social imitative play

Restricted behavior, interests, or activities (other than stereotypies):
- Preoccupation with restricted patterns of interest
- Inflexible adherence to specific, nonfunctional routines or rituals
- Preoccupation with parts of objects

It is uncommon for the diagnosis of autism to be made on the sole appearance of stereotypies in an infant or child. Most children with ASD will come to medical attention because of the manifestation of other social or communicative impairments, usually prior to the appearance of stereotypies. Moreover, ASD stereotypies commonly have a different clinical presentation compared with those in a normally developing child. The number of stereotypic movements may be increased, compared with the usual single stereotypic behavior in a normally developed child. ASD children commonly have numerous different movements and behaviors occurring in random order, or noticed during specific environmental interactions. Most types of stereotypic movement cannot be used to differentiate autistic from non-autistic children or adults, but some stereotypies such as atypical gazing at fingers or abnormal gait episodes (i.e., episodes of pacing, spinning, and skipping) are largely limited to autistic children.

Stereotypies in ASD children and adults may be difficult to differentiate from obsessive-compulsive behavior as well as complex tics. Adolescents with ASD have increased prevalence of tics as well as Tourette syndrome.

EVIDENCE AT A GLANCE 2

The prevalence of stereotypies secondary to developmental abnormalities is related to the type and severity of the condition. During a 15 minute video recording of ASD children, stereotypies were noted to occur in 71% of children with low functioning ASD and 63% of children with high functioning ASD. In a study based on reported weekly occurrence, ASD and mentally retarded adults manifested stereotypies in 85% and 80%, compulsions in 78% and 56%, self-injurious behavior in 52% and 28%, and tics in 22% and 10%, respectively.

Epidemiology

The prevalence of stereotypic movements is high in normally developed children, most so in the third year of life. Stereotypic movements subside during the early childhood years, though a substantial portion of children experience stereotypies well into their late childhood years. Stereotypies occur more in boys; there is a higher male predominance, estimated at 3:2 to 3:1. A family history of similar behaviors is sometimes difficult to elicit, though one study showed 17% co-occurrence in first-degree relatives.

Stereotypies are common in children and adolescents diagnosed with autism or mental retardation, as well as socially isolated children and sensory deprived children with congenital deafness and blindness.

Differential diagnosis

Stereotypies may cause much parental concern as they are given erroneous diagnoses with more severe implications. It is important to identify these other conditions as treatment and prognosis may differ considerably.

The major differential diagnosis of stereotypic behavior is complex motor tics (see Table 12.1 and Table 12.2). Tics, like stereotypies, are brief, repetitive, unvoluntary movements common in the pediatric

Table 12.1 Conditions mimicking stereotypic movements

Tics
Compulsions
Mannerisms
Self-injurious behavior
Epileptic activity
Paroxysmal (kinesigenic, non-kinesigenic, exertional) dyskinesias
Psychogenic movement disorder

age. Tics may be simple movements or vocalizations, or they may be complex, involving numerous muscle groups, and may be similar in appearance to stereotypies. There are, however, many clues to differentiate stereotypic movements from tics. Tics are noted later in life compared with stereotypies. The age of onset of tics is usually 6–7 years of age, rarely prior to the age of 5 (although tics in children as young as 2 years have been described). Tics may be transient in nature, occurring for brief periods of days to weeks only to subside spontaneously. Stereotypies tend to be a condition noted over months and sometimes years. If persistent, chronic tics may increase during later childhood or young adolescence, an age in which stereotypies usually subside. Tics usually come in groups, and a child will have numerous different tics appearing in random order, waxing and waning over time, compared with the rather steady appearance of one stereotypic movement in a given child. Tics have a rostro-caudal prevalence, with facial movements predominating, specifically eye, nose, and mouth involvement, and lesser extremity involvement. Tics involving the extremities tend to be asymmetric rather than the bilateral appearance of upper extremity complex stereotypies.

Complex tics tend to be more coordinated sequential movements that may resemble normal motor activity giving a semi-purposeful or purposeful appearance (i.e., gesturing, touching, grooming), although non-purposeful complex tics are noted (i.e., head shaking or truncal posturing). This is in contrast to the non-purposeful appearance of stereotypic movements. Although complex tics tend to be longer than simple tics, they rarely exceed a few seconds in duration. When tics are frequent, they may seem to be prolonged; however, there will usually be a brief pause between sequential tics. Stereotypic movements last for several

Table 12.2 Differentiating tics from stereotypies

	Tics	Stereotypies
Age of onset	Usually >5 years	<3 years
Transient episodes	Transient tic disorder common	Usually lasting for months to years
Severity over time	Most severe at 10–12 years	Subside during late childhood
Number of different movements	Variable, usually more than one	Usually one
Consistency over time	Random, changing	Stable appearance
Symmetry	Less common	Usually
Complex movement appearance	Semi-purposeful or purposeful	Non-purposeful
Duration	Few seconds	Several seconds, minutes
Subjective description	Intrusive, annoying, premonitory urge	Enjoyable, part of imaginary play
Suppression	Brief	Able for long periods
Precipitant	Stress, anxiety	Excitement, boredom
Family history	Common	Less common

seconds and sometimes minutes, and seem to be a continuous movement throughout their occurrence. Tics may be felt by the child to be intrusive, annoying, or irritating, and may interfere with daily activities while occurring. Older children describe a localized sensation or some form of discomfort, called a "premonitory urge" as a harbinger of the tic, performed by the child in an unvoluntary manner in order to eradicate the sensation. They are able to suppress the need to tic for brief periods of time, until the urge "overcomes" the voluntary suppression and the need to tic reappears. Stereotypies are usually felt by the child as non-intrusive, fun, or purposeless, with no local premonitory sensation. They are able to stop the movement when asked to do so for extended periods of time. Tics appear or increase in severity with periods of stress or sudden anxiety. Stereotypies are usually not related with stress in normally developed children. Finally, tics have a strong familial occurrence, less common in stereotypies.

Compulsive behavior may be repetitive and seemingly purposeless activity mimicking stereotypic movements. However, compulsions are readily differentiated from stereotypies as the obsessive thought process driving the compulsive behavior is severely intense and intrusive in nature, they are difficult to suppress, and distracting or denying their performance might elicit anxiety.

Mannerisms are sometimes confused with common stereotypies and habits. Mannerisms are unique, voluntary, idiosyncratic gestures or movements that occur in a specific individual in relation to specified activity. They do not appear at random and do not have the suppressible appearance of stereotypies. Examples of mannerism might be ritualistic activity of a baseball player prior to batting, grunting sounds vocalized by a tennis player, or facial grimacing of a musician during performance.

Head nodding deserves its own differential diagnosis. It has been described as the clinical feature of the rare "bobble doll syndrome," associated with posterior fossa lesions and malformations in young children. Ocular abnormalities (i.e., strabismus, nystagmus, or oculomotor apraxia) should be excluded. Abnormal head posturing may be noted at this age group with paroxysmal torticollis, spasmus nutans, as well as Sandifer syndrome.

Self-injurious behavior (SIB) is uncommon in the normally developed child. It is more often found in individuals with neurodevelopmental disabilities such as autism, blindness, or mental retardation, as well as inborn errors of metabolism or genetic conditions such as Lesch–Nyhan syndrome, neuro-acanthocytosis syndromes, Cornelia de Lange syndrome, or Prader–Willi syndrome. Some SIBs are repetitive in nature and resemble stereotypic movements, such as head banging, self hitting or biting, lip or hand chewing, skin picking or scratching, and hair pulling. These behaviors may be considered to be subset of stereotypic behavior; however, SIB are unique in their predilection to disabled individuals, the intensity of the behavior, the harmful nature of some activities, their rather brief distractibility, and their appearance relative to stress and anxiety. The treatment of individuals with SIB may be challenging and prognosis is guarded.

Epilepsy is always a concern with repetitive automatic behavior in children. The preservation of consciousness and the immediate cessation of stereotypic movement upon distraction differentiate it from epileptic automatisms.

Children with paroxysmal dyskinesia may be thought to have stereotypies. They present at a young age with repeated episodes of variable degrees of chorea and/or dystonia, lasting from seconds to minutes and occurring up to many times daily. They are triggered by sudden movement, exertion, stress, or fatigue.

Functional movement disorders (FMD) are caused by psychological factors rather than a neurologic etiology, and may include a wide array of movement and posturing patterns. Abnormal posturing or high-amplitude hand tremor might be reminiscent of stereotypic hand flapping, head nodding, or other stereotypies. Distractibility, being a key factor in diagnosis of FMD, is noted with stereotypies as well. However, FMDs tend to occur at an older age, and are rare (although not unheard of) below the age of 8 years. A child or adolescent suddenly presenting with bilateral distractible hand flapping is much more likely to have FMD rather than a stereotypy.

Prognosis

In contrast to common belief, stereotypies are not short-lived. Follow-up studies of normally developing children have shown that stereotypies tend to subside gradually during late childhood. Many children will gradually conceal the movements and perform them in private settings or incorporate them into daily routine. However, a significant number of children have persistent movements well into adolescence. In a follow-up study, 21% of normally developed children reported having stereotypies for more than 10 years. Disability in a normally developed child presenting with stereotypies might be caused by co-morbid conditions. These include reported attention deficit hyperactivity disorder, developmental coordination disorder,

obsessive-compulsive disorder, tic disorders, speech and language disorders, and sleep disorders.

Management

Stereotypies are considered as causing little interference with daily living and usually do not cause psychosocial problems in the normally developed child. However, they may cause significant parental anxiety, as parents might tend to perceive the movements as intrusive for the child's behavior and are concerned with the social impact of the movements, especially in the school-aged child. Interestingly, peers may not consider the stereotyped movement to be abnormal, and consider it to be part of the child's normal movement repertoire. Parental concerns should be addressed during office visits.

Behavior modification interventions may be tried in the older child with persistent movements. One small study showed a reduction of movement over a period of one year in 6- to 14-year-old children treated with a combination of habit reversal and differential reinforcement of other behaviors. Although anecdotal use of benzodiazepines, neuroleptics, and clonidine have been described, no large studies investigating these interventions for suppression of stereotypies have been performed, and this avenue should be discouraged in the normally developed child. Several studies have been conducted with serotonin reuptake inhibitors and show a small effect on repetitive behaviors in ASD. Small studies also support the use of dopamine-blocking agents, such as olanzapine, and divalproex, but larger studies are needed.

Further Readings

Bodfish JW, Symons FJ, Parker DE, Lewis MH. Varieties of repetitive behavior in autism: comparisons to mental retardation. *J Autism Dev Disord* 2000; **30**: 237–143.

Carcani-Rathwell I, Rabe-Hasketh S, Santosh PJ. Repetitive and stereotyped behaviours in pervasive developmental disorders. *J Child Psychol Psychiatry* 2006; **47**: 573–581.

Edwards MJ, Lang AE, Bhatia KP. Stereotypies: a critical appraisal and suggestion of a clinically useful definition. *Mov Disord* 2012; **27**: 179–185.

Evans DW, Leckman JF, Carter A, Reznick JS, Henshaw D, King RA, Pauls D. Ritual, habit, and perfectionism: the prevalence and development of compulsive-like behavior in normal young children. *Child Dev* 1997; **68**: 58–68.

Goldman S, Wang C, Salgado MW, Greene PE, Kim M, Rapin I. Motor stereotypies in children with autism and other developmental disorders. *Dev Med Child Neurol* 2009; **51**: 30–38.

Harris K, Mahone EM, Singer H. Nonautistic motor stereotypies: clinical features and longitudinal follow-up. *Pediatr Neurol* 2008; **38**: 267–272.

Jankovic J. Stereotypies. In: Jankovic J, Fahn S., Principles and Practice of Movement Disorders. Philadelphia: Churchill Livingstone Elsevier; 2007: 443–450.

Kurlan R. A clinically useful definition of stereotypies. *Mov Disord* 2013; **28**: 404.

Leekam S, Tandos J, McConachie H, Meins E, Parkinson K, Wright C, Turner M, Arnott B, Vittorini L, Le Couteur A. Repetitive behaviours in typically developing 2-year-olds. *J Child Psychol Psychiatry* 2007; **48**: 1131–1138.

Meige H, Feindel E. *Tics and Their Treatment*, transl. by Wilson SAK. London: Sidney Appelton; 1907: 264–266.

Miller JM, Singer HS, Bridges DD, Waranch HR. Behavioural therapy for treatment of stereotypic movements in nonautistic children. *J Child Neurol* 2006; **21**: 119–125.

Muthugovindan D, Singer H. Motor stereotypy disorders. *Curr Opin Neurol* 2009; **22**: 131–136.

Singer HS. Stereotypic movement disorders. *Handb Clin Neurol* 2011; **100**: 631–639.

13

Paroxysmal Movement Disorders

Christina L. Vaughan, MD

Hospice and Palliative Medicine Program, University of California San Diego/Scripps Health, La Jolla, California, USA

Introduction

Paroxysmal neurological conditions that result in abnormal hyperkinetic movements generally fall under the categories of migraine, cerebral ischemia, epileptic seizure, metabolic derangement, psychiatric condition, or movement disorder. Temporary loss of consciousness is an important distinguishing characteristic that differentiates most other etiologies from movement disorders. An electroencephalogram (EEG) is helpful to differentiate seizures from other etiologies of paroxysmal events that may or may not be associated with loss of consciousness. The diagnosis of epilepsy is usually straightforward, especially when precise and detailed personal and eyewitness accounts of the prodrome, onset, evolution, and recovery period after the event are obtained. Non-epileptic paroxysmal movement disorders are rare extrapyramidal diseases, and identification requires detailed history taking and physical examination. However, the challenge of a paroxysmal disorder lies in its intermittent pattern, which may require prolonged periods of observation. Sometimes home video recordings are necessary for diagnosis.

This chapter focuses predominantly on primary hyperkinetic paroxysmal movement disorders that occur during wakefulness in adults: with emphasis on the paroxysmal dykinesias, episodic ataxias, but also including brief coverage of myoclonus, startle syndromes, oculogyric crisis, and functional (psychogenic) syndromes. Many movement disorders can present episodically (see Table 13.1) and will be addressed elsewhere. The phenomenology of the movements must first be classified, but with the caveat that bizarre movements do not necessarily indicate a functional etiology.

Paroxysmal dyskinesias

Paroxysmal choreodystonic disorders or paroxysmal dyskinesias are a heterogeneous group of movement disorders typified by recurrent attacks of abnormal involuntary movements (see Table 13.1). The diagnosis is largely based on the history—the patients are generally completely normal between attacks, and the movements include athetosis, ballismus, chorea, dystonia, or a combination of these. Currently, the paroxysmal dyskinesias are classified by their triggers and on the basis of the duration and frequency of the attacks, effectiveness of medication, and associated syndromes. Those occurring in wakefulness are classified into three categories according to the precipitant, duration of attacks, and etiology: (1) paroxysmal kinesigenic dyskinesia (PKD), in which attacks are brief and provoked by sudden voluntary movements; (2) paroxysmal non-kinesigenic dyskinesia (PNKD), in which attacks occur spontaneously; and (3) paroxysmal exertion-induced dyskinesia (PED), in which attacks are induced by prolonged exercise. Table 13.2 outlines the major differences between these categories. Paroxysmal dyskinesias can be sporadic, familial (autosomal dominant inheritance), or secondary to

Non-Parkinsonian Movement Disorders, First Edition. Edited by Deborah A. Hall and Brandon R. Barton.
© 2017 John Wiley & Sons, Ltd. Published 2017 by John Wiley & Sons, Ltd.
Companion website: www.wiley.com/go/hall/non-parkinsonian_movement_disorders

Table 13.1 Paroxysmal movement disorders during wakefulness

I) Paroxysmal dyskinesias
   a. Primary
      i. Paroxysmal kinesigenic dyskinesia (PKD)
      ii. Paroxysmal non-kinesigenic dyskinesia (PKND)
      iii. Paroxysmal exercise-induced dyskinesia (PED)
   b. Secondary
      i. Multiple sclerosis
      ii. Post-traumatic
      iii. Tumor or a vascular lesion
      iv. Metabolic derangements
      v. Central nervous system infections
      vi. Anoxic brain injuries
      vii. Basal ganglia calcifications
      viii. Kernicterus
      ix. Antiphospholipid syndrome
      x. Arnold–Chiari malformation with syringomyelia
      xi. Parasagittal meningioma
      xii. Progressive supranuclear palsy
      xiii. Spinal cord injury
II) Epilepsy/seizure
III) Episodic ataxias
IV) Action and intention tremors
V) Action dystonia
VI) Action myoclonus
VII) Akathetic movements
VIII) Startle syndromes/hyperekplexia
IX) Stereotypies
X) Tics
XI) Hemifacial spasm
XII) Oculogyric crisis
XIII) Functional movement disorders

other disorders. PKD is the most common type, with an estimated prevalence of 1 in 150,000. PNKD has an estimated prevalence of one in a million and paroxysmal exercise-induced dyskinesia is even less often encountered. Lack of familiarity with these disorders and the normal neurological examination between attacks frequently causes diagnostic delays and may also contribute to underestimates of prevalence. Lifestyle modification to avoid precipitating factors is important in the management of paroxysmal dyskinesias. Drugs such as acetazolamide, anticholinergics, levodopa, and tetrabenazine have been inconsistently successful.

Paroxysmal kinesigenic dyskinesia

Paroxysmal kinesigenic dyskinesia (PKD) is a rare, typically autosomal dominant disorder, characterized by kinesigenic triggers, duration of attacks <1 minute, preserved consciousness, absence of structural diseases or epileptiform activity, and beneficial effect of phenytoin or carbamazepine (100 mg twice a day). PKD onset is usually between 5 and 15 years of age. Although the term "kinesigenic dyskinesia" is used, other triggers are possible, such as startle and the intention to move. In PKD, an "aura," such as an unusual cephalic or epigastric sensation, may precede the attacks, further adding to the diagnostic confusion. The threshold for attacks is reduced by anxiety and stress. The movements often include dystonic postures, with or without dyskinesias.

Approximately a quarter of PKD cases are sporadic; however, PKD is considered to be an autosomal dominant condition with variable penetrance and most of the reported cases are familial. In some families, infantile convulsions were occasionally observed in the same pedigree, hence the labeling of ICCA syndrome (infantile convulsions with choreoathetosis), which led to the belief that the underlying pathophysiological mechanism was due to a sodium channelopathy. Several groups have recently identified mutations in the proline-rich transmembrane protein 2 (*PRRT2*) gene as the cause of PKD and ICCA. Despite the presence of this mutation in affected family members, the clinical manifestations can vary. There is limited research regarding the function of *PRRT2*, but mutations in this gene may appear to cause neuronal hyperexcitability. The prognosis of PKD is favorable and the patients typically have excellent responses to antiepileptic drugs.

★ TIPS AND TRICKS

Diagnosis of paroxysmal kinesigenic dyskinesia (PKD)

- An identified kinesigenic trigger for the attacks
- Short duration attacks (<1 minute)
- No loss of consciousness or pain during attacks
- Age of onset between 5–15 years
- Normal interictal neurological examination
- Exclusion of other organic diseases
- Control of attacks with carbamazepine or phenytoin

Paroxysmal non-kinesigenic dyskinesia

Paroxysmal non-kinesigenic dyskinesia (PNKD) is a rare movement disorder that can mimic epilepsy. It is distinguished from PKD by less frequent, but longer lasting attacks. The attacks are not induced by sudden movement but can occur spontaneously. PNKD usually manifests in childhood, and is slightly more common in males (1.4:1). Most cases are familial, but sporadic cases have been reported. One mutation has been identified in the gene encoding myofibrillogenesis regulator-1 (*MR-1*) on chromosome 2q35, also known as DYT8. In addition, two other loci have been identified: *PNKD2* on chromosome 2q31 and another on chromosome 1p that is associated with spasticity. Clinically, patients with or without mutation in *MR-1* manifest symptoms in childhood or early adolescence, although the *MR-1* negative cases have a more variable age at onset. All patients exhibit chorea and dystonia, but the *MR-1* positive cases also have speech involvement. Attacks typically begin in one limb, but often spread to all limbs and the face. Patients may sometimes lose the ability to communicate during attacks, but they do not lose consciousness. The frequency of attacks is between one a week to several in a lifetime, the attacks tend to diminish with age, and their duration and intensity varies. In the *MR-1* positive cases, the attacks are typically triggered by alcohol, caffeine, exercise, or emotional stress. Other possible triggers can include changes in temperature, micturition, defecation, menses, pregnancy, starvation, and certain medications such as dopamine agonists. The episodes in *MR-1* positive cases are prevented or aborted by sleep. Both subtypes seem partially responsive to benzodiazepines, although this effect can subside in *MR-1* negative cases. Antiepileptic medications have limited, if any, utility, and PNKD has been noted to be refractory to medical management. Several reports have shown that pallidal deep brain stimulation may be successfully utilized in patients with refractory PNKD.

Paroxysmal exertion-induced dyskinesia

Paroxysmal exertion-induced dyskinesia (PED) attacks usually begin between 1 to 16 years of age and are triggered by longer lasting physical activity like walking or running for perhaps 10–15 minutes. The movements are usually dystonic and occur in the body part involved in the exercise and last for 5–30 minutes after ceasing the exercise. Either side can be affected at different attacks, and only rarely do attacks become generalized. Neurological examination between attacks does not typically reveal abnormal findings. PED is usually idiopathic (familial or less commonly sporadic) and only rarely due to an acquired cause. PED can be associated with mutations in the glucose transporter gene, *GLUT1*, responsible for glucose transport across the blood-brain barrier, and it has been suggested that the dyskinesias results from an exertion-induced energy deficit causing episodic dysfunction in the basal ganglia. When PED is familial, the mode of inheritance is autosomal dominant with incomplete penetrance. An association with familial epilepsy has been reported, although rarely. Linkage analysis in a family with "Rolandic epilepsy, paroxysmal exercise-induced dyskinesia, and writer's cramp syndrome" revealed a cluster of genes at the pericentromeric region of chromosome 16, near the paroxysmal kinesigenic dyskinesia locus. Acetazolamide, levodopa, and trihexiphenidyl have been reported to be effective in small series or individual cases.

Table 13.2 Paroxysmal dyskinesias

	Paroxysmal kinesigenic dyskinesia (PKD)	Paroxysmal non-kinesigenic dyskinesia (PNKD)	Paroxysmal exercise-induced dyskinesia (PED)
Etiology	Inherited, sporadic, secondary	Inherited, sporadic, secondary	Inherited, sporadic, secondary
Inheritance	Autosomal dominant; loci chromosome 16q; *PRRT2* mutation	Autosomal dominant; myofibrillogenesis regulator-1 (*MR-1*) gene positive mutation: chromosome 2q35	Autosomal dominant or recessive Linkage chromosome 16 or glucose transporter (*GLUT1*) gene mutation
		Autosomal dominant; *MR-1* gene negative mutation	
Gender ratio (M:F)	4:1	1.4:1	1:1
Age at onset (years)	5–15	<1–12	1–16
		1–23	
Attack trigger	Sudden movement, startle, hyperventilation	Alcohol, caffeine, stress	Prolonged exercise
Attack duration	<5 min, usually <30 s	2 min–3 h	5 min–2 h
		2 min–3 h	
Attack frequency	1–20/d—rarely (<5 in life)	3/d–2/yr	1/d–2/mo
		3/d–2/yr	
Treatment	Carbamazepine, phenytoin	Benzodiazepines (clonazepam)	Acetazolamide
		Benzodiazepines (clonazepam)	

Source: Adapted from Jankovic 2009.

Secondary causes of paroxysmal dyskinesias

In clinical practice, in patients with a family history and age of onset before 20 years, no investigations are required, except for genetic studies. In patients older than 20 years and without a family history, secondary causes need to be pursued, and neuro-imaging and laboratory studies are necessary to rule out multiple sclerosis, which can present with paroxysmal dystonias, head trauma, tumor, or a vascular lesion such as a lacunar stroke causing hemiballismus. Metabolic derangements should also be considered, especially hypo- and hyper-glycemia, hyperglycinemia, and hypercalcemia. Other reported secondary causes have included peripheral trauma, central nervous system infections, anoxic brain injuries, thyrotoxicosis, basal ganglia calcifications, kernicterus, Arnold–Chiari malformation with syringomyelia, parasagittal meningioma, methylphenidate therapy, progressive supranuclear palsy, and spinal cord injury. PED can sometimes be an initial manifestation of dopa-responsive dystonia and in rare cases has been seen as the sole presenting symptom of young-onset Parkinson disease. Sometimes these secondary cases have features of both kinesigenic and non-kinesigenic dyskinesia, and patients with secondary paroxysmal dyskinesias appear more likely to have baseline neurological defects present between paroxysmal episodes than patients with primary paroxysmal dyskinesia.

Episodic ataxias

Episodic ataxia (EA) is a rare familial disorder characterized by brief attacks of generalized ataxia with normal or near normal neurological function between attacks. Inheritance is autosomal dominant. EA is characteristically present in childhood or adolescence and presents as ataxia and myokymia (type 1, potassium channelopathy) or vertigo, ataxia and occasionally syncope (type 2, calcium channelopathy). In EA1, the attacks are brief, triggered by startle and are associated with subtle myokymias in the face or hands. Patients with EA1 can have paroxysmal kinesigenic dyskinesias as well, and interictal myokymia is a sign of EA1. EA1 was linked to missense mutations on chromosome 12p13 in the gene encoding for the voltage-gated potassium channel, *KCNA1*. In EA2, the attacks last for hours to days, are induced by stress or exertion, and usually downbeat nystagmus is present. Vertigo is more frequent in EA2. EA2 typically results from nonsense mutations in the *CACNA1A* gene, on chromosome 19p13.2, which encodes the alpha1A subunit of the P/Q-type calcium channel. In both subtypes, dysarthria, tremor, or visual disturbances may be present in some cases during episodes. These events are commonly diagnosed as epilepsy and EEG recordings can reveal sharp and slow waves. Additionally, epileptic seizures can occur, further confusing the diagnosis. Both EA1 and EA2 are ion channel disorders and respond to acetazolamide and the potassium channel blocker 4-aminopyridine. More recently, other forms of episodic ataxia have been described, and include EA3 to EA6 (see Table 13.3).

Myoclonus

Myoclonus is a common movement disorder and can be classified based on its clinical characteristics, pathophysiology, or cause. Grouped by clinical features, myoclonus can be considered spontaneous, action, or reflex and all may be paroxysmal. This is reviewed in Chapter 4.

Startle syndromes

Startle syndromes are a heterogeneous group of disorders, comprising hyperekplexia, startle epilepsy, and neuropsychiatric syndromes that are distinguished by an abnormal motor response to startling events. Careful history taking is usually sufficient to accurately differentiate these entities. Hyperekplexia usually begins from early childhood and manifests as an exaggerated startle response with forced closure of the eyes and an extension of the extremities followed by a generalized stiffness and collapse. It can be mistaken for cataplexy in patients with narcolepsy, or atonic or tonic epileptic seizures. More minor forms of hyperekplexia display an exaggerated startle response without tonicity and collapse and may be confused with functional syndromes. Hyperekplexia may be (1) hereditary, due to a genetic mutation in the alpha-1 subunit of the glycine receptor on chromosome 5; (2) sporadic; or (3) symptomatic, secondary to widespread cerebral or brainstem damage. Treatment of the severity of the startle response and degree of hypertonicity is usually accomplished with clonazepam.

Table 13.3 Episodic ataxias*

	EA1	EA2	EA3	EA4	EA5	EA6
Chromosome	12p13	19p13.2	1q42			
Gene	Potassium channel, KCNA1	alpha1A subunit of the P/Q-type calcium channel CACNL1A4			CACNB4	SLC1A3
Age at onset	Childhood, early adolescence		Childhood/ variable	Early adulthood		Childhood
Clinical features	Interictal myokymia +/− paroxysmal kinesigenic dyskinesia, interictal myokymia	Intermittent attacks of ataxia, dysarthria, nausea, vertigo, downbeat nystagmus	Vestibular ataxia, tinnitus, interictal myokymia	"Periodic vestibulocerebellar ataxia": recurrent attacks of ataxia, vertigo, diplopia	Ataxia and seizures; recurrent episodes of ataxia with vertigo	Ataxia, slurred speech
Attack trigger	Startle	Stress or exertion	Stress, fatigue, movement, and arousal after sleep			Fever
Attack duration	Seconds–minutes	Minutes–days	<30 minutes			
Treatment	Phenytoin, acetazolamide	Acetazolamide, potassium channel blocker 4-aminopyridine	Acetazolamide		Acetazolamide	

*EA, episodic ataxia

Oculogyric crisis

Oculogyric crisis (OGC) is an acute dystonia that can occur after administration of high-potency dopamine receptor-blocking agents, commonly within 72 hours. OGC is characterized by sustained spasmodic deviation of the eyes, most often upward though may be lateral, downward, or oblique. The most frequently reported associated features include backward and lateral flexion of the neck, a wide-open mouth, tongue protrusion, and ocular pain. Occasionally, such episodes are preceded by prodromal symptoms such as restlessness, agitation, malaise, or a fixed stare. Although the exact mechanism of OGC is unknown, there is evidence that it might be caused by an imbalance between reduced dopaminergic and increased cholinergic and GABAergic activity. The mainstay of treatment and prevention of acute dystonia is with anticholinergic medication.

Functional syndromes

These are debilitating conditions with persistent fluctuating abnormal movements that cannot be attributed to any known structural or neurochemical disease. Most functional movement disorders fulfill psychiatric criteria for a somatoform disorder, usually conversion or other somatization disorder, although sometimes they can be associated with a factitious disorder or malingering. These cases present a particular diagnostic challenge, as identification has been one of exclusion because there is no single clinical feature or specific laboratory test that leads to a definitive diagnosis. Tremor is the most common functional phenomenology, followed by dystonia, and these tend to fluctuate significantly or occur in paroxysms. Features that support a functional etiology include abrupt onset, with maximal disability from the beginning; spontaneous remissions; self-inflicted injuries; multiple somatizations; obvious psychiatric disturbances; and functional disability out of proportion to the physical examination. On examination, movements may disappear with distraction, commence with suggestion, or be associated with give-way weakness, functional patterns of sensory loss, embellished responses to a stimulus, or bizarre gait patterns that, despite the dramatic movements, do not result in falls. Functional tremor is usually highly variable in frequency, amplitude, and direction and is best assessed with the entrainment test. The entrainment test entails first establishing that when deliberately finger-tapping independently, each hand taps at a different frequency, yet when tapping concurrently the two hands become entrained together with matching frequencies demonstrating the difficulty to voluntarily tap simultaneously with two hands at slightly different frequencies. Organic dystonia tends to be action-induced, especially at the beginning, whereas functional dystonia often begins as a fixed posture. Episodes of twisting facial movements that deviate the mouth to one side tend to be functional, as organic facial dystonia usually does not move the mouth sidewise. Functional myoclonus may be difficult to distinguish from organic causes without the use of physiology; the contraction is always >50 ms, and usually abates and stops with distraction. Psychotherapy is the most effective treatment approach, though the longer the duration of functional symptoms, the more refractory the movements are to treatment.

Further Readings

Bhatia KP. Familial (idiopathic) paroxysmal dyskinesias: an update. *Seminars Neurol* 2001; **21**(1): 69–74.

Bhatia KP. Paroxysmal dyskinesias. *Mov Disord* 2011; **26**(6): 1157–1165.

Blakeley J, Jankovic J. Secondary paroxysmal dyskinesias. *Mov Disord* 2002; **17**(4): 726–734.

Bruno MK, Hallett M, Gwinn-Hardy K, et al. Clinical evaluation of idiopathic paroxysmal kinesigenic dyskinesia: new diagnostic criteria. *Neurology* 2004; **63**(12): 2280–2287.

Demirkiran M, Jankovic J. Paroxysmal dyskinesias: clinical features and classification. *An Neurol* 1995; **38**(4): 571–579.

Hallett M, Weiner WJ, Kompoliti K. Psychogenic movement disorders. *Parkinsonism Related Disord* 2012; **18**(suppl 1): S155–157.

Houser MK, Soland VL, Bhatia KP, Quinn NP, Marsden CD. Paroxysmal kinesigenic choreoathetosis: a report of 26 patients. *J Neurol* 1999; **246**(2): 120–126.

Jankovic J, Demirkiran M. Classification of paroxysmal dyskinesias and ataxias. *Adv Neurol* 2002; **89**: 387–400.

Karakis I, Cole AJ, Hoch DB, Sharma N. Extrapyramidal epilepsy. *Epileptic Disord* 2011; **13**(2): 181–184.

Van Rootselaar AF, Schade van Westrum S, Velis DN, Tijssen MA. The paroxysmal dyskinesias. *Pract Neurol* 2009; **9**(2): 102–109.

14

Uncommon Movement Disorders and Movement Disorder Mimics

Nina Browner, MD

National Parkinson Foundation Center of Excellence, University of North Carolina at Chapel Hill, North Carolina, USA

Introduction

Despite modern advances in technology, the recognition and diagnosis of uncommon hyperkinetic movements still relies heavily on pattern recognition of characteristic features. Although unusual, they all have distinct presentations. Because the etiology of these movement disorders is heterogeneous, they are organized into alphabetical order and their pathophysiology is reviewed individually. Abnormal involuntary movements (dyskinesias) are usually caused by brain damage or dysfunction. Occasionally, however, lesions of the spinal cord, spinal root, cervical or lumbar plexus, or even peripheral nerves can cause a variety of dyskinesias. Peripheral injury as a cause of some movement disorders has been previously described in belly dancer's dyskinesias, hemifacial spasm, and "jumpy stump" syndrome after limb amputation and can potentially play a role in development of painful legs and moving toes syndrome.

✥ SCIENCE REVISITED

Movement disorders induced by peripheral injury

Peripheral injury as a cause of some movement disorders is a controversial topic within the movement disorders community. The mechanisms postulated include injury-related structural reorganization of the local neuronal circuitry by axonal sprouting following nerve injury, resulting in disinhibited intraspinal reflex pathways or hyperexcitable motor neurons. Some have suggested that the disorder is due to alteration of either cortical or subcortical central nervous system function. Proponents of the concept that peripheral trauma can induce a centrally mediated movement disorder often use the example of the post-amputation stump movements to support this concept, postulating that peripheral injury alters the processing of afferent sensory input to central cortical and subcortical structures and leads to central reorganization. Criteria for movement disorders related to trauma should include (1) the injury must be severe enough to cause local symptoms that persist for at least two weeks or require medical attention within two weeks of the injury, (2) the onset of the movement disorder must have occurred within a few days or months (up to one year) after the injury, and (3) the onset of the movement disorders must have been anatomically related to the side of the injury.

Alien hand/limb syndrome

Alien hand/limb syndrome (AHS) is characterized by involuntary movement of a limb in conjunction with a failure of the patient to recognize the ownership of

Table 14.1 Differentiation of types of alien limb syndrome

AHS type	Lesion	Limb affected	Typical movements
Callosal-frontal AHS	Dominant frontal lobe	Dominant	1. Grasping, groping, and other positive exploratory behaviors 2. Frontal release signs present
Callosal AHS	Anterior corpus callosum	Non-dominant	1. Hand apraxia 2. Oppositional intermanual conflict 3. Frontal release signs absent
Posterior AHS	Posterior corpus callosum	Either dominant or non-dominant	1. Non-purposeful 2. Non-conflictual 3. Include arm levitation and finger writhing

one's limb, in some cases with estrangement from or personification of the limb itself (i.e., recognizing the alien limb as a separate entity and/or giving it a name). There are many descriptions provided by the patients: a feeling that one's body part is foreign, loss of control over that body part, personification of the affected body part, and autonomous activity that is perceived as outside voluntary control. Most commonly the hand is affected, although any limb or combination of limbs may fulfill the alien limb criteria. In cases of alien hand, the hand acts at odds with the patient's will, creating a sense of loss of bimanual coordination and in some cases an intermanual conflict when hands act at cross purposes. Accompanying signs include rigidity, cortical sensory findings, apraxia, and neglect. The ipsilateral lower extremity is often subtly involved as well. The observed behavior is so odd that often the patient's complaint is initially dismissed as functional.

During the history, a verbally expressed feeling that the movements are not under self-control and personification of the arm raise an alert for the diagnosis of alien limb. The two major diagnostic criteria for AHS are the patient's complaint that the limb feels foreign and the presence of complex involuntary movements of the limb that cannot be classified as any identifiable movement disorder.

Depending on the anatomical lesion and clinical presentation, AHS has been classified into three separate syndromes: callosal-frontal, callosal, and posterior AHS. The major differences between the syndromes are outlined in Table 14.1, although patients often defy exact classification. Multiple etiologies of AHS are described in the literature, such as callosal or thalamic infarcts, tumors, infections, Creutzfeldt–Jacob disease, demyelinating disease, corticobasal degeneration, or even callosotomy. Neuroimaging studies are most helpful in detecting a lesion that causes AHS. The majority of cases implicate parietal lobe dysfunction contralateral to the affected limb, usually in the right brain.

Rehabilitation treatment is targeted toward the specific needs of the patient and education for compensatory strategies of AHS. Visualization of the planned movement, distraction of the affected limb, and maintaining a slow/steady pace with activities may decrease the frequency of AHS movements, allowing improvement in patient's activities of daily living. Usually medications are not effective for treatment of AHS, although recently there has been one report of AHS improvement with clonazepam and botulinum toxin injections. Spontaneous improvement of the AHS symptoms and recovery is common in vascular lesions.

☆ TIPS AND TRICKS

Diagnosis of alien limb syndrome
Upon examining the patient with alien limb, other frontal release signs or neurological deficits, including hemiparesis, hyperreflexia, Babinski sign, and parkinsonism should be noted. Pure alien limb syndrome without additional neurological findings is very uncommon. Neuroimaging, preferably brain MRI, is helpful in identifying potential lesions in the dominant medial frontal lobe, anterior corpus collosum, non-dominant parietal-occipital area, or

generalized unilateral cortical atrophy at the posterior parietal areas, suggestive for corticobasal degeneration. In some cases, glucose metabolism positron emission tomography (^{18}FDG PET) scans are beneficial to identify the areas of decreased metabolism in the above-mentioned anatomical regions. The scans may be especially helpful in identifying early corticobasal degeneration, with glucose hypometabolism in contralateral parietal and frontal cortical regions.

Belly dancer dyskinesia

The term "belly dancer dyskinesia" refers to a form of focal involuntary movements affecting the abdominal wall. The clinical characteristics of this unusual dyskinesia are variable, but usually consist of writhing movements and contractions of the abdominal muscles reminiscent of the undulating movements of a belly dancer. Along with the abdominal wall movements, oscillatory movements of the umbilicus are described. The abdominal wall movements are slow, rhythmic, and writhing, unlike the regular, rhythmic jerks described in segmental myoclonus. The movements are present equally when laying at rest as when standing or walking, unlike the abdominal muscle spasms of axial torsion dystonia. These movements cannot be voluntarily suppressed, but may be influenced by respiratory maneuvers. For example, deep inspiration and breath holding may suppress the movements.

Such response to respiratory maneuvers in some patients can be explained by involvement of the diaphragm and is associated with diaphragmatic flutter. The flutter is characterized by contraction of one or both domes of the diaphragm at the frequency of 1–8 Hz superimposed on normal tidal breathing. The diaphragmatic movements depress the abdominal contents during each descent, leading to repetitive propulsion and retraction of the anterior abdominal wall, creating jerky motions. Additional muscle groups including intercostal, scalene, paraspinal, and abdominal muscles may be recruited and may contribute to the observed abdominal wall movements. The movements are intermittent and fluctuate during the breathing cycle.

Onset is usually gradual. Many, but not all, patients, have a history of preexisting trauma to the abdominal wall or abdominal surgical procedures. There are single case reports for the following: tardive etiology, basal ganglia lesion in the setting of hyponatremia-induced pontine and extrapontine myelinosis, and functional movement disorder.

Screening of the diaphragm for abnormal movements should be performed as part of the assessment of isolated abdominal dyskinesias, with the fluttering of the diaphragm best observed on video fluoroscopy. Alternating contractures of the recti and oblique muscles are described on EMG. Investigations such as spinal and abdominal imaging should be performed, but they usually fail to reveal any local abnormalities to explain the movement disorder.

Prognosis is unfavorable as there is no known effective treatment. The clinical course may therefore be long-lasting or permanent.

Jumpy stumps

The movements consist of jerking or spasm of the amputation stump. These are alternating flexion and extension or abduction and adduction of the stump. It can involve either upper or lower extremity stumps. The motor phenomena are typically associated with severe lancinating pain, consistent with the phantom limb sensory experience, although cases without pain have been described. The movements can occur spontaneously, but commonly they are triggered by a voluntary movement of the stump or sensory stimulation of the stump.

The epidemiology is hard to estimate, given the rarity of the phenomenon, but incidence has been estimated at approximately 1% of amputations. Transient jerking of the amputation stumps in the post-operative period is common, but cases of pathologic "jumpy stumps" are associated with a delayed onset and persist over many years. No other risk factors, except for amputation, have been described as a risk factor for this movement disorder.

In most cases treatment is unsatisfactory. Some anecdotal reports can be found where baclofen (20–40 mg/d), doxepin, topiramate and gabapentin (900 mg/d) were successfully used to treat the movement disorder. Local and epidural anesthesia may be temporally effective, although multiple other interventions including diazepam, carbamazepine, lumbar sympathetic blockage, intrathecal saline, and direct injections of saline into the sciatic nerve failed to alleviate either the pain or the movements. In addition, some patients report relief by putting pressure on the stump, squeezing the stump, or applying counterstimulation on the opposite side of the body.

Painful legs and moving toes

Painful legs and moving toes (PLMT) is characterized by pain in one or more limbs that is accompanied by repetitive, non-rhythmic digit movements. Predominantly lower extremities are involved, although there were some reports of painful arm and moving hand as well as mouth and tongue involvement. Patients report pain as stabbing, tingling, burning, shooting, or lancinating and it severity ranges widely among patients. The pain precedes the movement disorder sometimes by months or even years. The digit movements are a constant, chaotic combination of flexion/ extension or abduction/adduction and usually can be voluntarily suppressed for a short period or by applying pressure to the sole of the foot. Although the movement aspect of PLMT tends to attract attention, patients are much more distressed by the pain in the extremity, except for complaints related to moving digits rubbing on footwear. Clinical characteristics of PLMT patients are summarized in Table 14.2.

Based on the electromyography (EMG) results, peripheral neuropathy accounts for the common identifiable cause of the pain in PLMT, of which the majority of cases are due to small fiber neuropathy, trauma, and radiculopathy. Some cases of PLMT can be temporally linked to procedures: epidural injection, myelography, or toe surgery. There are some reports of developing PLMT after cessation of neuroleptics or cessation of anxiolytics. Then again, in about one-third of patients, it is hard to identify cause for the pain. Neurological examination can be either normal or show some mild neurological symptoms related to underlying neuropathy (asymmetric or symmetric): sensory peripheral neuropathy, reduced vibration sense, reduced or absent reflexes (typically ankle jerks), mild distal limb weakness, and occasionally hyperreflexia and impaired rapid alternating movements.

Treatment results for the pain and movements are overall disappointing. PLMT is predominantly a debilitating pain syndrome, and most patients require pain management rather than treatment of the movement of their affected digits. Despite targeting the pain with a vast array of drugs, few patients report gratifying pain relief. There are some anecdotal reports of partial pain relief with a combination of gabapentin, levodopa, and lorazepam. A few patients benefit from localized

Table 14.2 Clinical characteristics of patients with painful legs and moving toes and associated lesions

Clinical characteristics	Hassan et al. $N=76$	Dressler et al. $N=18$	Comments
Age of onset	58 (24–86)	60.3 (28–76)	Adults 30–80 years
Male : Female ratio	26:50	3:15	Predominantly females
Bilateral : unilateral	25:51	10:8	Could be unilateral or bilateral initially, eventually up to 4% of cases becomes bilateral

Lesions identified: location	Hassan et al. $N=76$	Dressler et al. $N=18$	Comments
Cryptogenic	32	3	Cryptogenic, peripheral neuropathy, radiculopathy, and peripheral trauma are the main causes
Peripheral neuropathy	21	3	
Cauda equina/radiculopathy	8	8	
Peripheral trauma	8	4	
Peroneal/tibial mononeuropathy	3	0	
Other	4	0	
Spinal cord	0	0	

therapy (epidural corticosteroid or local tibial nerve blockade) or physical therapies (transcutaneous electrical nerve stimulation, massage, cold soaks, chiropractor-delivered therapy, or acupuncture). Surgical intervention (spinal laminectomies and fusions) are not helpful and may even worsen the pain. There appears to be no evidence that this syndrome spontaneously resolves over time. Overall, most of the patients' symptoms stay the same over a period of 5–7 years. Although the phenomenology of the movement and the prominence of the discomfort due to pain may raise the question about a functional nature of this disorder, the movements of PLMT are almost impossible to perform voluntarily because of the pattern of recruitment and the excessive voluntary motor unit firing rate on EMG. None of the cases in large series of PLMT patients had red flags for functional disorders, such as multiple somatic complaints, variability in presentation, history of physical or sexual abuse, or non-epileptic seizures.

Myokymia

Myokymia refers to involuntary, spontaneous, localized, transient, or persistent quivering muscle movements. It affects a few muscle bundles within a single muscle, but is usually not extensive enough to cause movement at a joint. The movements are slow, "worm-like" and undulating, usually prolonged, and involve a larger area of muscle than fasciculations. They are not worsened by movement or certain positions, and they persist during sleep.

Myokymia often occurs in normal individuals, causing persistent focal twitching of the muscle, commonly the orbicularis oculi. It is exacerbated by fatigue, anxiety, or caffeine. Myokymia also appears in a various disease states that are associated with an abnormality somewhere along the motor axon: demyelination of the nerve, toxins (e.g., rattlesnake toxin or gold salts), edema, decreased blood levels of ionized calcium, and other factors.

Myokymia may be generalized or focal, with focal myokymia being more common. Focal facial myokymia may be due to irritation of the fasciculus of the VII cranial nerve within the brainstem by a multiple sclerosis plaque (common presentation) or a brainstem lesion such as pontine glioma or syrinx (infrequent presentation). About 15% of patients with Guillain–Barré syndrome are described to have bilateral facial myokymia associated with mild bilateral face weakness; in these cases, the myokymia appears in the first three weeks of the illness and persists up to one month. Focal facial myokymia is usually transient, but may persist for long periods when it is due to channelopathy or a structural lesion such as pontine glioma or syrinx. Focal limb myokymia is particularly characteristic of radiation damage to a nerve or plexus, and it is rarely associated with nerve compression syndromes or Guillain–Barré syndrome.

Generalized myokymia is often associated with autonomic changes (hyperhydrosis or changes in bowel/bladder control). There are many causes for generalized myokymia, and they are briefly described in Table 14.3.

A thorough neurological evaluation in patients with myokymia would help identify cases associated with structural lesions. A neuroimaging study with contrast is essential in evaluation of focal facial myokymia. For limb or generalized myokymia, EMG is often used. On EMG, continuous repetitive brief discharges of groups of 2–6 motor unit potentials are recorded, recurring rhythmically or semi-rhythmically at 5–60 Hz usually several times per second. Following each burst there is a short period of electrical silence, with repetition of the same burst at regular intervals. Myokymic discharges may or may not be accompanied by the clinical myokymia.

> ### ⬡ SCIENCE REVISITED
>
> Although an abnormality along the motor axon has been thought to be the etiology of myokymia, recent evidence suggests abnormalities in axonal voltage-gated potassium channels (VGKCs). Thus, currently, myokymia is not considered a peripheral injury-induced movement disorder.

Treatment of myokymia is focused largely on the underlying etiology. Most patients with facial or focal limb myokymia are not particularly disturbed by the myokymia itself. Instead, it is the accompanying symptoms of the particular neurological or medical condition that are the cause of myokymia that is the major concern to patients and their caretakers. Patients with radiation plexopathy require no intervention. Myokymia seen in acute or chronic polyradiculoneuropathy usually improves with immunomodulatory therapy. Botox injections also

Table 14.3 Forms of generalized myokymia

Idiopathic generalized myokymia (neuromyotomia or Isaac's syndrome)	A disorder with insidious onset characterized by generalized muscle stiffness and persistent contractions of extremity, trunk, and bulbar muscles due to underlying continuous muscle fiber activity. Exercise transiently enhances the contractions approximately 30 seconds beyond the voluntary effort. It is associated with hyperhidrosis, auto-antibodies directed at the voltage-gated potassium channel (VGKC), and can be seen with other immunological disorders.
Hereditary episodic ataxia with myokymia EA-1	Autosomal dominantly inherited syndrome mapped on chromosome 12p with missense mutation in the KCNA2 gene. The attacks of ataxia with tremor last up to 15 minutes, are precipitated by kinesigenic stimulus such as exertion or startle, and are responsive to azetazolamide. The myokymia may lead to generalized stiffness or be simply contraction of distal muscles.
Morvan's syndrome	A rare autoimmune disorder causally associated with auto-antibodies directed at the voltage-gated potassium channel (VGKC), with myokymia, insomnia, and hyperhidrosis.
Generalized myokymia and muscle cramping without peripheral neuropathy	Hereditary form of generalized myokymia associated with muscle stiffness without any associated ataxia or peripheral neuropathy and responsive to carbamazepine and phenytoin. Nerve conduction velocities are normal.
Myokymia and ataxia with continuous muscle discharges	A congenital degenerative disease characterized by clubfoot, joint contractions, cerebellar ataxia, rest tremor, myokymia, and increased creatine kinase levels.
Myokymia and impaired muscle relaxation with continuous muscle discharge	A disorder of peripheral nerves characterized by generalized muscle twitching, weakness, stiffness, cramping, and hyperhidrosis, persistent during sleep and initial fatigue, followed by increasing strength with continued effort. Nerve conduction velocities are reduced.

provide short-term relief for focal myokymia. Phenytoin and carbamazepine have proved to be effective in treating patients with generalized myokymia, specifically patients with continuous muscle fiber activity described in Isaac's syndrome (see Table 14.3). High therapeutic drug levels usually are required to reach satisfactory control of symptoms. EMG can objectively document the disappearance of myokymic discharges. Generalized myokymia associated with immune-mediated conditions, namely myasthenia gravis, thymoma, and various types of peripheral neuropathies, shows improvement with plasma exchange, IVIG treatment, and immunosuppressants such as prednisone.

Myokymia

There is now considerable evidence available that an abnormality of axonal voltage-gated potassium channels (VGKCs) is the basis of the myokymic discharges occurring in several of the myokymic syndromes, and thus generalized myokymia is considered to be autoimmune channelopathy. Presence of the generalized myokymia in patients with other autoimmune disorders also proves humoral autoimmune pathogenesis of the disorder. It is speculated that the plasma exchange causes an interference with the function of the voltage-dependent potassium channels, thus creating relief in some patients with generalized myokymia.

Startle/hyperekplexia

A startle response is a brief motor response, usually a jerk, elicited by an unexpected auditory or, occasionally, tactile, visual, or vestibular stimulus. A normal startle response to auditory stimuli typically involves the upper part of the body, readily habituates, and is almost entirely extinguished after four to six stimuli.

In contrast, in pathological startle syndromes, movements are of greater amplitude, more widely distributed, and habituate poorly. Startle syndromes form a heterogeneous group of disorders with three categories: hyperekplexia, stimulus-induced disorders, and neuropsychiatric syndromes.

Stimulus-induced disorders

The stimulus-induced disorders cover a broad range of epileptic and non-epileptic disorders. Startling stimuli can induce responses other than startle reflexes, such as startle-induced epilepsy, startle-provoked epileptic seizures, and pyridoxine-dependent epilepsy. Startle-induced stiffness other than hyperekplexia is mainly seen in stiff-person syndrome. Stiff-person syndrome is an autoimmune disorder characterized by progressive axial stiffness and intermittent spasms, primarily evoked by unexpected stimuli. The stiffness in stiff-person syndrome is nearly continuous, contrasting sharply with stiffness in adult hyperekplexia that only occurs after a startle and lasting 1–2 seconds. Exaggerated startle reflexes have been reported in stiff-person syndrome and the diagnostic workup in stiff-person syndrome includes an EMG of the long back muscles showing continuous muscle activity. Patients with cataplexy show a loss of muscle tone due to unexpected stimuli rather than an increase in tone. Cataplexy is commonly induced by laughter, but may occasionally occur after being startled. It is of interest that patients with narcolepsy can have an excessive startle reflex. Additional information from electroencephalography (EEG) and video can help, as many stimulus-induced disorders now have an identified gene defect. Anti-epileptic drugs, including benzodiazepines, are frequently employed as the best treatment option.

Neuropsychiatric syndromes

Neuropsychiatric syndromes with exaggerated startle reflex are on the borderland of neurology and psychiatry, and their etiology is poorly understood. These syndromes include startle-induced tics, culture-specific disorders such as Latah and the "Jumping Frenchmen of Maine," and functional startle syndromes and anxiety disorders. They all involve non-habituating exaggerated startle evoked by loud noises or by being poked forcefully in the side. After a startle reflex, various other responses might be seen, including "forced obedience" (involuntary, immediate obedience to commands), echolalia, and echopraxia. No specific startle motor pattern has been identified, but additional symptoms, such as copying behavior, variable recruitment patterns, and the presence of a second "orienting" response on the electromyography (EMG) testing help steer the diagnosis toward these disorders. Clinical evidence indicates that patients with voluntary or functional jerks have a mean latency in excess of 100 ms and an inconsistent startle pattern. In the clinical setting, the patient's history and a (home) video recording, together with genetic and electrophysiologic testing, can help classify these challenging disorders.

REVISITING SCIENCE

Startle reflex

The startle reflex is present from 6 weeks of age and persists for life. Recordings of the startle reflex reveal two subsequent responses: the "early" response, also known as the "muscular tension reflex," and a second "late" response, also described as the "what-is-it?" or "orienting response." The "early" response is a bilaterally synchronous shock-like set of movements: forceful closure of the eyes, rising of bent arms over the head, and flexion of the neck, trunk, elbows, hips, and knees. This pattern, which can be seen particularly after auditory startling stimuli, has been interpreted as the rapid accomplishment of a defensive stance. The first part of startle reflex originates in the caudal brainstem and is roughly uniform from time to time and between individuals. The second "what-is-it?" or "orienting response" occurs after a period of decreased activity following the first response, with a latency of 400–450 ms, lasting 3 or more seconds. The organism is orienting toward the stimulus source, including postural adjustments with emotional and voluntary behavioral components; the response is therefore more variable.

Hyperekplexia

Hyperekplexia (HPX) means "to startle excessively" and refers to an exaggerated motor startle reflex combined with stiffness. Hyperekplexia can be split

Table 14.4 Features in distinguishing different types of hyperekplexia

Features	Hereditary	Sporadic	Symptomatic
Clinical features	Short-lasting startle-related stiffness and continuous stiffness in the neonatal period	Late-onset HPX without stiffness in the neonatal period	Excessive startle reflex associated with symptomatic lesion
Family history	Positive	Negative	Negative
Hallmark	Head retraction response	Attacks of tonic neonatal cyanosis	Neurological signs and symptoms that points to damage to the brainstem.
MRI brain	N/A	N/A	Brainstem; basal ganglia abnormalities
Genetic testing	*GLRA1 mutation or GLRB, GPHN, ARHGEF9 involvement*	Negative	Negative
Neurophysiology findings	N/A	N/A	Polymyographic startle-EMG study should be done to determine whether the abnormal response can be classified as a startle reflex

up into a "major" and "minor" forms. The major form is characterized by (1) excessive startle reflexes starting at birth and lasting throughout life, (2) startle-induced falls due to generalized stiffness after a startle reflex that lasts a few seconds causing patients to fall forward "as stiff as a stick" while fully conscious, and (3) continuous stiffness in the neonatal period. The minor form, which is restricted to excessive startle reflexes with no stiffness or falls, has no known genetic cause or underlying pathophysiological substrate. By etiology, the HPX can be divided into hereditary, sporadic, and symptomatic forms. Features helpful to distinguish between different types of HPX are presented in Table 14.4.

Family history and additional clinical and radiological information provide the most important signs to distinguish between hereditary, sporadic, and symptomatic HPX. Preserved consciousness distinguishes it from epileptic seizures. The distinction between sporadic and symptomatic hyperekplexia can be difficult when thorough investigations show several neurological abnormalities, but a defined neurological syndrome is lacking.

In patients with the minor form, additional brainstem abnormalities point toward a symptomatic form, and imaging should be done. Examples of symptomatic HXP: postanoxic encephalopathy, occlusion of posterior thalamic arteries, post – traumatic, paraneoplastic, brainstem stroke, hemorrhage or glioma. Such condition as multiple sclerosis, lateral sclerosis, medulla compression and multiple system atrophy have described startle as a symptom. In patients with a non-symptomatic minor form, the cause remains difficult to establish and a polymyographic startle-EMG study should be done to determine whether the abnormal response can be classified as a startle reflex. The line between these minor forms of hyperekplexia and neuropsychiatric causes of excessive startling is vague, but the presence of behavioral-psychiatric symptoms should help.

Hereditary HPX is inherited commonly in an autosomal dominant or autosomal recessive and rarely X-linked pattern with mutations in the glycine receptor, alpha 1 (*GLRA1*) gene. On history and exam, apart from startling, falls, and stiffness, a patient with hereditary HPX has other noteworthy signs. One feature is the head-retraction response, which consists of a brisk, involuntary backward jerk of the head after the top of the nose or the middle portion of the upper lip is slightly tapped with a reflex hammer. This is a hallmark of

HPX in stiff newborns, but has also been described in children with cerebral palsy. Additional features include periodic limb movements in sleep and hypnagogic myoclonus, sudden-infant death, epilepsy, motor delay in the first year of life with subsequent catch-up, congenital dislocation of the hips, spastic paraparesis, and mild intellectual disability. Some individuals with this condition have a low tolerance for crowded places and loud noises. Standard tests of serum, urine, and cerebrospinal fluid, electroencephalography, CT, and MRI reveal no abnormalities. This form of HPX has a genetic basis: approximately 80% of hereditary HPX is caused by mutations in the *GLRA1* gene, encoding different parts of the inhibitory glycine receptor, leading to the production of a receptor that cannot properly respond to glycine. As a result glycine is less able to transmit signals in the spinal cord and brainstem.

Sporadic HPX can be defined as HPX without a positive family history and without an established neurological cause, which accounts for the excessive startle reflex. The symptoms of sporadic cases closely resemble the triad of the major form of hereditary HPX. However, one clinical difference from hereditary HPX is that these patients commonly have described attacks of tonic neonatal cyanosis. These tonic attacks are rarely seen in patients with the *GLRA1* mutation and can be stopped by the Vigevano maneuver, which consists of forced flexion of the head and legs toward the trunk. Sporadic HPX symptoms in the minor form of hereditary HPX form a heterogeneous group, which can best be summarized as acquired idiopathic or late-onset HPX without other neurological signs.

Symptomatic HPX is an excessive startle reflex associated with focal neurological signs and symptoms, usually pointing to lesions to the brainstem. Symptomatic HPX is quite rare; reported causes mainly involve brainstem or cerebral damage. Since all cases of symptomatic HPX concern late-onset HPX, without stiffness in the neonatal period, they are therefore clinically categorized as the minor form of HPX.

Diagnosis of HPX

When dealing with a case of exaggerated startle, an extensive history must be taken. A useful beginning is to distinguish whether startling stimuli induce hyperstartling or another response. If the response is a startle reflex, major and minor forms of hyperekplexia should be considered. Falling and stiffness provide useful clues: short-lasting startle-related stiffness and continuous stiffness in the neonatal period form the most reliable clinical criteria for the major form. Together with a positive family history and a positive head-retraction response, hereditary hyperekplexia is very likely, so screening for mutations in GLRA1 should be done. If the GLRA1 gene shows no mutation in familial and sporadic cases of major forms of hyperekplexia, screening of other genes (e.g., GLRB, GPHN, ARHGEF9) should be considered.

Family history and additional clinical and radiological information provide the most important signs to distinguish between hereditary, sporadic, and symptomatic HPX. The preserved consciousness distinguishes it from epileptic seizures. The distinction between sporadic and symptomatic hyperekplexia can be difficult when thorough investigations show several neurological abnormalities, but a fitting neurological syndrome is lacking.

In patients with the minor form additional brainstem abnormalities point toward a symptomatic form, and imaging should be done. Examples of symptomatic HXP include postanoxic encephalopathy, occlusion of posterior thalamic arteries, post-traumatic, paraneoplastic, brainstem stroke, hemorrhage, or glioma. Such conditions as multiple sclerosis, lateral sclerosis, medulla compression, and multiple system atrophy include startle as a possible symptom. In patients with a non-symptomatic minor form, the cause remains difficult to establish and a polymyographic startle-EMG study should be done to determine whether the abnormal response can be classified as a startle reflex. The line between these minor forms of hyperekplexia and neuropsychiatric causes of excessive startling is vague, but the presence of behavioral-psychiatric symptoms should help.

Treatment of HPX

Clonazepam is the first-choice therapy for any type of HPX. The dose of Clonazepam 1 mg per day yields improvement in stiffness and decreases the magnitude of motor startle reflexes in the major hereditary form.

Further Readings

Albers JW, Allen AA, 2nd, Bastron JA, Daube JR. Limb myokymia. *Muscle Nerve* 1981; **4**(6): 494–504.

Auger RG, Daube JR, Gomez MR, Lambert EH. Hereditary form of sustained muscle activity of peripheral nerve origin causing generalized myokymia and muscle stiffness. *Ann Neurol* 1984; **15**(1): 13–21.

Bakker MJ, van Dijk JG, van den Maagdenberg AM, Tijssen MA. Startle syndromes. *Lancet Neurol* 2006; **5**(6): 513–524.

Browne DL, Gancher ST, Nutt JG, Brunt ER, Smith EA, Kramer P, et al. Episodic ataxia/myokymia syndrome is associated with point mutations in the human potassium channel gene, KCNA1. *Nat Genet* 1994; **8**(2): 136–140.

Dressler D, Thompson PD, Gledhill RF, Marsden CD. The syndrome of painful legs and moving toes. *Mov Disord* 1994; **9**(1): 13–21.

Feinberg TE, Schindler RJ, Flanagan NG, Haber LD. Two alien hand syndromes. *Neurology* 1992; **42**(1): 19–24.

Graff-Radford J, Rubin MN, Jones DT, et al. The alien limb phenomenon. *J Neurol* 2013; **260**: 1880–1888.

Gutmann L. Myokymia and neuromyotonia. *J Neurol* 2004; **251**(2): 138–142.

Haq IU, Malaty IA, Okun MS, Jacobson CE, Fernandez HH, Rodriguez RR. Clonazepam and botulinum toxin for the treatment of alien limb phenomenon. *Neurologist* 2010; **16**(2): 106–108.

Hassan A, Mateen FJ, Coon EA, Ahlskog JE. Painful legs and moving toes syndrome: a 76-patient case series. *Arch Neurol* 2012; **69**(8): 1032–1038.

Iliceto G, Thompson PD, Day BL, Rothwell JC, Lees AJ, Marsden CD. Diaphragmatic flutter, the moving umbilicus syndrome, and "belly dancer's" dyskinesia. *Mov Disord* 1990; **5**(1): 15–22.

Jankovic J. Can peripheral trauma induce dystonia and other movement disorders? yes! *Mov Disord* 2001; **16**(1): 7–12.

Jankovic J. Peripherally induced movement disorders. *Neurol Clin* 2009; **27**(3): 821, 32, vii.

Kulisevsky J, Marti-Fabregas J, Grau JM. Spasms of amputation stumps. *J Neurol Neurosurg Psychiatry* 1992; **55**(7): 626–627.

Lee W, Day TJ, Williams DR. Clinical, laboratory and electrophysiological features of Morvan's fibrillary chorea. *J Clin Neurosci* 2013; **20**(9):1246–9.

Newsom-Davis J, Mills KR. Immunological associations of acquired neuromyotonia (Isaacs' syndrome): report of five cases and literature review. *Brain* 1993; **116** (Pt 2): 453–469.

Tijssen MA, Schoemaker HC, Edelbroek PJ, Roos RA, Cohen AF, van Dijk JG. The effects of clonazepam and vigabatrin in hyperekplexia. *J Neurol Sci* 1997; **149**(1): 63–67.

Tijssen MA, Shiang R, van Deutekom J, Boerman RH, Wasmuth JJ, Sandkuijl LA, et al. Molecular genetic reevaluation of the Dutch hyperekplexia family. *Arch Neurol* 1995; **52**(6): 578–582.

Weiner WJ. Can peripheral trauma induce dystonia? no! *Mov Disord* 2001; **16**(1): 13–22.

Part 3

Other Disease Syndromes

15

Tardive Syndromes

Stephanie Lessig, MD

Department of Neurosciences, University of California San Diego, La Jolla, California, USA

Introduction

Tardive syndromes refer to abnormal movements caused by long-term use of dopamine-blocking agents. These can include the classic tardive dyskinesia as well as tardive dystonia, akathisia, myoclonus, tics, tremor, and parkinsonism. Treatment of these disorders includes removal of the offending agent if possible, along with prescription of other medications that target decreasing these potentially disabling movements.

Definition

"Tardive" from "tardy" denotes the "late" symptoms that are a "later" complication of agents that block the dopamine system. The phrase "tardive dyskinesia" is often used to describe tardive syndromes that include several movement disorders (Table 15.1). These are characterized by a variety of abnormal, involuntary, hyperkinetic movements. The common offending agents are the antipsychotics, but any medication with dopamine-blocking properties can cause movement disorders, including the anti-nausea medication metoclopramide.

According to the International Congress of Movement Disorders (1990), in order to be classified as a tardive syndrome, disorders must:

1) have clinical features of a movement disorder, characterized by abnormal, involuntary movements,

2) be caused by exposure to dopamine receptor-blocking agents (DRBA) within 6 months of onset of symptoms, and

3) last at least one month after stopping the offending agent.

According to the *Diagnostic and Statistical Manual of Mental Disorders*, 4th edition (DSM-IV), patients must have had exposure to DRBAs for one month if the patients are over age 60, whereas the American Psychiatric Task Force (1992) definition requires three months of exposure. Lists of agents reported to cause tardive syndromes are provided in Tables 15.2 and 15.3.

Pathophysiology

Tardive syndromes are caused by blockage of postsynaptic dopamine receptors. There are five subtypes of dopamine receptors in the brain (named D1–D5). Agents known to cause tardive syndromes have in common the ability to block D2-receptors to varying degrees. Although there are medications other than DRBA reported to cause dyskinesias (Table 15.2), for the purpose of this chapter the discussion will be limited to syndromes caused by DRBAs.

Despite the causal relationship of neuroleptic agents and tardive syndromes, the pathophysiology is not well understood. It is thought to be a combination of pre- and postsynaptic hypersensitivity to

Non-Parkinsonian Movement Disorders, First Edition. Edited by Deborah A. Hall and Brandon R. Barton.

© 2017 John Wiley & Sons, Ltd. Published 2017 by John Wiley & Sons, Ltd.

Companion website: www.wiley.com/go/hall/non-parkinsonian_movement_disorders

Table 15.1 Types of tardive syndromes

Withdrawal emergent syndrome
Dyskinesia ("classic" or "oral–bucchal–lingual")
Dystonia
Akathisia
Myoclonus/tics/tremor
Parkinsonism

the dopamine system, as well as influence of abnormalities in striatal GABA-containing neurons and striatal cholinergic interneurons. However, little has been discovered to distinguish patients who develop tardive syndromes from those who do not.

⚗ SCIENCE REVISITED

Described below is a sample of studies suggesting abnormalities in patients who develop TD:

CSF studies: CSF GABA was found to be reduced in five patients with schizophrenia with TD who were matched with schizophrenics on neuroleptics without TD (Thaker et al., 1987).

PET: A prospective study of patients receiving antipsychotics demonstrated those who developed TD had relative hypermetabolism in the temporolimbic, brainstem, and cerebellar regions with hypometabolism in the parietal and cingulated gyrus (Szymanski et al., 1996).

Genetics: A meta-analysis of genetic studies has supported the view that a polymorphism in the D3 receptor gene has a higher risk of developing TD (Bakker et al., 2006).

Clinical features

The first tardive syndrome described was tardive dyskinesia (TD), in patients treated with antipsychotics for schizophrenia. Original descriptions included repetitive, almost rhythmic movements of the mouth region. These have subsequently been reported to occur in 20–40% of patients treated with DRBAs. As other tardive symptoms have been recognized, these original dyskinesias are often termed "classic tardive" or "oral–buccal–lingual

dyskinesias." This is still the most common phenomenology seen in tardive syndromes, with parkinsonism being the next most common, followed by dystonia and akathisia.

Risk factors

Use of typical neuroleptic agents at higher dose and longer duration are most commonly linked to development of tardive syndromes, with 5% of patients developing a tardive syndrome for each year of treatment. In addition, age seems to play a role, with older patients being more likely to develop these disorders. Other reported risk factors include female sex, African American race, a preexisting mood disorder, cognitive impairment, substance abuse, diabetes, and HIV-positive status.

Tardive syndromes

Tardive dyskinesia ("classic TD")

The original description of movements induced by DRBAs included rapid, progressive, stereotyped movements of the oral–buccal–lingual (OBL) area that can resemble chewing. Movements are voluntarily suppressible by patients, or reduced when patients are engaged in activities such as talking and chewing. They usually do not interfere with normal function, and patients often do not notice their chewing unless attention is drawn to it.

On examination, perioral and oral movements are most frequently observed. When the patient is asked to extend the tongue, irregular, writhing movements can be observed. In addition to OBL movements, there can be repetitive movements of the distal limbs that resemble piano playing. When seated or standing, the patient may exhibit rocking motions or flexion/extension of the thighs resembling stamping. These latter movements may represent chorea or akathisia, also related to DRBA use.

Tardive dystonia

Dystonia is defined as sustained, co-contraction of agonist and antagonistic muscles, causing abnormal posturing of the affected body part. Tardive dystonia commonly occurs in younger adults and is the common cause of secondary dystonia. This disorder can occur anywhere from

Table 15.2 Dopamine-blocking medications known to cause tardive syndromes

Phenothiazides	Chlorpromazine	Pyrimidinone	Risperidone
Thioxanthenes	Triflupromazine	Benzisothiazole	Ziprasidone
Butyrophenones	Thioridazine	Benzisoxazole	Iloperidone
Diphenylbutylpiperidine	Mesoridazine	Substituted benzamides	Metoclopramide
Dibenzazepine	Trifluoperazine	Indolones	Tiapride
Thienobenzodiazepine	Prochlorperazine	Quinolones	Supiride
	Perphenazine		Clebopride
	Chlorprothixene		Remoxipride
	Thiothixene		Veralipride
	Haloperidol		Amisulpride
	Droperidol		Molindone
	Pimozide		Aripiprazole
	Loxapine		
	Olanzapine		

Table 15.3 Non–dopamine-blocking medications reported to cause tardive syndromes

Anticholinergics	Benzhexol, biperiden, ethopropazine, orphenadrine, procylindine
Antidepressants	Phenelzine, fluoxetine, sertraline, trazodone, amitriptyline, amoxapine, doxepin, imipramine
Anxiolytics	Alprazolam
Antiepileptics	Carbamazepine, ethosuximide, phenobarbital, phenytoin, valproic acid
Bipolar medications	Lithium
Anti-parkinsonian medications	Bromocriptine, levodopa, ropinirole, pramipexole
Calcium channel blockers	Flunarizine, cinnarizine
N-acetyl-4-methoxytryptamine	Melatonin

days to years after DRBA exposure. The prevalence in patients exposed to neuroleptics is much higher than that seen in the general population for idiopathic torsion dystonia. As in primary dystonia, there can be an associated "sensory trick" (geste antagoniste), where tactile stimulation of a specific area relieves the movement and is at times unrelated to the movements themselves. However, specific dystonic patterns may be different from idiopathic torsion dystonia. The common neck or cervical tardive dystonia position is retrocollis (backward movement), as opposed to the torticollis (turning), or laterocollis (lateral shift of the head) seen in idiopathic dystonia. When trunk muscles are involved, tardive dystonia presents more frequently with opisthotonus (extension/arching of the back) rather than the lateral twisting seen in idiopathic dystonia. The extremities are infrequently involved in adults in either condition; however, the upper limbs may appear internally rotated with elbows extended and wrists flexed in tardive dystonia. Also, in tardive dystonia, voluntary action tends to reduce the movement, whereas in idiopathic torsion dystonia, movement is often exacerbated with activity. Respiratory and pharyngeal muscles can also be affected in tardive dystonia, with an irregular breathing pattern observed (respiratory dyskinesias). This is generally not life-threatening, though has been reported to cause acute shortness of breath, hypoxia, and aspiration.

Tardive akathisia

Akathisia is defined as an unpleasant internal sensation, commonly of the lower extremities, that is relieved by voluntary motions of the affected part. Akathisia causes patients to have a restless type of appearance, and they may be seen rocking, grunting, or moaning. It often coexists with classic TD and is particularly resistant to treatment (see below).

Tardive myoclonus/tics/tremor

These are other movement disorders seen after exposure to DRBAs but not as commonly. Their appearance is largely indistinguishable from other etiologies of these movements.

Withdrawal emergent syndrome

Withdrawal can be observed when neuroleptics are acutely withdrawn after long-term use. It is commonly seen in children, though it has been reported in adults. Movements are more choreic (dance-like) in appearance, and occur in the limbs, neck, and trunk more than in the oral–buccal–lingual muscles (as opposed to classic TD). These movements typically disappear completely after three months. Reinstitution of neuroleptic treatment can suppress the movements; subsequent gradual taper of these agents usually avoids recurrence.

Parkinsonism

This is a dose-dependent movement disorder found with exposure both to DRBAs and dopamine-depleting agents such as reserpine and tetrabenazine. Classic signs, indistinguishable from idiopathic Parkinson disease (PD), can be observed, including asymmetric tremor, rigidity, and bradykinesia. Occurrence does seem to be more frequent with advancing age, as seen with PD. Patients can persist with symptoms despite long-term neuroleptic discontinuation, bringing into question the proposed term of tardive parkinsonism (versus neuroleptic-induced parkinsonism). It is unclear whether this is a true tardive syndrome, or whether Parkinson disease pathology may in fact play a role in these patients.

Differential diagnosis of tardive syndromes

While, by definition, tardive syndromes result from prior neuroleptic exposure, this can be less clear when symptoms appear longer after such exposure, or when symptoms are prolonged despite discontinuation of the offending agents. Other neuropsychiatric conditions can also mimic the movements, or initially present with psychosis requiring subsequent neuroleptic exposure, masking the true diagnosis. Two examples of these would include Huntington disease or Wilson disease. Knowledge of the typical movements of Huntington disease (chorea, which also has associated gait and eye movement abnormalities not seen in TD) or Wilson disease (dystonia, which is often oromandibular unlike that seen in TD) can distinguish these conditions. (For symptoms that support investigation for an alternative diagnosis, see Tips and Tricks below.)

Treatment

The best treatment of choice for tardive syndromes is prevention, with avoidance of DRBAs if possible, and patients should be warned about this potential side effect. Once the syndrome develops, discontinuation or decrease of the offending agents should be considered; however, this may not be possible in cases of psychosis. Also, at times, symptoms initially worsen with reduction of neuroleptic agents, and the medication must be reduced slowly if possible. Acute withdrawal of neuroleptics can be potentially life-threatening. If symptoms continue to be disabling despite limitation of the offending agents, other treatments may be considered

Dopamine agents

Ironically, dopamine-depleting agents are the agents of choice for tardive dyskinesia, and often, other tardive syndromes. They are thought to be useful as they deplete presynaptic stores of amines rather than block postsynaptic receptors. The two commonly used drugs for this class are reserpine and tetrabenazine, although reserpine is less available currently. Due to their anti-dopaminergic properties, the most common side effects include orthostatic hypotension, depression, and parkinsonism. Orthostasis is best avoided by slow introduction of these agents, from between 0.125 and 0.25 mg daily of reserpine increased by 0.25 mg weekly (though doses of 5–8 mg per day may be required), or 25 mg daily of tetrabenazine increased by 25 mg weekly. Patients with concomitant depression will likely have this exacerbated by use of these agents. Parkinsonism can occur with prolonged use, and may require drug discontinuation.

The atypical antipsychotics clozapine and quetiapine are known to have less potential to cause tardive syndromes. Though these both have D2 blocking properties, there is less affinity for the D2 receptor than that seen with other antipsychotics. Clozapine and quetiapine can also be used for psychosis in place of other, more typical agents, to allow potential removal of the offending DRBAs. It remains unclear whether these agents can be used as an actual treatment for TD, as evidence for this has been at the case report level. Other dopaminergic agents, including Parkinson disease medications such as dopamine agonists, monoamine oxidase inhibitors, and levodopa have not been shown to be useful in treating tardive syndromes, and risk the induction of underlying psychosis.

GABAergic medications

Given the more favorable side effect profile, particularly for long-term use, agents that work on the GABA (gamma-aminobutyric acid, a predominantly inhibitory neurotransmitter) system can also be used. Baclofen can be tried, starting at doses of 5–10 mg per day and increasing to 60–80 mg per day in divided doses of three times per day. Sedation is the most common side effect. Ataxia, confusion, and in severe cases hallucinations can also occur. Coma, respiratory depression, and seizures can occur in overdose or acute withdrawal. Benzodiazepines may also be beneficial, usually either clonazepam, in doses of 0.5 mg daily and increased by 0.5–1 mg per week, or diazepam. Sedation is the common side effect, and tolerance can develop with prolonged use.

Other agents

Anticholinergic agents, such as benztropine or trihexyphenidyl, are also commonly used, though with variable efficacy in classic tardive dyskinesia. With tardive dystonia and parkinsonism, however, anticholinergics may be quite useful. Doses include benztropine 0.5 mg starting twice per day and increased as tolerated. Trihexyphenidyl can be given in doses starting at 1 mg twice per day, with doses of up to 30 mg per day needed at times, if tolerated. Side effects are similar to those seen with cardiac agents used for their anticholinergic properties, and include dry mouth, sedation, orthostasis, urinary retention, and visual blurring. In elderly patients, confusion and frank psychosis can also occur. Several other agents have been investigated for use in TD, though with inconsistent results, including the NMDA antagonist amantadine, as well as antioxidant therapies with tocopherol (vitamin E) and pyridoxine (vitamin B6). Ginkgo biloba has also been investigated in schizophrenic patients with tardive symptoms and found to be effective.

For tardive dystonia, as well as in other tardive syndromes, intramuscular botulinum toxin treatments can also be used. Botulinum toxin works to weaken muscle contractions, thereby reducing the dystonic movements. There are four types of botulinum toxin available, though most widely used is onabotulinum toxin A. Doses vary depending on the muscles injected. Deep brain stimulation has also been tried in tardive dystonia in refractory cases, as well as for other tardive syndromes. (For an overview of the treatment of tardive syndromes, see Tips and Tricks below.)

⭐ **TIPS AND TRICKS**

Treatment of tardive syndromes
Slow taper of the offending agents is the treatment of choice for tardive syndromes, with clozapine or quetiapine substituted in cases of psychosis. If this is not possible or disabling symptoms persist despite discontinuation, a dopamine-blocking agent such as reserpine or tetrabenazine can be used, which should be titrated slowly to avoid side effects. In tardive dystonia or parkinsonism, anticholinergics are the treatment of choice. Baclofen or clonazepam may also be used or added if other agents are not tolerated or contraindicated. In severe cases of tardive dystonia, botulinum toxin injections or deep brain stimulation may be considered.

Summary

Tardive syndromes are a variety of movement disorders that can be caused by use of DRBAs. While different phenomenologies are commonly recognized, more work needs to be done to understand patients at risk of developing these symptoms. As the cause of the movements is iatrogenic, avoidance or judicious use of these agents is the only true way to prevent the development of these syndromes. However, if tardive syndromes occur, there are medications (including dopamine-depleting agents, anticholinergics, and GABAergic agents) that can be helpful in treating these disorders. If severe, more invasive measures such as botulinum toxin treatments and deep brain stimulation can be attempted. Further understanding of how DRBAs cause these syndromes will hopefully lead to development of agents as effective as DRBAs without such untoward side effects.

Further Readings

Bakker PR Van Harten PN, VanOs J: Antipsychotic-induced tardive dyskinesia and the Ser9Gly polymorphism in the DRD3 gene: a meta analysis. *Schizophr Res* 2006; **83**(2–3): 185–192.

Bhidayasiri R, Boonyawairoj S. Spectrum of tardive syndromes: clinical recognition and management. *Postgrad Med J* 2011; **87**(1024): 132–141.

Bhidayasiri R, Boonyawairoj S. Spectrum of tardive syndromes: clinical recognition and management. *Postgrad Med J* 2011; **87**(1024): 132–141.

Bhidayasiri R, Fahn S, Weiner WJ, et al. Evidence-based guideline: treatment of tardive syndromes. Report of the Guideline Development Subcommittee of the American Academy of Neurology. *Neurology* 2013: **81**(5): 463–469.

Dyskinesia APATfoT. Tardive Dyskinesia: A Task Force Report of the American Psychiatric Association. Washington, DC: American Psychiatric Press, 1992.

Fahn S, Jankovic J, eds. The tardive syndromes. Principles and Practice of Movement Disorders, 479–518. Philadelphia: Churchill Livingstone Elsevier, 2007.

Jankovic J, Clarence-Smith K. Tetrabenazine for the treatment of chorea and other hyperkinetic movement disorders. *Expert Rev Neurother* 2011; **11**(11): 1509–1523.

Soares KJ, McGrath JJ. The treatment of tardive dyskinesia: a systematic review and meta-analysis. *Scizophr Res* 1999; **39**: 1–16.

Soares-Weiser K, Maayan N, McGrath J. Vitamin E for neuroleptic-induced tardive dyskinesia. *Cochrane Database Syst Rev* 2011; **2**: CD000209.

Syzmanski S, Gur RC, Gallacher F, et al. Vulnerability to tardive dyskinesia development in schizophrenia: an FDG-PET study of cerebral metabolism. *Neuropsychopharmacology* 1996; **15**: 567–575.

Thaker GK, Tamming CA, Alps LD, et al: Brain gamma-aminobutyric acid abnormality in tardive dyskinesia. *Arch Gen Psychiatry* 1987; **44**: 522–529.

16

Heavy Metal Accumulation Diseases

Khashayar Dashtipour, MD, PhD and Janice Fuentes, MD

Department of Neurology, Movement Disorders, Loma Linda University School of Medicine, Loma Linda, California, USA

Introduction

The description of "heavy metals" has been used in research and in legislation related to chemical hazards that may cause teratogenic or pathophysiological sequelae. Many different characterizations have been suggested. Prior definitions were based on density, some on atomic number or atomic weight, and some on chemical properties or toxicity. A popular classification of metals and semimetals (metalloids) is associated with contamination and potential toxicity or ecotoxicity. There are thirty-five metals that are known to have occupational or residential exposure; twenty-three of these are heavy elements or "heavy metals." These elements can be found in our diet and in our environment. They are essential for our health and are involved in numerous biochemical pathways; however, the majority may cause toxicity resulting in acute or chronic pathophysiological changes.

Heavy metal toxicity and metabolic errors can cause an array of systematic and neurological dysfunction. Toxicity can lead to changes in energy levels, blood composition, the function of vital organs such as the kidneys, liver, and lung. Long-term exposure may result in similar phenotypes seen in chronic neurological diseases associated with muscle and neurological degenerative processes such as Alzheimer disease, Parkinson disease (PD), muscular dystrophy, and multiple sclerosis. Toxic levels of heavy metals can be found in our living, recreational, and work domains. Many public health efforts have taken place to inform the public to take protective measures against potential exposures. In the United States, heavy metal toxicity is relatively uncommon; however, exposures may be identified by epidemiological data or clinical manifestations. A thorough history and clinical recognition of the toxic signs are vital when these exposures occur. Identification of exposure can be time sensitive and may result in permanent dysfunction or be potentially fatal. Therefore testing for heavy metals is essential when there is clinical suspicion. Only nine out of the twenty-three heavy metals mentioned above have been found to be associated with movement disorders (Table 16.1) and will be discussed below.

Arsenic

Arsenic and its composites are used in the manufacturing industry of glass, computer chips, wood preservatives, pesticides, herbicides, and insecticides. Arsenic contamination of groundwater is a global problem in underdeveloped countries or after infrastructure damage.

Chronic arsenicosis is a multisystem disorder and can be present with a wide range of symptoms associated with cancer, genotoxicity, and cellular disruption. The neurotoxic effect of arsenic is associated with changes in the function of brain cell membranes caused by generation of reactive oxygen species (ROS) and nitrogen oxide (NO). The neurological manifestation of arsenic toxicity varies from peripheral nerve involvement to encephalopathy.

Non-Parkinsonian Movement Disorders, First Edition. Edited by Deborah A. Hall and Brandon R. Barton.
© 2017 John Wiley & Sons, Ltd. Published 2017 by John Wiley & Sons, Ltd.
Companion website: www.wiley.com/go/hall/non-parkinsonian_movement_disorders

Table 16.1 Heavy metals associated with movement disorders

Heavy metals	Movement disorders symptoms/syndromes
Arsenic	Alteration in finger tapping, tremor, and hand–eye discoordination
Bismuth	Myoclonus, tremor, ataxia
Copper	Tremors, dystonia, chorea, ataxia, aceruloplasminemia, Wilson disease
Iron	Neurodegeneration with brain iron accumulation, neuroacanthocytosis
Lead	Parkinsonism, cerebellar ataxia
Manganese	Parkinsonism, dystonia, monotone speech, tremor, rigidity, forward-leaning gait, problems with dexterity and balance
Mercury	Tremor, ataxia, dysarthria, choreoathetosis, masked facies, and myoclonus
Thallium	Tremor, ataxia, chorea, and athetosis.
Zinc	Staggering gait

Some patients can manifest with abnormal movements such as alteration in finger tapping, tremor, and hand–eye discoordination. Finally, a possible role of arsenic as one of the environmental factors in the etiology of PD has been suggested.

> ☆ TIPS AND TRICKS
>
> Arsenic levels can be measured in blood, urine, fingernails, and hair. Twenty-four-hour urine tests are the most reliable for acute arsenic exposure. Fingernail and hair testing are used to measure chronic exposure. Hair testing can be recommended in those who have not dyed their hair for at least two months as the dyes can contaminate the hair samples.

Treatment

Chelation therapy with British anti-lewisite (BAL), dimercaptosuccinic acid (DMSA), and D-penicillamine are the primary drugs used to remove arsenic. Supportive care with abundant fluids increases the elimination of arsenic, facilitating treatment. In some cases of acute toxicity, hemodialysis, gastric lavage, whole bowel irrigation and the use of supportive measures may also be necessary.

Bismuth

Bismuth and its compounds are used in cosmetics, pigments, and a few pharmaceuticals, notably Pepto-Bismol®. Bismuth poisoning mostly affects the kidney, liver, and bladder. Melanosis of the vagina, erythema, oral lesions, skeletal problems, nephrotoxicity, hepatotoxicity, methaemoglobinaemia, encephalopathy, and bowel dysfunction are the distinct abnormalities that have been linked to the ingestion of bismuth compounds. Bismuth neurotoxicity occurs after repeated ingestion of the compound. Bismuth neurotoxicity presents with a prodromal phase consisting of a neuropsychiatric deficit, followed by an acute phase with encephalopathy and finally recovery. Patients may manifest with various abnormal movements during the acute phase of the toxicity such as myoclonus, tremor, ataxia, and even seizures. The outcome of the severe cases can result in coma and death.

> ☆ TIPS AND TRICKS
>
> Bismuth levels can be obtained from blood, urine, and CSF.
>
> EEG in patients convulsing due to bismuth toxicity typically shows frontotemporal slow waves and sometimes spike-and-wave activity. CSF shows elevated bismuth levels and increased 5-hydroxyindoleacetic acid (5-HIAA) levels. 5-HIAA is the main metabolite of serotonin in the human body.

Treatment

Bismuth toxicity treatment is best performed by the metal chelator dimercaprol, which increases renal clearance and improves the clinical signs of encephalopathy.

Copper

The major applications of copper are in electrical wiring, roofing, plumbing, and industrial machinery. Copper at low concentration is used as a bacteriostatic agent, fungicide agent, and a wood preservative. Copper is essential for life and is required for cellular respiration, neurotransmitter biosynthesis, pigment formation, and connective tissue strength. Either a deficiency or an excess of copper can result in serious consequences. Copper concentrations are highest in the liver, muscle, and bone. In humans, copper is absorbed in the gut, and then transported to the liver bound to albumin. After processing in the liver, copper is distributed to other tissues by the protein ceruloplasmin, which carries the majority of copper in blood and undergoes enterohepatic circulation. Some excess copper may be excreted via bile, which carries some copper out of the liver.

> ### SCIENCE REVISED
>
> Copper is an important metal for a functional catalytic center. The catalytic activity of enzymes play essential parts in neurobiology and pathogenesis, including ceruloplasmin, copper/zinc superoxide dismutase, dopamine hydroxylase, cytochrome-*c* oxidase, and hephaestin.

In copper deficiency, the decline of the cell's metabolic activity may lead to permanent neurological impairment. Also copper may be involved in free radical production, which could result in mitochondrial damage, DNA breakage, and neuronal injury. Copper is present throughout the brain and is prominent in the basal ganglia, hippocampus, cerebellum, numerous synaptic membranes, and in the cell bodies of cortical pyramidal and cerebellar granular neurons. Copper is implicated directly or indirectly in the pathogenesis of numerous neurological diseases, including aceruloplasminemia, Alzheimer disease, ataxic myelopathy, amyotrophic lateral sclerosis, Huntington disease, Menkes disease, occipital horn syndrome, PD, prion disease, and Wilson disease.

Copper-related diseases associated with movement disorders

Aceruloplasminemia

Aceruloplasminemia is an autosomal recessive neurodegenerative disease. Iron accumulates in the retina and basal ganglia by mutations in the ceruloplasmin gene. Ceruloplasmin contains 95% of the copper in plasma, and studies have shown that ceruloplasmin functions as a ferroxidase. Failure to incorporate copper into apoceruloplasmin results in an unstable apoprotein that is rapidly degraded. The clinical symptoms of aceruloplasminemia include parkinsonism, tremors (resting, postural, or action tremor), facial and neck dystonia, chorea, ataxia (gait ataxia or dysarthria), blepharospasm, grimacing, and psychiatric disturbance including depression and cognitive dysfunction.

Wilson disease

Wilson disease is an autosomal recessive disorder caused by the loss-of-function mutations in the copper transport gene *ATP7B*. This consequently causes liver disease, neuropsychiatric symptoms, and basal ganglia degeneration. There is impairment in the ability of copper to be incorporated into ceruloplasmin. The loss of *ATP7B* causes the rapid degradation of apoceruloplasmin in the plasma, resulting in reduced copper-carrying capacity. There is simultaneous impairment in the excretion of copper into bile. This leads to hepatic copper accumulation and damage, elevated levels of non-ceruloplasmin-bound copper in the plasma and ultimately, copper overload in extrahepatic tissues. Copper accumulation in the basal ganglia leads to neurologic abnormalities that usually present in the second or third decade as (1) an akinetic-rigid syndrome resembling parkinsonism, (2) a generalized dystonic syndrome, or (3) postural and intention tremor with ataxia, titubation, and dysarthria (pseudosclerosis). The tremor is classically a slow, high-amplitude proximal tremor with the appearance of "wing-beating" when the arms are elevated and the hands placed near the nose. In addition to liver and brain, the eye is also a primary site of copper deposition in Wilson disease. Eye movements can be distorted with slow saccades and occasionally ophthalmoplegia.

Iron

Iron is the most important element for almost all types of cells. Iron is involved in the normal function of neuronal tissues. It is an essential cofactor of the enzyme tyrosine hydroxylase required for the synthesis of myelin and the neurotransmitters dopamine, norepinephrine, and serotonin. Iron-related neurodegenerative disorders can result from both iron accumulation in specific brain regions or defects in its metabolism and/or homeostasis. Iron accumulation has been shown to lead to neuronal death. Available iron interacts with molecular oxygen and generates reactive oxygen species (ROS) through Fenton and Haber–Weiss reactions, which leads to oxidative stress inducing lipid peroxidation, nucleic acid modification, protein misfolding and aggregation, and cell dysfunction and death. Mitochondrial dysfunction has also been raised as a common cause for a number of neurodegenerative diseases. Iron-related neurodegenerative disorders can result from both iron accumulation in specific brain regions or defects in its metabolism and/or homeostasis.

Iron-related diseases associated with movement disorders

Huntington disease (HD)

HD is a neurodegenerative disorder characterized by progressive motor, cognitive, and psychiatric deterioration. In HD, increased iron levels have primarily been observed in the basal ganglia. In addition, ferritin-Fe levels are increased in the striatum of early clinical HD patients as measured by magnetic resonance imaging (MRI). Iron levels increase during the early stage in HD and continue to increase with age, which suggests that iron may play a role in the progression of the disease; however, the mechanisms involved in this process are not yet understood. It has been postulated that in HD, iron accumulates due to the neuronal loss and is most likely a secondary effect of the disease. (See Chapter 6 on chorea for more information on HD.)

Parkinson disease (PD)

PD is a progressive disorder that manifests with resting tremor, bradykinesia, rigidity, and eventually gait and postural dysfunction. PD is characterized by the loss of substantia nigra dopaminergic neurons and the deposition of intracellular inclusion bodies known as Lewy bodies. Several studies have confirmed that in PD, an increase of iron in the substantia nigra possibly leads to nigrostriatal dopamine neuron degeneration resulting in the production of ROS, causing lipid peroxidation. Iron accumulation may also enhance α-synuclein aggregates, causing the death of dopaminergic neurons.

There are still some conflicting reports regarding the role of iron in PD.

Neuroacanthocytosis (NA)

NA syndromes are characterized by cognitive and psychiatric features within the context of a progressive movement disorder, occurring from mutations in a number of genes (Table 16.2). NA syndromes are a group of rare neurodegenerative diseases that include chorea-acanthocytosis (ChAc), McLeod syndrome (MLS), Huntington disease-like 2 (HDL2), and pantothenate kinase associated neurodegeneration (PKAN). These diseases primarily affect the basal ganglia and are associated with central and peripheral nervous system abnormalities. Phenotypically, they may result in chorea, dystonia, bradykinesia, seizures, oral dyskinesia, muscle weakness, cognitive impairment, and psychiatric symptoms. One feature shared by NA is the hematological association of acanthocytes, which are spiky red cells with an undefined membrane dysfunction.

Neurodegeneration with brain iron accumulation (NBIA)

NBIA is composed of a group of rare inherited neurodegenerative diseases characterized by a progressive movement disorder and accumulation of iron in the basal ganglia, often the globus pallidus (Table 16.3). NBIA diseases include aceruloplasminemia, fatty acid hydroxylase-associated neurodegeneration (FHAN), mitochondrial membrane protein-associated neurodegeneration (MPAN), neuroferritinopathy, pantothenate kinase-associated neurodegeneration (PKAN), and phospholipase-A2 associated neurodegeneration (PLAN). The NBIA disorders are defined by brain magnetic resonance imaging showing signal changes that correspond to iron deposition in the basal ganglia.

Lead

Common causes of lead toxicity are ingestion of paints, pottery, and inhalation of leaded gasoline, flour contamination, exposure to lead stearate, and contamination from automobile batteries. Lead is quickly absorbed in the bloodstream and may affect the nervous, hematopoietic, reproductive, urinary tract, and immune systems. Lead has a long half-life leading to a rapid accumulation. In addition, lead

Table 16.2 Neuroacanthocytosis syndromes

Disease	Genetics	Age of onset	Pathophysiology	Neurological features	Additional features
Chorea-acanthocytosis (ChAc)	AR	Late teens-early adulthood	Mutation of gene *VPS13A* that produces the protein chorein. This protein has been associated with sorting and trafficking.	Parkinsonism, chorea, orofacial dystonia, tics, self-mutilation, epilepsy, myopathy, neuropathy	Cognitive/behavioral changes
Huntington disease-like 2 (HDL2)	AD	Any age but typically in adulthood	CTG/CAG expansion mutation located within *Junctophilin-3* on chromosome 16q24.3. Prominent cortical and striatal atrophy and intranuclear inclusions.	Parkinsonism, chorea, dystonia, dementia	Cognitive/behavioral changes, psychiatric features
McLeod syndrome (MLS)	X-linked	Mid-late adulthood	Variety of mutations in the gene *XK* including single nonsense and missense mutations, nucleotide mutations at or near the splice junctions of introns of *XK*, and different deletion mutations affecting cellular membrane protein.	Parkinsoninsm, chorea, dystonia, tics, epilepsy, myopathy, neuropathy	Cognitive/behavioral changes, psychiatric symptoms, cardiomyopathy, hepatosplenomegaly
Pantothenate kinase-associated neurodegeneration (PKAN)	AR	Any age but typically in childhood	Mutation in the gene *PANK2* that codes for protein pantothenate kinase 2, a regulatory enzyme in biosynthesis of coenzyme A from vitamin B5.	Parkinsoninsm, chorea, dystonia, tremors, hemiballism, gait disturbances, optic atrophy, dementia	Pigmentary retinopathy, cognitive impairment

Table 16.3 Neurodegeneration with brain iron accumulation (NBIA) diseases

Disease	Genetics	Age of onset	Pathophysiology	Neurological features	Additional features	MRI findings
Aceruloplasminemia	AR	Adulthood	Mutations in the *CP* gene, which codes for the protein ceruloplasmin that is involved in iron transport and processing	Chorea, dystonia, ataxia tremors, blepharospasm, dementia	Retinal degeneration, anemia, diabetes mellitus	T1- and T2- weighted images reveals hypointensity reflecting iron accumulation in the brain (striatum, thalamus, dentate nucleus)
Fatty acid hydroxylase-associated neurodegeneration (FHAN)	AR	Childhood	Mutations in the *FA2H* gene, which codes for the protein fatty acid 2-hydroxylase. This protein catalyzes the synthesis of 2-hydroxysphingolipids.	Dystonia, ataxia, spastic paraplegia or quadriplegia, seizures, dysphagia, dysarthria	Optic atrophy, strabismus, nystagmus	T2- weighted images reveals hypointensity, reflecting iron accumulation in the globus pallidus, progressive atrophy of the cerebellar hemispheres, vermis, pons, medulla, and spinal cord and thinning of the corpus callosum.
Mitochondrial membrane protein-associated neurodegeneration (MPAN)	AR	Childhood	Mutations in *C19orf12* gene	Parkinsonism, dystonia, spasticity, dysarthria, optic atrophy, neuropathy	Psychiatric features	T2-weighted images reveals iron accumulation in the globus pallidus, and substantia nigra
Neuroferritinopathy	AD	Mid-late adulthood	Mutations in the *FTL* gene, which provides instructions for making the ferritin light chain that is one part (subunit) of the protein ferritin.	Parkinsonism, chorea, dystonia, spasticity, tremor, ataxia, dysarthria, dysphagia, dementia	Behavioral changes	T2-weighted images reveals hyperintensity in the caudate, globus pallidus, putamen, substantia nigra, and red nuclei, followed by cystic degeneration in the caudate and putamen.

Disorder	Inheritance	Age of onset	Molecular basis	Clinical features	Additional features	Neuroimaging
Pantothenate kinase-associated neurodegeneration (PKAN)	AR	Any age but typically in childhood	Mutation in the gene *PANK2* that codes for protein Pantothenate kinase 2, a regulatory enzyme in biosynthesis of coenzyme A from vitamin B5.	Parkinsoninsm, chorea, dystonia, tremors, hemiballism, gait disturbances, optic atrophy, dementia	Pigmentary retinopathy, cognitive impairment	T2-weighted image reveals marked hypointensity in the globus pallidi with high signal intensity foci (eye-of-the-tiger appearance).
Phospholipase-A2 associated neurodegeneration (PLAN)	AR	Childhood	Mutations of the gene *PLA2G6* that codes for the protein phosholipase-A2. This protein catalyze the cleavage of fatty acids from the sn-2 position of phospholipids.	Dystonia, chorea, ataxia, neuropathy, severe hypotonia, seizures, optic atrophy	Cognitive impairment	Most patients have optic atrophy, cerebellar cortical atrophy, and gliosis. T2-weighted images show hypointensity in the globus pallidus and substantia nigra consistent with iron accumulation.

excretes at a slow rate via the urinary and gastrointestinal tract. Lead is neurotoxic in the CNS, primarily affecting the frontal cortex, hippocampus, and cerebellum. Headaches, poor attention span, irritability, and loss of memory can be some of the initial complaints by patients with lead toxicity. Acute encephalopathy is one the most dangerous manifestations when blood lead levels are more than 100 μg/dl. The symptoms of the acute encephalopathy presentation include persistent vomiting, ataxia, seizures, papilledema, impaired consciousness, and coma. Lead toxicity has also been associated with a variety of movement disorders such as parkinsonism and cerebellar ataxia. The peripheral nervous system can be affected as well, causing peripheral motor neuropathy. Hyperintensities are common findings on MRI from cerebral calcifications. Chelation treatment such as dimercaprol and succimer enhance urinary excretion.

Manganese

Manganese is an essential trace nutrient, which is stored mainly in the bones, liver, and kidneys. Manganese also has a role in the brain where it binds to manganese metalloproteins and especially to glutamine synthetase in astrocytes. Manganese toxicity is highest in miners, welders, smelters, in individuals receiving parenteral nutrition, in acquired hepatocerebral degeneration (AHD), or in drug addicts exposed to ephedrine-containing potassium permanganate via dust, fume inhalation, or intravenously injected self-prepared methcathinone hydrochloride (ephedrone), which is synthesized from pseudoephedrine hydrochloride, a potent oxidant. Excessive oxidative stress is one possible mechanism for neurotoxicity of manganese. Neuronal and cell death can be caused by manganese, and its contribution to free radicals.

In the early stages, manganese toxicity may cause psychiatric features such as depression, mood swings, compulsive behaviors, hallucinations, and psychosis, previously referred to as "manganese madness" or "locura manganica." In the later stages of toxicity, patients may present with signs of movement disorders including parkinsonism and dystonia. Other signs include weakness; monotone and slowed speech; masked/grimacing facies; rigidity; a characteristic gait called cock-walk, which is manifested by walking on the toes with elbows flexed and the spine erect; inability to walk backward without falling; and general problems with dexterity and balance. Tremor, when present, tends to be postural or kinetic rather than resting as seen in PD. Hypermanganesemia has also been associated with an autosomal-recessive dystonic syndrome: a homozygous mutation in the SLC30A10 gene, which encodes for a manganese transporter, has been found to be responsible for a dystonia-parkinsonism, hypermanganesemia, cirrhosis, and polycythemia syndrome. Hypermanganesemia detected from peripheral blood samples in patients with SLC30A10 mutations is usually much higher than in other causes of hypermanganisemia. Patients with SLC30A10 mutations have a variety of clinical symptoms including young-onset generalized dystonia, paraparesis without dystonia, late-onset asymmetric parkinsonism, and early postural instability. Treatment with chelation therapy such as calcium sodium edetate and oral iron can improve disability and prevent cirrhosis and mortality.

Manganese toxicity may be diagnosed from the blood manganese–iron ratio or by brain MRI. MRI typically shows increased signal intensity on T1-weighted images of the globus pallidus and basal ganglia. In contrast to PD, fluorodopa PET scans are normal in patients with manganese parkinsonism. B-CIT SPECT, however, may be abnormal, indicating degeneration of presynaptic dopaminergic terminals in some patients with manganese parkinsonism. Clinical symptoms of manganism may persist or progress months to years later, but the imaging findings normalize approximately six months after cessation of exposure.

> ★ **TIPS AND TRICKS**
>
> DaTSCAN (dopamine transporter imaging) is normal in parkinsonism due to secondary hypermanganesemia and patients with SLC30A10 mutations. Hypermanganesemia in SLC30A10 mutations and Wilson disease are the only potentially treatable inherited metal storage disorders described to date.

Mercury

Mercury is used in thermometers, barometers, manometers, sphygmomanometers, float valves, mercury switches, and other devices. Mercury poisoning can also result from exposure to water-soluble forms of Hg such as mercuric chloride or methylmercury, inhalation of mercury vapor, or eating seafood contaminated with mercury. The organs most frequently affected by mercury in chronically exposed subjects are the nervous system, kidneys, and mucosal surfaces of the mouth. Acute exposure to mercury has been shown to result in psychotic reactions characterized by delirium, hallucinations, and suicidal tendency. Chronic exposure may lead to the constellation of neurological symptoms, including peripheral neuropathy, sleep disturbances, psychological problems, and a variety of movement disorders such as tremor, ataxia, dysarthria, choreoathetosis, parkinsonian masked facies, and myoclonus. Tremor from mercury toxicity is a fine resting tremor that initially involves the hands and later spreads to the eyelids, lips, and tongue. The difference between mercury tremor and parkinsonian tremor is that the resting tremor in mercury is faster than the one seen in PD. The tremor mostly occurs when the patient is emotionally stressed and exacerbated with movement, but otherwise is absent or is very minimal; however, several studies have documented that mercury and manganese have been associated with secondary parkinsonism.

Treatment

Currently available drugs for acute mercurial poisoning include chelators N-acetyl-D, L-penicillamine (NAP), BAL, 2,3-dimercapto-1-propanesulfonic acid (DMPS), and dimercaptosuccinic acid (DMSA).

Thallium

Soluble thallium salts are highly toxic and were historically used in rat poisons and insecticides. Many thallium compounds are colorless, odorless, and tasteless. Thallium is absorbed through the skin. This heavy metal poses environmental and occupational threats as well as therapeutic hazards because of its use in medicine. Thallium has been used in the treatment of syphilis, malaria, tuberculosis, and diseases of the scalp; however, the use of thallium has been discontinued as a result of the high toxicity. Currently, a thallium isotope is used to image the myocardium and tumors. The exact mechanism of thallium toxicity remains unknown. Several mechanisms may be associated with thallium effect in humans, including impaired glutathione metabolism, oxidative stress, and disruption of potassium-regulated homeostasis. Thallium toxicity causes a variety of symptoms, including gastroenteritis, loss of appetite, hair loss, abnormal nail growth (e.g., the appearance of Mees' lines), cardiac complications, and breathing difficulties that often culminate in death. Thallium is also neurotoxic affecting the central and peripheral nervous system. Thallium toxicity in the CNS has been associated with localized areas of edema and vascular engorgement in cerebral hemispheres and brain stem. There are chromatolytic changes in neurons in the motor cortex, third nerve nuclei, substantia nigra, and globus pallidus. There is no evidence of inflammatory reaction. In the peripheral nerves, axonal degeneration has been found with secondary degeneration of the myelin sheath. Involvement of the nervous system can cause a variety of clinical manifestations such as behavioral changes, somnolence, hallucinations, headache, damage to the optic nerve that leads to visual impairment, neuropathy, pseudobulbar paralysis, seizures, coma, and even death. Movement disorders associated with thallium toxicity may include tremors, ataxia, chorea, and athetosis.

> ### ★ TIPS AND TRICKS
>
> Generally, elevated levels in the urine, blood, and saliva are better indicators of poisoning than thallium content in the hair.

Treatment

Thallium toxicity does not respond to traditional chelation therapy. In the first couple of hours after thallium poisoning, the treatment consists of gastric lavage, and emesis is induced in order to prevent further absorption of thallium into the body. Hemodialysis or hemoperfusion are also used to remove thallium from the blood serum. Additionally, treatment with potassium chloride may promote renal excretion of thallium. Ferric hexacyanoferrate, $(Fe^4[Fe(CN)^6]^3)$ also known as Prussian blue, iron blue, Chinese blue, Paris blue,

Brunswick blue, and Turnbull's blue, has been the most common antidote for thallium poisoning.

Zinc

Zinc plays a key role in the maintenance of human health. Zinc is an essential component of hundreds of proteins and metalloenzymes, including alkaline phosphatase, carbonic anhydrase, lactate dehydrogenase, carboxypeptides, DNA and RNA polymerases found in body tissues. Zinc is also involved in the regulation of the DNA transcription, cell proliferation, neurogenesis, synaptogenesis, neuronal growth, and neurotransmission. The signs and symptoms of zinc toxicity include neurological, respiratory, gastrointestinal, cardiovascular symptoms, and even death. Alterations in brain zinc status can lead to the pathogenesis of diseases related to development, mood disorders such as depression and anxiety, neurodegeneration and dementia, such as that observed in Alzheimer disease. Most recently, it was discovered that adult neurogenesis in the brain is dependent on zinc, a finding that has widespread implications for hippocampal function including learning and memory and control of emotion and mood. A specific cerebellar involvement consists of staggering gait, which might occur secondary to zinc toxicity. The antioxidant enzyme Cu-Zn superoxide dismutase (SOD) is said to be very sensitive to changes in the plasma Zn/Cu ratio, and alterations in SOD activity with zinc supplementation may result in excess free radicals that are damaging to the cell membrane. The common pathway for the elimination of zinc is in the stool and only small amounts are passed in the urine. The recommended treatment for zinc toxicity is removal of the source of zinc, chelation therapy such as calcium EDTA and supportive therapy.

Further Readings

Bradley B, Singleton M, Po ALW. Bismuth toxicity— a reassessment. *J Clin Pharm Therapeut* 1989; **14**: 423–441.

Cersosimo MG, Koller WC. The diagnosis of manganese-induced parkinsonism. *NeuroToxicology* 2006; **27**: 340–346.

Choi DW, Koh JY. Zinc and brain injury. *Ann Rev Neurosci* 1998; **21**: 347–375.

Cvjetko P, Cvjetko I, Pavlica M. Thallium toxicity in humans. *Archiv Indust Hygiene Toxicol* 2010; **61**, 111–119.

Danks DM. Copper deficiency in humans. *Ann Rev Nutrition* 1988; **8**: 235–257.

Fosmire G J. Zinc toxicity. *Am J Clin Nutrition* 1990; **51**: 225–227.

Greenberg S, Briemberg H. A neurological and hematological syndrome associated with zinc excess and copper deficiency. *J Neurol* 2004; **251**: 111–114.

Hart RP, Rose CS, Hamer RM. Neuropsychological effects of occupational exposure to cadmium. *J Clini Exper Neuropsychol* 1989; **11**, 933–943.

Liang YX, Sun RK, Sun Y, Chen ZQ, Li LH. Psychological effects of low exposure to mercury vapor: application of a computer-administered neurobehavioral evaluation system. *Environ Res* 1993; **60**: 320–327.

Maret W, Sandstead HH. Zinc requirements and the risks and benefits of zinc supplementation. *J Trace Elem Med Biol* 2006a; **20**: 3–18.

Nierenberg DW, Nordgren RE, Chang MB, Siegler RW, Blayney MB, Hochberg F, Toribara TY, Cernichiari E, Clarkson T. Delayed cerebellar disease and death after accidental exposure to dimethylmercury. *New Eng J Med* 1998; **338**: 1672–1676.

Olanow CW. Manganese-induced parkinsonism and Parkinson's disease. *Ann NY Acad Sci* 2004; **1012**: 209–223.

Rodriguez VM, Jimenez-Capdeville ME, Giordano M. The effects of arsenic exposure on the nervous system. *Toxicol Lett* 2003; **145**: 1–18.

Sinczuk-Walczak H, Szymczak M, Halatek T. Effects of occupational exposure to arsenic on the nervous system: clinical and neurophysiological studies. *Int J Occup Med Environ Health*, 2010; **23**: 347–355.

Snyder RD. The involuntary movements of chronic mercury poisoning. *Archiv Neurol* 1972; **26**: 379–381.

Supino-Viterbo V, Sicard C, Risvegliato M, Rancurel G, Buge A. Toxic encephalopathy due to ingestion of bismuth salts: clinical and EEG studies of 45 patients. *J Neurol Neurosurg Psychiatry* 1977; **40**: 748–752.

Thomas M, Hayflick SJ, Jankovic J. Clinical heterogeneity of neurodegeneration with brain iron accumulation (Hallervorden–Spatz syndrome) and pantothenate kinase-associated neurodegeneration. *Mov Disord* 2004; **19**: 36–42.

Tuschl K, Mills P, Parsons H, Malone M, Fowler D, Bitner-Glindzicz M, Clayton P. Hepatic cirrhosis, dystonia, polycythaemia and hypermanganesaemia—a new metabolic disorder. *J Inherit Metab Dis* 2008; **31**: 151–163.

Ward RJ, Dexter DT, Crichton RR. Chelating agents for neurodegenerative diseases. *Curr Med Chem* 2012; **19**: 2760–2772.

17

ICU Intensive Care Unit Movement Disorder Emergencies

Florence C. F. Chang, MBBS, FRACP[1] and Steven J. Frucht, MD[2]

[1]Neurology Department, Westmead Hospital, Wentworthville, NSW, Australia
[2]Mount Sinai Medical Center, New York, USA

Introduction

Hyperkinetic movement disorder emergencies can occur either de novo or as an acute exacerbation of a preexisting movement disorder. Hyperkinetic movement disorders like neuroleptic malignant syndrome, serotonin syndrome, NMDA receptor encephalitis, and status dystonicus often require admission to the intensive care unit for control of the movement disorder, airway management, and prevention of rhabdomyolysis with associated organ failure. It is important to recognize hyperkinetic movement disorder emergencies, as failure of timely diagnosis leads to significant morbidity and mortality. Movement disorder emergencies can present acutely to the emergency department, to a neurologist's clinic, or may be encountered during inpatient consultations. The diagnosis is made following a detailed history with emphasis on precipitating factors and focusing on phenomenology of the movement disorder during physical examination. The phenomenology helps guide and narrow down the list of differential diagnoses (Table 17.1).

In general, there is a lack of randomized clinical trials comparing therapies for movement disorder emergencies, due to the acute nature and low incidence of such emergencies. Treatment strategies are therefore based on retrospective case series and expert opinion. For hyperkinetic movement disorder emergencies, the initial focus is on providing critical supportive measures like airway protection, prevention of rhabdomyolysis (and subsequent renal failure), and treatment of hyperthermia, in addition to provision of adequate analgesia. After securing the airway, temporizing measures to reduce hyperkinetic movements can be initiated. For example, sedation with benzodiazepines in a controlled setting (i.e., intensive care unit or ICU) is a frequent strategy. If this doesn't reduce the hyperkinetic movements, short acting general anesthetics like propofol are useful in adults, but best avoided in children because of the risk of fatal metabolic acidosis (Cautions and Warnings). Neuromuscular blockade can be instituted if sedation and general anesthesia don't work. Non-depolarizing neuromuscular blockers are preferred (atracurium) over depolarizing agents, which can worsen rhabdomyolysis. Once the hyperkinetic movements improve with temporizing measures, disease-specific therapy such as pharmacotherapy or deep brain stimulation (for status dystonicus) can be started. Usually disease-specific therapy, which requires long term escalation, does not work as quickly as temporizing measures.

> ### ☆ TIPS AND TRICKS
>
> Supportive measures are the initial focus
>
> - Airway protection—endotracheal intubation, sedation and mechanical ventilation

Non-Parkinsonian Movement Disorders, First Edition. Edited by Deborah A. Hall and Brandon R. Barton.
© 2017 John Wiley & Sons, Ltd. Published 2017 by John Wiley & Sons, Ltd.
Companion website: www.wiley.com/go/hall/non-parkinsonian_movement_disorders

- Rhabdomyolysis—IV hydration, prevention of renal failure, monitoring electrolytes and serum creatine kinase
- Hyperthermia—cooling
- Pain—adequate analgesia

Temporizing measures

- Reduction of hyperkinetic movement in an intensive care unit setting: sedation with benzodiazepine, general anesthetic, neuromuscular blockers

Transition from temporizing measures to disease-specific therapy after improvement

- Disease-specific therapy
- Pharmacotherapy
- Consider deep brain stimulation for status dystonicus

☝ CAUTION AND WARNINGS

- Propofol infusion syndrome consists of rhabdomyolysis, metabolic acidosis, hyperkalemia, lipemia, renal failure, hepatomegaly, and cardiovascular collapse, which is common in children and those treated with long-term propofol and IV corticosteroids.
- Non-depolarizing neuromuscular blockers are preferred (atracurium) over depolarizing agents, which can worsen rhabdomyolysis.

The hyperkinetic movement disorder emergencies covered by this chapter include NMDA encephalitis, neuroleptic malignant syndrome, serotonin syndrome, status dystonicus, airway emergencies, tic status, drug induced akathisia, non-epileptic myoclonus, and acute hemiballism and hemichorea.

NMDA receptor encephalitis

This syndrome was first described in 2005, and in 2007 was found to be associated with the presence of N-methyl-D-Aspartate (NMDA) receptor auto-antibodies and ovarian teratoma. NMDA receptor encephalitis is now the second most common immune-mediated encephalitis, after acute disseminated encephalomyelitis. It mostly affects children and adults below the age of 50. It is a stepwise, progressive illness that presents with psychosis, memory deficit, seizures, and poverty of speech. The symptoms then progress into a reduced level of consciousness, catatonia, abnormal movements, autonomic disturbance, and hypoventilation. The abnormal movements are characteristically oro-buccal–lingual dyskinesia. Other associated phenomenology includes limb and trunk choreoathetosis, oculogyric crisis, dystonia, rigidity, and opisthotonic postures (see Video 17.1). A dissociative state is common (i.e., resistance to eye opening yet unresponsive to painful stimuli) and is thought to be secondary to NMDA receptor antagonism, as a similar clinical picture is observed after NMDA receptor antagonist use (ketamine and phencyclidine).

NMDA receptor encephalitis may or may not be associated with ovarian teratoma. The presence of ovarian teratoma is more frequent in adults than children, as well as in patients with African rather than Caucasian ethnicity. Early in the disease course, MRI brain and cerebrospinal fluid (CSF) can be normal. If the scan is abnormal, it typically shows mild to transient FLAIR or T2 hyperintensity in the hippocampi, cerebellum, or cerebral cortex. CSF examination shows pleocytosis with CSF-specific oligoclonal bands. CSF NMDA receptor antibodies are positive in all cases, but these should be measured in serum to monitor the effect of treatment, as positive treatment response is associated with a decline in NMDA receptor antibody titer.

The initial treatment involves searching for an underlying ovarian teratoma and immunotherapy: corticosteroids: methylprednisolone intravenous 1 g/d for 5 days with intravenous immunoglobulin (0.4 g/kg per day for 5 days) or plasma exchange (less well tolerated in children) as first-line therapy. Since immunotherapy effectiveness is synergistic with ovarian teratoma removal, it is important to search for an underlying ovarian teratoma, which contains the antigenic epitope that stimulates NMDA receptor antibody production. If age appropriate for women, a transvaginal ultrasound or pelvic ultrasound usually visualizes most ovarian masses. MRI or CT of the pelvis is useful if greater resolution is required. In men, testicular ultrasound for teratoma is recommended. In patients whose ultrasound is unremarkable but their clinical scenario fits well with the described clinical syndrome, exploratory laparoscopy and blind oophorectomy has been reported as successful treatment. Resection of the teratoma often leads to recovery in

Table 17.1 Movement disorder emergencies and associated phenomenology

Acute onset chorea/ hemiballism	*Vascular*—cerebrovascular accident, cavernous angioma. *Metabolic*—chorea gravidarum, hyperosmolar nonketotic hyperglycemia, hyperthyroidism, polycythemia rubra vera *Infectious*—Sydenham's chorea, toxoplasmosis, HIV encephalitis, tuberculoma *Structural*—lesion in basal ganglia, cerebellum, subthalamic nucleus, or thalamus *Inflammatory*—multiple sclerosis, sarcoidosis, antiphospholipid syndrome, systemic lupus erythematosus, NMDA encephalitis *Drugs*—anticonvulsants, oral contraceptives, cocaine, amphetamines, levodopa, alcohol
Acute onset tremor	Neuroleptic malignant syndrome, serotonin syndrome, drug-induced or psychogenic tremor
Acute onset myoclonus	*Metabolic*—uremic or hepatic encephalopathy *Toxic*—serotonin syndrome, tricyclic antidepressants, opiates, imipenem, quinolones, fourth-generation cephalosporins, gabapentin, triptans, monoamine oxidase inhibitors, amphetamine, cocaine Post-anoxic myoclonus Epileptic myoclonus
Acute onset dystonia	Device failure of preexisting deep brain stimulator Drug induced—dopamine receptor antagonists, clonazepam, dopamine-depleting agents
Acute exacerbation of tics	*Drug induced*—stimulants, dopamine antagonist reduction or cessation Infection Exacerbation of concomitant psychiatric disorder
Acute orofacial/limb dyskinesia	NMDA encephalitis Drug induced—levodopa

inverse order of symptom development. However, improvement may be prolonged, and most patients require a three- to four-month inpatient admission either in intensive care or under close supervision for behavioral disturbances, followed by months of physical and behavioral rehabilitation.

Patients who do not have associated teratomas tend to be refractory to first-line immunotherapy and need aggressive second-line immunotherapy, such as cyclophosphamide ($750\,mg/m^2$ given with first dose of rituximab following by monthly cycles) or rituximab ($375\,mg/m^2$ weekly for 4 weeks) or both. Clinical response to immunotherapy is followed by reduction in both CSF and serum NMDA receptor antibody titer, and immune therapy can be reduced once this occurs. Up to 25% of patients without a teratoma relapse months to years after the initial presentation. Therefore it is important to periodically monitor symptoms and consider adding mycophenolate mofetil or azathioprine for at least 1 year after initial immunotherapy is discontinued. In addition, periodic screening for ovarian teratoma for at least 2 years after the recovery from encephalitis is recommended.

★ **TIPS AND TRICKS**

- NMDA receptor encephalitis can potentially be missed. For example, a patient with NMDA receptor antibody with new onset psychosis and treatment with typical antipsychotics, followed by rigidity, autonomic instability, rhabdomyolysis can mimic neuroleptic malignant syndrome (NMS), but does not respond to NMS treatment.
- Oro-facial or limb dyskinesia, consisting of semi-rhythmic choreoathetotic movements during period of altered consciousness, is associated with NMDA receptor encephalitis.
- Diagnostic workup should include MRI brain, CSF, and serum NMDA receptor antibody and pelvic imaging to look for ovarian teratoma.
- First line immunotherapy should be started after diagnostic workup is sent and before the results of antibody tests return.

Neuroleptic malignant syndrome

Neuroleptic malignant syndrome (NMS) follows exposure to dopamine receptor antagonists or dopamine-depleting agents. Typical and atypical neuroleptics, tetrabenazine, droperidol, prochlorperazine, metoclopramide, sertraline, and promethazine may trigger NMS. According to the DSM-IV diagnostic criteria, following the offending drug exposure, patients develop muscle rigidity and fever with at least 2 of the following clinical signs and features: diaphoresis, labile blood pressure, tachycardia, incontinence, dysphagia, mutism, tremor, leukocytosis, or raised serum creatine kinase. Serum iron level is often low. NMS occurs typically 24 to 48 hours after the offending drug exposure or adjustment of dosage. The pathophysiologic mechanism is secondary to abrupt changes in the central dopamine transmission. It progresses for 48 to 72 hours and lasts an average of 1 to 2 weeks. NMS is rare, but fatal if undiagnosed and untreated, due to renal failure from rhabdomyolysis, respiratory failure secondary to aspiration pneumonia, or decreased chest wall compliance. Therefore it should be considered in the differential diagnosis of mental status change in the perioperative period.

★ TIPS AND TRICKS

A trial of intravenous benztropine or diphenhydramine is useful to differentiate between acute dystonic reaction and NMS. Acute dystonic reaction resolves within minutes of benztropine or diphenhydramine administration, whereas it has no effect on NMS.

Treatment of NMS involves early aggressive ICU admission, stopping the neuroleptic or causative agent, and considering treatment with antipyretics and dopaminergic agents such as levodopa or dopamine agonists. Dantrolene has Class III evidence as a treatment for NMS.

⚗ SCIENCE REVISITED

Dantrolene reduces muscle rigidity via inhibition of the ryanodine receptor, a major calcium release channel of the skeletal muscle sarcoplasmic reticulum. It acts as a muscle relaxant and prevents further rhabdomyolysis.

The duration of pharmacological treatment depends on the half-life of the offending agent, but generally treatment is continued for 7–10 days. If the neuroleptic agent is required for psychosis control and is reintroduced too early (within 2 weeks), it can cause recurrence of NMS. Most patients tolerate reintroduction of a neuroleptic 2 weeks after recovery from NMS. Electroconvulsive therapy can be used as an alternative to neuroleptic therapy if acute control of psychosis is required. IV pulse methylprednisolone has class I evidence for its efficacy in reducing the course of the disease (see Table 17.2).

Serotonin syndrome

Serotonin syndrome is a syndrome that occurs secondary to an increase in serotonin activity in the central nervous system. It is mediated by the 5-hydroxytryptamine 1A (5HT1A) receptor in the brainstem and spinal cord. Serotonin syndrome can be caused by any drug that enhances serotoninergic transmission, through mechanisms of inhibition of metabolism, direct receptor activation, inhibition of uptake, or via increasing the serotonin precursor. The cause is commonly selective serotonin reuptake inhibitor overdose or an interaction between monoamine oxidase inhibitor (MAOI) and serotonergic agents. Serotonin syndrome has been reported after a combination of serotonin reuptake inhibitors with protease inhibitors, reverse transcriptase inhibitors, L-tryptophan, monoamine oxidase inhibitors, meperidine, clomipramine, moclobemide, ziprasidone, MDMA "ecstasy," or lithium. Predisposing factors such as acquired liver disease, pulmonary disease, and cardiovascular disease leads to a decrease in the metabolism of serotonergic drugs; hence they predispose an individual to serotonin syndrome.

Serotonin syndrome consists of: confusion, agitation, coma, tachycardia, hyperthermia, hyperreflexia, rigidity, tremor, incoordination, and myoclonus. The presence of clonus (inducible, spontaneous, or ocular), myoclonus, agitation, diaphoresis, tremor, and hyperreflexia is more sensitive and specific for the diagnosis of serotonin syndrome, as opposed to NMS. Rigidity and hyperthermia of greater than 38.0 °C suggests severe serotonin toxicity and likelihood of progression to respiratory failure. The lack of prominent hypertension distinguishes it from MAO inhibitor overdose or tyramine "cheese

Table 17.2 Medications used for NMS: dosage, contraindications and side-effect profile (class III evidence)

Medication	Dose	Contraindications	Side effects
Dantrolene	1 to 2.5 mg/kg Intravenous and repeat after 5 minutes until tonic contractions resolve, Maximum 10 mg/kg/d	Liver failure	Hepatotoxicity, muscle weakness, phlebitis, gastric discomfort, and respiratory failure
Bromocriptine*	2.5 to 5 mg every 6–8 hours oral or via nasogastric tube Maximum 40 mg/d	Severe cardiovascular condition	Weakness, hypotension, headache, nausea
Amantadine	100 mg daily via NG tube, then titrate to 200 mg every 12 hours	Liver failure, congestive cardiac failure, seizures	Hypotension, edema, skin rash
Apomorphine†	2 mg every 3 hours for 3 days via subcutaneous injection, 2 mg every 6 hours for 2 additional days	Hypersensitivity to sulphur compounds	Severe nausea, angina, injection site reaction, somnolence

*Relieves hypothermia by its dopaminergic effects on the anterior hypothalamus. It should be continue for 10 days after control of symptoms and tapered slowly. Symptoms improve in 24–72 hours with a reduction in serum creatine kinase.

†Apomorphine is useful if there's difficulty in administering oral D2 agonists such as bromocriptine or amantadine. Preloading with domperidone is required to prevent severe nausea and vomiting.

reaction" (hypertensive crisis secondary to MAO inhibitor interaction with tyrosine rich food). The mortality from serotonin syndrome is high if unrecognized and left untreated.

The severity of symptoms determines the treatment, as mild cases are self-limiting once the offending drug is stopped and the patient may not necessarily require inpatient hospitalization (Table 17.3). The moderate to severe cases will need intensive care unit admission. Drugs like clonazepam, diphenhydramine, and benztropine are useful for alleviating tremor and rigidity, but they don't counteract serotonin syndrome. Stopping the offending drug and starting lorazepam, cyproheptadine, or chlorpromazine is useful for symptom control and provides directed therapy. Bromocriptine and dantrolene are not useful therapies and may worsen serotonin syndrome. Propranolol was used in the past but can abolish tachycardia, which is a useful guide to determine the efficacy and duration of treatment. Propofol, rocuronium, intubation, ventilation, and cooling with a hypothermic blanket has successfully treated life-threatening serotonin syndrome. If the serotonin syndrome is secondary to interaction between an irreversible monoamine oxidase inhibitor and a serotoninergic drug, one should wait at least 4 weeks after stopping an irreversible monoamine oxidase inhibitor before restarting a serotoninergic drug. It takes 4 weeks for the monoamine oxidase enzyme to replete.

> ☆ **TIPS AND TRICKS**
>
> - Rigidity and hyperthermia of greater than 38.0 C suggests severe serotonin toxicity and likelihood of progression to respiratory failure.
> - Myoclonus helps distinguish serotonin syndrome from NMS. The lack of prominent hypertension distinguishes it from MAO inhibitor overdose or tyramine "cheese reaction."
> - If the serotonin syndrome is secondary to interaction between an irreversible monoamine oxidase inhibitor and a serotoninergic drug, one should wait at least 4 weeks after stopping an irreversible monoamine oxidase inhibitor before restarting a serotoninergic drug. It takes 4 weeks for the monoamine oxidase enzyme to replete.

Table 17.3 Medications for serotonin syndrome: dosages, contraindication, and side effects

Medication	Dose	Contraindications	Side effects
Lorazepam	1 to 2 mg intravenous every 5 minutes until light sedation*	Liver failure	Somnolence
Cyproheptadine	12 mg initially, then 2 mg every hour oral Maximum 32 mg per day	No major contraindications	Somnolence, hepatotoxicity
Chlorpromazine†	50 to 100 mg intramuscular injection	No major contraindications	Hypotension

*Under a setting where close airway monitoring and protection is available.
†Useful therapy in patients who require acute parenteral therapy.

Status dystonicus (dystonic storm)

Status dystonicus is defined as increasingly frequent and severe episodes of generalized dystonia, requiring urgent hospital admission. Patients often have underlying primary or secondary generalized dystonia. Tonic muscle spasm is the most common form, characterized by sustained muscle contractions or postures. The phasic form, characterized by rapid and repetitive dystonic movement, is more common in secondary dystonia and female patients. Precipitating factors include initiating a chelating agent for patients with Wilson disease, intercurrent infection, trauma, deep brain stimulator (DBS) device failure, or discontinuation of medications for dystonia. Mortality rate is high, with up to 10% dying secondary to renal failure from rhabdomyolysis and respiratory failure. Patients require intensive care unit monitoring of respiratory and airway status, and serial serum creatine kinase, electrolyte, and serum creatinine measurements. As this is a rare condition, there is no definitive treatment data on optimal treatment strategy.

The following recommended therapy is based on reports of large case series (Table 17.4). The first-line treatments are medications targeting dystonia. For example, a combination of: anticholinergics (e.g., trihexiphenidyl), dopamine-depleting agents (e.g., tetrabenazine), baclofen, and/or benzodiazepines are useful. However, in a large case series and literature review, first-line therapy is only effective in 10% of cases, and often patients require ICU for second-line treatment. Dopamine receptor antagonists are less used due to the risk of inducing tardive dyskinesia. If the patient displays airway compromise secondary to bulbar or respiratory complications, second-line treatment involves ICU admission

and sedation with water soluble, fast acting benzodiazepines like midazolam (30–100 ug/kg/h) accompanied by intubation and artificial ventilation for airway protection. Occasionally, when deep sedation is ineffective, bilateral DBS surgery to the globus pallidus internus was shown in a large case series to be most effective, followed by intrathecal baclofen infusion (Video 17.2).

> ★ **TIPS AND TRICKS**
>
> - Patients with airway compromise require intensive care unit admission, sedation, intubation, and artificial ventilation.
> - Anticholinergics, baclofen, and dopamine-depleting agents are successful in 10% cases.
> - Status dystonicus refractory to medical therapy and deep sedation often responds to bilateral globus pallidus internus DBS surgery.

Airway emergencies

Airway compromise may occur in two clinical scenarios with movement disorders: (1) laryngeal adductor dystonia in dystonic conditions and (2) laryngeal abductor paralysis in multiple system atrophy.

Laryngeal adductor dystonia in dystonic conditions

Laryngeal adductor breathing dystonia occurs in both primary and secondary dystonia and rarely after exposure to neuroleptics. Primary spasmodic

Table 17.4 Medications used for status dystonicus: dosages, contraindication, and side effects

Medication	Dosage	Contraindications	Side effects
Trihexyphenidyl	2 to 8 mg 3 times a day oral or via nasogastric tube	No major contraindications	Dry mouth, blurred vision, tachycardia, urinary retention
Baclofen	25 mg 3 times a day oral or nasogastric tube	Hypersensitivity to baclofen	Weakness, drowsiness, hypotonia
Tetrabenazine	12.5 to 50 mg 3 times a day oral or nasogastric tube	Active depression	Depression, sedation, parkinsonism, akathisia
Reserpine	0.1 to 0.25 mg twice a day oral or nasogastric tube	Active depression, severe renal failure, active gastrointestinal diseases	Depression, orthostatic hypotension, diarrhea, akathisia, parkinsonism, gastrointestinal hemorrhage
Haloperidol	2 to 5 mg every 4–8 hours oral or via nasogastric tube	Parkinson disease	Parkinsonism, akathisia, prolonged QT interval, sedation and orthostatic hypotension

dysphonia is task specific and occurs during speech and not during breathing; thus it does not cause airway compromise. In acute airway obstruction, emergency endotracheal intubation is performed with the backup of surgical team ready to perform emergency tracheostomy or cricothyroidotomy as endotracheal intubation will not be easy. In non-emergent airway obstruction, botulinum toxin injection to the thyroarytenoid muscle should be done sequentially, one side at a time, with a 2 weeks interval to avoid complete vocal cord paralysis.

Laryngeal abductor paralysis in multiple system atrophy

Multiple system atrophy is a progressive illness and laryngeal abductor paralysis can occur at any stage, but paralysis is more common in the advanced stages of the illness. Patients often have sleep apnea or nocturnal stridor leading up to impending fatal airway obstruction. Treatment of laryngeal abductor paralysis is the only independent determinant for survival in this condition, and the method of treatment depends on its severity. Severity is evaluated with a fiberoptic laryngoscopy. Low-grade paralysis is managed by continuous positive airway pressure ventilation at night. High-grade paralysis warrants surgical management such as tracheostomy, which is the most reliable procedure. Other

surgical options are arytenoidectomy, cord lateralization, and cordectomy.

Tic status

Tic severity varies during the course of tic disorders. Tic status is an increase in the frequency and severity of tics; enough to disrupt social, vocational or daily activities. For example, self-injurious tics, coprolalia, copropraxia, or violent neck tics, which can induce cervical myelopathy, are tic emergencies. Tic status can be precipitated by a change in medications, intercurrent illness, or worsened comorbid psychiatric illness. Stimulants like methylphenidate used to treat ADHD have been reported to exacerbate tics in case reports, although a randomized controlled study did not support this.

The first-line medication therapy is a rapid escalation of benzodiazepines (Table 17.5). Second-line therapy is dopamine-depleting agents, like tetrabenazine, with monitoring for worsening depression. Dopamine-depleting agents are preferred over dopamine receptor antagonists, which can cause tardive syndromes; for this reason, dopamine receptor antagonists are reserved as third-line medication therapy. Medications like guanfacine and clonidine are unlikely to stop tic status.

Botulinum toxin injection to accessible sites can be a useful adjunct for tic treatment. For example,

Table 17.5 Medications used for tic status: dosages, contraindications, and side effects

Medication	Dosage	Contraindications	Side effects
Clonazepam	0.5 to 5 mg twice a day orally	Significant liver disease, acute close angle glaucoma	Sedation
Tetrabenazine	12.5 to 50 mg 2–3 times a day orally	Active depression	Depression, sedation, parkinsonism, akathisia
Haloperidol	2 to 5 mg every 4–8 hours orally	Parkinson disease	Parkinsonism, akathisia, prolonged QT interval, sedation and orthostatic hypotension.
Reserpine	0.1 to 0.25 mg daily or twice a day orally	Active depression, severe renal failure, active gastrointestinal diseases	Depression, orthostatic hypotension, diarrhea, akathisia, parkinsonism, gastrointestinal hemorrhage
Botulinum toxin type A	2.5–10 units intramuscular injection in small muscles; 25–100 units in large muscles	No major contraindications	Weakness, dysphagia
Botulinum toxin type B	250–1000 units intramuscular injection in small muscles and 2500–10000 units in large muscles		

blinking and cervical tics can be successfully treated with botulinum toxin injection. There is one case report of successful control of coprolalia after botulinum injection to one vocal cord.

There is one small randomized crossover trial of DBS to the centromedian nucleus of the thalamus. It was performed on medication refractory tic status patients with a 37% improvement in tic severity. The improvement was persistent after one year, but there was no improvement in associated behavior or mood disturbance. DBS targeting the globus pallidus was assessed in a small open-labeled trial with four patients: it reported a similar improvement in tic severity. However, more randomized blinded controlled trials are needed before establishing DBS surgery as a proven effective management of medication refractory tic disorder.

Drug-induced akathisia

Akathisia is a subjective sense of restlessness associated with restless movements and inability to stay still. It is a clinical diagnosis, which is made following exposure to neuroleptics, dopamine-blocking agents, or anti-emetics. There are no laboratory tests that support the diagnosis. It is important to inform patients of this potential side effect when starting dopamine receptor blockers so that akathisia is not mistaken for anxiety or agitation due to a worsening preexisting psychiatric condition. The course is self-limited once the causative medication is stopped, except in tardive akathisia, which tends to persist indefinitely without treatment. Propranolol is used as first-line treatment (Table 17.6); however, its dosage is limited by side effects such as hypotension and bradycardia. Up 80 mg per day of propranolol may provide at least 50% reduction in akathisia. Other nonselective beta-blockers are less efficacious due to reduced ability to cross the blood-brain barrier. A randomized placebo-controlled trial of low dose mirtazapine or vitamin B6 (1200 mg per day) found both treatments to be efficacious compared to placebo and reduced the akathisia by 30–60%. 5-HT2A antagonists counteract the dopamine receptor blockade by increasing dopamine neurotransmission. Randomized placebo-controlled trials of 5-HT2A antagonists, like mianserin, reduce

Table 17.6 Medications used for akathisia: dosage, contraindications, and side effects

Medication	Dosage	Contraindication	Side effects
Propranolol	20 to 40 mg twice a day	Asthma, diabetes, cardiac conduction abnormality	Hypotension, bradycardia, depression
Mirtazepine	15 mg per day	History of seizures, MAO inhibitor use	Weight gain, asthenia, dry mouth
Mianserin	15 mg per day	History of seizures	Weight gain, asthenia, dry mouth, leukopenia, agranulocytosis

akathisia. Mild orthostatic hypotension and sedation were the only side effects. Similarly, trazodone, a 5-HT2A/2C antagonist, has been shown in a double-blind crossover trial, to reduce akathisia at a dose of 100 mg daily compared to placebo. Benzodiazepines, clonidine, and amantadine have not been shown to successfully reduce akathisia in placebo-controlled trials but can be helpful. Anticholinergics can be useful but have not been efficacious in double-blind placebo trials;.in addition, they are limited by the side-effect profile.

Non-epileptic myoclonus

Epileptic myoclonus treatment is different from non-epileptic myoclonus and is not covered by this chapter. Electroencephalography or surface EMG polymyography can differentiate between epileptic myoclonus and non-epileptic myoclonus, especially as clinical examination cannot differentiate the two.

SCIENCE REVISITED

Surface EMG polymyography classifies myoclonus based on its duration, stimulus sensitivity and distribution. Myoclonus of duration less than 50 ms is due to cortical or reticular reflex myoclonus, which are fragments of focal epilepsy. Other electrophysiological findings supporting myoclonus of cortical origin are as follows:

1) Cranial–caudal spread of myoclonus from cranial nerve innervated muscles to paraspinal and upper and lower extremity musculature.
2) Presence of premyoclonus EEG transient imaged using combined EEG and EMG digital recording with back averaging.

3) Presence of giant somatosensory evoked potentials (N1/P1 or N1/P2 amplitude greater than 10 uV measured at contralateral central region with ear-reference recording). This supports the finding of stimulus sensitive cortical myoclonus.

However, myoclonus with a duration of 50 to 300 ms arises from the brainstem, spinal cord, or peripherally and is classified as non-epileptic myoclonus.</bxb>

The common etiology of non-epileptic myoclonus is toxic metabolic encephalopathy or post-hypoxic encephalopathy. In these causes, the myoclonus is usually generalized or multifocal. Drugs such as general anesthetic agents (etomidate and enflurane), dopamine receptor blockers, opioids, imipenem, and quinolone antibiotics can cause myoclonus. The treatment is identification of the offending agent and its withdrawal. Post-hypoxic myoclonus occurs after survival from respiratory or cardiac arrest. Post-hypoxic myoclonus is typically disabling as it is more pronounced during action or intention.

There is a lack of controlled trials examining the efficacy of myoclonus pharmacotherapy and often multiple medication trials are needed (Table 17.7). Clonazepam, valproate, and recently levetiracetam have been used to control myoclonus of cortical origin. For both cortical and subcortical myoclonus, sodium oxybate or clonazepam is an effective therapy.

Acute chorea and hemiballism

Chorea is an involuntary, irregular, and unpredictable flowing movement that moves from one body part to another in a non-stereotyped fashion. Hemiballism is a large amplitude involuntary

Table 17.7 Medications used for myoclonus: dosage, contraindications, and side effects

Medication	Dosage	Contraindications	Side effects
Clonazepam	0.5 to 5.0 mg twice a day oral or via nasogastric tube	Sleep apnea, liver failure	Sedation, depression, hypotension
Sodium valproate	10 to 15 mg/kg twice a day oral or via nasogastric tube	Liver failure, hyperammonemia	Pancreatitis, rash, thrombocytopenia, liver function abnormalities
Levetiracetam	250 to 750 mg twice a day oral or intravenously	No major contraindications	Aggressive behavior, depression
Sodium oxybate	3 to 9 g oral daily, continue every 3–4 hours if symptoms persists	No major contraindications	Drowsiness, sleep disturbance, nausea

Table 17.8 Medications used for hemiballism/chorea: dosage, contraindications, and side effects

Medication	Dosage	Contraindication	Side effects
Tetrabenazine	12.5 to 50 mg 2–3 times a day orally	Active depression	Depression, sedation, parkinsonism, akathisia
Reserpine	0.1 to 0.25 mg daily or twice a day orally	Active depression, severe renal failure, active gastrointestinal diseases	Depression, orthostatic hypotension, diarrhea, akathisia, parkinsonism, gastrointestinal hemorrhage
Haloperidol	2 to 5 mg every 4–8 hours orally	Parkinson disease	Parkinsonism, akathisia, prolonged QT interval, sedation, and orthostatic hypotension

movement of the proximal joints. Hemiballism occurs commonly after a stroke in the subthalamic nucleus or accompanying hyperosmolar non-ketotic hyperglycemia. Hemiballism initially requires no more than non-pharmacological management such as padding or soft restraints to protect the limb from injury. It usually reduces to hemichorea or athetosis after a few days. Dopamine-depleting agents, such as tetrabenazine, are reserved for hemiballism that does not resolve (see Table 17.8). Tetrabenazine is preferred over reserpine due to its short half-life and lack of side effects, such as hypotension and diarrhea. The dopamine-depleting agents are preferred over dopamine receptor blockers because they do not carry the risk of engendering a tardive syndrome. If dopamine-depleting agents are contraindicated, dopamine receptor antagonists should be used for a short-term period, with the patient made aware of possible side effects such as tardive syndromes. Since hemiballism usually recedes over time, patients should be reassessed at three months later to evaluate the need for continuous pharmacological therapy. A small number of case reports show successful treatment with risperidone, topiramate, levetiracetam, gabapentin, and sertraline. Case series show inconsistent benefit with sodium valproate but improvement after botulinum toxin injection.

Further Readings

Ackermans L, Duits A, van der Linden C, Tijssen M, Schruers K, Temel Y, et al. Double-blind clinical trial of thalamic stimulation in patients with Tourette syndrome. *Brain* 2011; **134**(Pt 3): 832–844.

Caroff SN, Mann SC. Neuroleptic malignant syndrome. *Med Clin North Am* 1993; **77**(1): 185–202.

Dalmau J, Lancaster E, Martinez-Hernandez E, Rosenfeld MR, Balice-Gordon R. Clinical experience and laboratory investigations in patients with anti-NMDAR encephalitis. *Lancet Neurol* 2011; **10** (1): 63–74.

Dunkley EJ, Isbister GK, Sibbritt D, Dawson AH, Whyte IM. The Hunter serotonin toxicity criteria: simple and accurate diagnostic decision rules for serotonin toxicity. *Qjm* 2003; **96**(9): 635–642.

Fasano A, Ricciardi L, Bentivoglio AR, Canavese C, Zorzi G, Petrovic I, Kresojevic N. Status dystonicus: predictors of outcome and progression patterns of underlying disease. *Mov Disord* 2012; **27**(6): 783–788.

Kleinig TJ, Thompson PD, Matar W, Duggins A, Kimber TE, Morris JG, et al. The distinctive movement disorder of ovarian teratoma-associated encephalitis. *Mov Disord* 2008; **23**(9): 1256–1261.

Krause T, Gerbershagen MU, Fiege M, Weisshorn R, Wappler F. Dantrolene—a review of its pharmacology, therapeutic use and new developments. *Anaesthesia* 2004; **59**(4): 364–373.

Kurlan R. Treatment of ADHD in children with tics: a randomized controlled trial. *Neurology* 2002; **58**(4): 527–536.

Mariotti P, Fasano A, Contarino MF, Della Marca G, Piastra M, Genovese O, et al. Management of status dystonicus: our experience and review of the literature. *Mov Disord* 2007; **22**(7): 963–968.

Rosebush PI, Stewart TD, Gelenberg AJ. Twenty neuroleptic rechallenges after neuroleptic malignant syndrome in 15 patients. *J Clin Psychiatry* 1989; **50**(8): 295–298.

Sato Y, Asoh T, Metoki N, Satoh K. Efficacy of methylprednisolone pulse therapy on neuroleptic malignant syndrome in Parkinson's disease. *J Neurol Neurosurg Psychiatry* 2003; **74**(5): 574–576.

Silber MH, Levine S. Stridor and death in multiple system atrophy. *Mov Disord* 2000; **15**(4): 699–704.

Tsutsumi Y, Yamamoto K, Matsuura S, Hata S, Sakai M, Shirakura K. The treatment of neuroleptic malignant syndrome using dantrolene sodium. *Psychiatry Clin Neurosci* 1998; **52**(4): 433–438.

18

Functional or Psychogenic Movement Disorders

S. Elizabeth Zauber, MD

Department of Neurology, Indiana University School of Medicine, Indianapolis, Indiana, USA

Introduction

Functional movement disorders (FMD) pose diagnostic and therapeutic challenges for clinicians. Quality of life ratings in patients with FMD are similarly impaired compared to those of patients with chronic neurological diseases such as multiple sclerosis or Parkinson disease (PD). When incorrectly viewed of as a diagnosis of exclusion, patients with FMD may be asked to undergo prolonged testing, which delays diagnosis and increases patient frustration. However, harm can arise from not making a prompt diagnosis by exposing patients to unnecessary tests or invasive procedures, and by not providing potentially effective treatment in a timely manner. An earlier definitive diagnosis can improve outcomes for these patients. Accurate diagnosis relies on clinical judgment and a careful exam and history. This chapter outlines an approach to the exam and history that can aid in diagnosis and treatment of FMD.

Terminology

A lack of consensus about the best name for FMD adds to patient and physician misunderstanding about this topic. Most movement disorder neurologists favor "psychogenic" or "functional." The advantage of "functional" is that it does not imply a psychological etiology and thus may be more acceptable to patients. However, some organic disorders, like idiopathic dystonia, could be considered functional in the sense that there is not a structural cause. Critics of the term "functional" argue that "psychogenic" is more accurate. The term "psychogenic" is more commonly encountered in the literature, but we will use "functional" in this chapter as many experts now favor this term. Each neurologist should consider the pros and cons of these terms when discussing the diagnosis with patients (see section on treatment). Other terms that may apply but are less commonly accepted include: medically unexplained symptoms, stress reaction, or hysterical.

Diagnosis

Physicians often underdiagnose FMD out of concern that they may be missing an organic disorder. Patients undergo rounds of laboratory and imaging studies, ordered by physicians who have incorrectly viewed FMD as a diagnosis of exclusion. The correct approach to diagnosing a FMD is based on the presence of typical positive findings in the exam and history as noted below.

History

The most important historical clues that a movement disorder may be functional include a sudden onset or onset after minor injury, rapid progression to maximal disability, spontaneous remissions, or paroxysmal symptoms (Table 18.1). A history of acute stressors and/or abuse may be present, but the absence of these should not rule out the diagnosis. It is important to inquire about how symptoms affect activities and responsibilities, and to screen for a history of other somatizations.

Non-Parkinsonian Movement Disorders, First Edition. Edited by Deborah A. Hall and Brandon R. Barton.
© 2017 John Wiley & Sons, Ltd. Published 2017 by John Wiley & Sons, Ltd.
Companion website: www.wiley.com/go/hall/non-parkinsonian_movement_disorders

Table 18.1 History and examination findings suggestive of Functional Movement Disorders (FMD)

Historical clues to FMD	Exam findings in FMD
<ul><li>Sudden onset or onset after minor injury</li><li>Rapid progression to maximal disability or maximal disability at onset</li><li>Spontaneous remissions</li><li>Paroxysmal symptoms</li></ul>	<ul><li>Movements are inconsistent time or vary in frequency</li><li>Movements disappear with distraction</li><li>Extreme slowness</li><li>Nonorganic signs: give-way weakness, non-anatomical sensory loss</li></ul>

Source: Adapted from Gupta 2009.

✋ CAUTION

Diagnostic pitfalls in FMDs

- Presence or absence of obvious psychiatric disturbance is not helpful.
- "I could not make that type of movement so it must be organic."
- "This is an unusual movement disorder, so it must be functional."

Exam

The physical exam signs supportive of a FMD include movements that are inconsistent and vary in frequency over time, movements that disappear with distraction, or the presence of extreme slowness. Patients may also have other nonorganic signs like give-way weakness, speech changes, and non-anatomical sensory findings. The physician should pay close attention to the patient's movements and function throughout the encounter, not just during the exam. FMD are often internally inconsistent, meaning they are present with some activities but not all during the examination.

Psychological findings

The presence or absence of obvious psychiatric disturbance is not helpful in the diagnosis. Some patients with FMD do not have psychiatric symptoms and many patients with organic movement disorders do experience psychiatric symptoms as a result of their disease or in reaction to having a disease.

Pathophysiology

FMD share similarities with injury-feigning behavior in animals. This behavior allows the animal to be nurtured, and protects the animal from aggression. FMDs may serve a similar unconscious role in humans to signal disability, distress, and need for care. Research into FMD suggests patients have a mismatch between sensation and perception. In a study of functional tremor, patient's self-reported tremor occurred more often during the day than was actually noted on actigraphy. Functional neuroimaging studies have been useful in elucidating the mechanism of FMD. Since involuntary movements preclude the use of functional MRI, most studies, to date, have examined patients with functional weakness. Compared to controls, these patients show greater activation in limbic areas such as amygdala and cingulate, and less activation in motor control areas, when performing movements. It is likely that those findings of altered brain function are also relevant to patients with FMD.

Types of functional movement disorders

Based on pooled data, the frequency of different presentations of FMD seen at major academic centers with a movement disorders clinic includes the following: tremor (40%), dystonia (31%), myoclonus (13%), gait disorder (10%), parkinsonism (5%), and tics (2%). Many patients with FMD have more than one type of abnormal movement. For example, it is not uncommon for a patient with functional tremor to also have an abnormal gait. Each type of movement phenomenology is considered separately below, but in practice, several types of phenomenology may be present in one patient at a time, or may occur at different times during the examination in the same patient.

Tremor

Tremor is the most common phenomenologic presentation of a FMD. Functional tremor has several characteristic features that can distinguish it from PD tremor, essential tremor, and dystonic tremor (Table 18.2).

Table 18.2 Comparison of different types of tremor

	Functional tremor	Essential tremor	Parkinson tremor
Side of symptoms	Often unilateral	Bilateral	Asymmetric
Part of limb affected	Arms, wrists, hands	Hands, fingers	Arm, wrist, hands, fingers
Rest (R), posture (P), or action (A)	R = P = A	A > P >> R	R >> P > A

Location

The precise location of the tremor can provide diagnostic clues, as functional tremor affects wrists, hands, arms, but spares the fingers. Functional tremor is often, but not always, unilateral and commonly affects the dominant arm. Other tremor characteristics provide useful clues. For example, PD tremor usually causes a rest tremor that is more marked than postural or action tremor. Essential tremor is prominent with action, less severe with posture, and typically absent at rest. Functional tremor may occur at rest, posture, and action, with equal severity of each portion.

Variability

Variability is an important feature of functional tremor. The tremor may vary in direction, amplitude, or frequency over the course of the exam and history. Further, it may increase in severity as attention is drawn to it, such as during the examination portion of the clinical evaluation.

Distractibility

Often functional tremor will improve during mental concentration or during complex motor tasks like tandem gait testing. In contrast, parkinsonian tremor usually emerges or worsens during concentration or walking. Entrainment is the tendency for functional tremor frequency in one limb to change and mimic the frequency of voluntary tapping of contralateral extremity. In addition, engaging the contralateral extremity in a tapping or another repetitive motor task may result in a change in tremor frequency in the involved limb. A large enough change in tremor during entrainment tasks can be simply observed by the examiner, but smaller changes may require electrophysiologic studies. Occasionally, this type of contralateral distraction technique will cause the tremor to temporarily stop. Patients often notice this, and demonstrating these exam findings to the patient may be useful when explaining the diagnosis.

When testing for distractibility, internally paced movements are usually not as effective as externally paced or larger amplitude ballistic movements. An example of using ballistic movements is as follows: First, the patient holds both hands outstretched. The examiner then asks the patient to make a rapid large amplitude movement with the contralateral arm. The examiner looks for a pause in tremor of the ipsilateral arm, during the ballistic movement. In patients with midline tremor such as a head tremor, appendicular movements may not provide sufficient distraction. Instead, tongue movements or other midline movements should be engaged.

Functional dystonia

Functional dystonia is the second common type of functional movement disorder. Historically, organic dystonia was thought to be functional because of its unusual qualities, such as sensory tricks and task specificity. Since the presentations of organic dystonia can be unique, unusual, and varied, a diagnosis of functional dystonia should be made by a neurologist significantly experienced in the diagnosis of dystonia.

History

The characteristics that separate functional dystonia from organic dystonia are similar to other FMD. For example, a sudden onset disability that is maximal at onset, or presents with paroxysmal symptoms, is common in functional dystonia. An important distinction is that functional dystonia may produce fixed postures at rest, while organic dystonia is usually most prominent with action, and less marked at rest. Further, fixed postures are rare early in the course of organic dystonia. Muscle hypertrophy is common in organic dystonia but rare in functional dystonia. Response to treatment is poor (Table 18.3). Pain is uncommon in organic dystonia with the exception of cervical dystonia. However, pain is a common finding in functional dystonia. As in other FMD, functional dystonia may

Table 18.3 Comparison of functional dystonia versus nonfunctional dystonia

	Functional dystonia	Dystonia
Posture	Fixed	Mobile
Onset	Sudden onset	Gradual
Pain	Common	Rare except in cervical dystonia
Muscle hypertrophy	Rare	Common
Response to treatment	Poor	Good

Source: Adapted from Hawley 2011.

often follow peripheral trauma. The combination of onset after peripheral trauma and pain has led to controversy about whether or not the fixed dystonia associated with complex regional pain syndrome represents functional dystonia.

Functional dystonia movements are usually incongruous with organic dystonia both in the nature and location of the movement. For example, organic dystonia in adults usually starts in the head or neck or upper extremity. Onset of dystonia in the leg in an adult can occur as the initial presentation of PD, but in the absence of other signs of PD, such a presentation could raise the question of functional dystonia.

Exam

Similar to the diagnostic approach in functional tremor, neurologists should look for typical characteristics when diagnosing functional dystonia. For example, patients with organic tremor should not have other abnormalities on neurological exam; however, with functional dystonia, they might have nonorganic signs such as extreme slowness. The movements often fluctuate during the exam such that they increase when attention is drawn to them and reduce with distraction. The abnormal movements may be triggered by non-physiological stimuli such as pressing on a particular part of the body or by moving the contralateral limb. Muscles usually appear relaxed at rest, but active muscle contraction against passive movement can be detected, which is not typical for organic dystonia.

Parkinsonism

Functional parkinsonism is one of the least common presentations of FMD. Patients with functional parkinsonism have features that may resemble, but are clearly distinct from, PD. As in functional tremor, the

tremor of functional parkinsonism is variable in frequency, severity, and can be distractible. In PD, tremor typically increases when a patient is engaged in a mental task; in contrast, functional tremor or the tremor of functional parkinsonism typically lessens or disappears during mental concentration.

Exam

Slow movements as well as a decrement in amplitude characterize bradykinesia in PD. Decrement is defined as follows: when asked to perform rapid, repetitive movements, PD patients may produce a normal size movement for a few taps and then the subsequent taps become smaller. There may be pauses or hesitations in the movement. Patients with functional parkinsonism have slow movements, but there is no decrement. Further, the slowness in functional parkinsonism may be variable such that the patient performs some casual actions with normal speed, but then is very slow when finger taps or coordination are being directly tested. Often patients with functional parkinsonism will display dramatic effort, sighing when performing motor testing.

Rigidity may be absent in functional parkinsonism. When present, it may be distractible. Asking the patient to move the extremity contralateral to the one being tested can reduce rigidity. In PD, the opposite occurs, moving the contralateral extremity increases tone.

Postural stability is tested in PD by pulling a patient backward and asking the patient to recover his balance by taking a step. Early in PD, patients have normal postural reflexes and perform this test normally. Later in the course, patients may take additional steps or fail to catch their balance. In functional parkinsonism, some patients might have atypical responses to this test such as back arching or flailing without falling, and others may fall "like a log."

Imaging

Neuroimaging can provide additional information in functional parkinsonism. DaTscans are now commercially available in the United States and provide a quantitative assessment of pre-synaptic dopaminergic cells. Imaging alone cannot make the diagnosis of functional parkinsonism, which remains a clinical diagnosis, but a normal DaTscan can be a useful tool to support the diagnosis.

Special note Just as patients with seizures can develop non-epileptic events, patients with PD can develop functional tremor. Treatment of both a functional and organic movement disorder is challenging but can be accomplished.

Gait disorders

Gait disorders may occur alone or in combination with other FMD. Several types of functional gait can occur. In all cases the gait abnormalities are not supported by other neurological exam findings. Often functional gait dysfunction is uneconomical, meaning that excessive energy is required to maintain postures or gait. Examples of functional gait are as follows:

1) *Astasia-abasia:* The patient appears to fall to one side, but in the process actually demonstrate very good balance by leaning to one side while balancing on one foot. This is most often observed when testing tandem gait.
2) *Knee buckling:* The patient walks normally for a few steps, then one or both knees bend and the patient drops to the ground.
3) *Dragging:* The patient drags one leg despite normal strength testing.
4) *Cautious gait:* The patient totters as if "walking on ice."

Jerks/myoclonus

Functional myoclonus causes jerks both at rest and with action. It can affect a single body part or more likely the trunk or whole body. As in other FMD, the movements are often distractible and variable or may be exacerbated by non-physiological stimuli, such as checking tendon reflexes. Electrophysiological testing can be of particular use in distinguishing functional myoclonus from cortical myoclonus. However, this type of testing, which requires simultaneous EMG and EEG, is not commonly available, even in academic medical centers. A simpler approach is to measure the duration of myoclonus using surface EMG. Organic myoclonus of all types will produce a short duration (<75 ms) of muscle activity, whereas functional myoclonic movements will be longer in duration.

Paroxysmal disorders

Paroxysmal disorders overlap with non-epileptic behavioral events. Since they may not be present at the time of the office visit, it is important to review a video of an attack. Rarely organic movement disorders occur only intermittently; for example, paroxysmal non-kinesigenic dyskinesia and paroxysmal kinesigenic dyskinesia may manifest in discrete attacks of symptoms, and often manifest initially at a young age. However, these conditions cause stereotyped movements of a relatively short duration. FMD commonly last longer than their organic counterparts, produce more variable movements, and have more adult onset.

Psychiatric diagnoses

Many patients with functional movement disorders have either conversion disorder or somatoform disorder. Rates of malingering are thought to be low. The common comorbid psychiatric disorders are depression and anxiety, with close to half of patients having a lifetime history of these disorders. Personality disorders are also common in patients with FMD. The number of patients with FMD who have a history of childhood abuse, about 5–15%, is greater than the general population, but still only affects a minority of patients with FMD.

Treatment

Conveying the diagnosis to patients is one of the most important aspects of treatment. If the diagnosis is not communicated in a compassionate manner, patients are unlikely to accept the diagnosis and proceed with treatment. Patient acceptance of the diagnosis is imperative for successful treatment.

Talking to patients about the diagnosis

Different methods of approaching the diagnosis exist, but the following is the suggested method of the author. Key concepts should be conveyed when relaying this diagnosis. First, the physician should communicate that he or she *knows what this is*. Next, that he or she believes the movements are *real* and *involuntary*. The neurologist should provide reassurance that there are *no signs of a progressive neurodegenerative* or life-threatening disorder. Last, because the nervous system has not been damaged, the condition is *potentially reversible*. Some argue that it is not necessary or productive for the neurologist to point to a psychological reason for the FMD. By comparison, some neurologists don't tell people at a first visit *why* the brain has reduced levels of dopamine in PD, only that the symptoms of PD come from a lack of dopamine in the brain. Similarly, in the setting of FMD it is sufficient to say that the nervous system is not functioning properly, that this is a common and reversible problem.

Some neurologists find it helpful to ask about feelings of panic or dissociation at onset of symptoms. They may then talk to patients about how these feelings at onset have led to the nervous system malfunctioning. Alternatively, some physicians may want to discuss the connection between mind and body, for example, someone who is nervous may have "butterflies in their stomach" and could be told "The stomach is not diseased, but the mind is causing physical symptoms." In an attempt to communicate the difference between a functional and structural problem, some neurologists use the analogy of a computer, stating that FMD is a software problem, rather than a hardware problem. It is important to stress to patients that you believe their movements to be involuntary. The risk in discussing a possible psychological etiology is that patients feel the doctor is saying the condition is "all in their heads," that they may feel the neurologist is not taking their symptoms seriously.

One common pitfall is to tell patients that the FMD has developed as a result of stress. Often patients do not feel stressed, either because they have converted the psychological reaction into a physical one or because the FMD developed at a time in their life that was relatively free of stress. It is important to *give the condition a name*, as family and friends will want to know. If they do not have a name, family and friends may continue to think that no one knows what is causing the movements, and encourage the patient to seek other opinions and further diagnostic tests. Another approach is to *show patients their signs*. It is not uncommon for a neurologist to discuss how the physical exam findings led to the diagnosis of an organic disorder. The same approach can be used in FMD and may help patients accept the diagnosis.

Multidisciplinary approach

Patients should continue to receive care from their primary care physician, neurologist, physical therapist, and psychiatrist. However, none of these clinicians has the expertise to treat patients with FMD alone. Historically, patients were admitted to an inpatient neurology unit where physical therapy, psychiatry, and neurology could all evaluate the patient quickly and collaboratively. While insurance changes usually no longer allow for all patients to be hospitalized, this multidisciplinary model should, when possible, be employed in the outpatient setting.

Psychotherapy

Unfortunately, it is not uncommon for a patient to agree to see a psychiatrist but then be told there is "nothing wrong" and that they need to go back to neurologist. Many psychiatrists and psychologists do not have enough experience or training in FMD. The neurologist should communicate to the mental health professional that they are *not asking the psychiatrist/psychologist to diagnose a FMD*, but are asking them to determine if there are any past or present events that may either impair recovery or that may be contributing to cause the FMD. Good communication between the neurologist and psychiatrist is essential. Lack of consensus between neurologist and psychiatrist can significantly interfere with the patient's recovery. There are no clinical trial data available to support the use of one type of psychotherapy over another. Most of the literature to support the use of psychotherapy comes from other functional conditions. Several clinical trials in progress are examining the efficacy of cognitive behavioral therapy and psychodynamic psychotherapy in the treatment of FMD.

Rehabilitation

Physical therapy and/or occupational or speech therapy should be offered, as this is effective for many patients. Physical therapy is particularly important in functional dystonia to maintain the range of motion. Physical therapy can also be useful from a psychological perspective because it gives the patient a non-psychological reason for improvement.

Pharmacotherapy

Medicines should only be used to treat underlying psychiatric or inciting medical issues. Neurologists should avoid the use of drugs to treat the movements. In particular, antipsychotics should be avoided given their potential to produce involuntary movements as part of a tardive syndrome, unless required for psychiatric care. Some patients may be reluctant to take antidepressants, especially if they are not accepting of a psychological origin of their symptoms. However, they may be open to taking an antidepressant in order to feel better and be more able to participate in physical therapy or other therapies needed to improve the FMD.

Alternative treatments

Patients often seek alternative therapies to treat FMD. For example, transcranial magnetic stimulation, hypnosis, biofeedback, TENS and acupuncture all have the potential to improve symptoms in some patients, although the literature regarding many of these therapies is not robust or lacking completely.

Prognosis

Very few studies have specifically examined the long-term outcomes of FMD. However, several patterns are noted. Patients who have the best prognosis have a shorter duration of symptoms, younger age, a clearly definable and treatable psychiatric disorder, or symptoms precipitated by a clear stressor. A poor prognosis has been associated with longer disease duration (over a year), the presence of a personality disorder, family invested in sick role, or pending legal issues.

Conclusions

FMD are commonly encountered in neurological practice. Specific historical clues and exam findings, outlined in this chapter, can alert physicians to the possibility of a FMD and aid in early diagnosis.

Treatment is most likely to be successful when initiated early, and when a multidisciplinary approach is employed, including neurology, psychiatry, and rehabilitation. Patients with a clearly identifiable stressor or treatable psychiatric disorder have the best prognosis. Unfortunately, many patients develop long-term disability from persistent symptoms. Ongoing research into the mechanisms of FMD may aid in future diagnostic and treatment options.

Further Readings

Bhatia KP, Schneider SA. Psychogenic tremor and related disoders. *J Neurol* 2007; **254**: 569–574.

Czarnecki K, et al. Functional movement disorders: successful treatment with physical therapy rehabilitation protocol. *Parkinsonism Relat Disord* 2012; **18**: 247–251.

Gupta A, Lang AE. Psychogenic movement disorders. *Curr Opin Neurol* 2009; **22**: 430–436.

Hallett M, et al. *Psychogenic Movement Disorders: Neurology and Neuropsychiatry*. Philadelphia: Lippincott Williams Wilkens, 2006.

Hallett M, et al. *Psychogenic Movement Disorders: And Other Conversion Disorders*. New York: Cambridge University Press, 2011.

Hawley JS, Weiner WJ. Psychogenic dystonia and peripheral trauma. *Neurology* 2011; **77**(5); 498–502.

Jankovic J. Diagnosis and treatment of psychogenic parkinsonism. *JNNP* 2011; **82**: 1300–1303.

McKeon A, et al. Psychogenic tremor: long term prognosis in patients with electrophysiologically-confirmed disease. *Mov Disord* 2008; **24**: 72–76.

Parees I, et al. Believing is perceiving: mismatch between self-report and actigraphy in psychogenic tremor. *Brain* 2012; **135**: 117–123.

Psychogenic Movement Disorders. Teaching course presented at Movement Disorders Society Congress, Dublin, June 2012.

Schrag A, Lang AE. Psychogenic movement disorders. *Curr Opin Neurol* 2005; **18**: 399–404.

Stone J, Edwards M. Trick or treat: showing patients with functional (psychogenic) motor symptoms their physical signs. *Neurology* 2012; **79**: 282–284.

Part 4

Additional Resources

19

Genetics of Movement Disorders

Deborah A. Hall, MD, PhD

Department of Neurological Sciences, Section of Movement Disorders, Rush University Medical Center, Chicago, Illinois, USA

Introduction

The genetics of movement disorders is a topic that is much broader than can be represented within a chapter of this length. In fact, today, genetic advances are so frequent that this chapter will be out of date before it arrives to print. For these reasons, the reader is referred to some online references. Online Mendelian Inheritance in Man (OMIM) at www.omim.org is a database that can be searched by gene or disease name and provides several links. The availability of testing for clinical or research purposes can be found on www.genetests. org, which is also linked on the OMIM site. The US National Institutes of Health has a home page http://ghr.nlm.nih.gov that covers basic genetic concepts in addition to genetic disorders. This chapter will cover the movement disorders included in this textbook, organized primarily by major phenomenology. When the gene is already discussed in a prior chapter, it will be noted for the reader.

Inheritance of genetic disorders will not be reviewed here, but the references above may be helpful to the reader interested in a refresher of autosomal, X-linked, or mitochondrial inheritance patterns. Movement disorders, which reflect neurological disorders in general, are caused by all of these modes of inheritance.

Essential tremor

Genes that are causal or increase risk for essential tremor (ET) are limited, both in number and significance. A mutation in the fused in sarcoma (*FUS*) gene was discovered in a Franco-Canadian family and in four additional ET patients, but has not been confirmed in other families or population studies. This gene may be a rare cause of monogenic ET. Two genome-wide association studies have been performed in ET with single nucleotide polymorphisms (SNP) identified in two genes. These SNPs may risk factors for ET, but replication and follow-up studies are needed. These two genes are *LINGO1*, which is involved in the regulation of neuroregeneration, and *SLC1A2*, which encodes the major glutamate reuptake transporter in the brain.

Myoclonus

Given the extensive list of causes of myoclonus, the consideration of genetic testing with this phenotype can be exhaustive. The etiologies of non-epileptic cortical myoclonus are covered in Table 4.2 in the myoclonus chapter. Basal ganglia degenerative disorders that are genetic include neurodegeneration with brain iron accumulation (NBIA), Wilson disease, and Huntington disease (HD). The former two are

Non-Parkinsonian Movement Disorders, First Edition. Edited by Deborah A. Hall and Brandon R. Barton.
© 2017 John Wiley & Sons, Ltd. Published 2017 by John Wiley & Sons, Ltd.
Companion website: www.wiley.com/go/hall/non-parkinsonian_movement_disorders

reviewed in the heavy metal accumulation diseases chapter (Chapter 16) and the latter in the chorea chapter (Chapter 6). Inherited prion disease, including Gerstmann–Straussler–Scheinker disease and fatal familial insomnia, are associated with mutations in the prion protein (*PRNP*) gene and manifest in autosomal dominant transmission. Point mutations in *PRNP* segregate with the familial prion diseases and are also associated with Creutzfeldt–Jakob disease. Many of the inherited ataxias, detailed in the ataxia chapter (including Tables 8.3 and 8.4), have myoclonus as part of the phenotype, such as in Friedreich ataxia, ataxia-telangiectasia, the spinocerebellar ataxias (SCAs), and dentatorubral-pallidal luysian atrophy (DRPLA).

Inborn errors of metabolism are less frequent causes of myoclonus, are predominantly autosomal recessive, and manifest in childhood. Lafora body disease is caused by mutations in the epilepsy progressive myoclonic 2 (*EPM2A or EPM2B*) genes and due to polyglucosan inclusions in cells of the brain, liver, muscle, and skin; patients have dementia or regression, myclonus, and seizures. Neuronal ceroid lipofuscinosis has a similar phenotype with the addition of blindness and is caused by mutations in *EPM1* that leads to lipoprotein accumulation in lysosomes in the brain, eccrine glands, skin, muscle, and gut. Sialodoses are also lysosomal storage disorders characterized by a cherry-red spot, myoclonus, and seizures and are caused by a mutation in the neuraminidase (*NEU1*) gene. Mitochondrial disorders, especially myoclonus epilepsy and ragged-red fiber (MERRF) syndrome, frequently include myoclonus with a host of other symptoms. MERRF can be caused by mutations in several mitochondrial genes: *MTTK, MTTl1, MTTH, MTTS1, MTTs2, MTTF*. These disorders tend to follow maternal inheritance patterns characteristic of mitochondrial disorders, but patients may also have mutations in nuclear-encoded mitochondrial genes and show Mendelian inheritance patterns. There are several other more rare disorders that cause both progressive myoclonic epilepsy and progressive myoclonic ataxia, and the reader is referred to the myoclonus references for more detail.

Tics

Although multiple genes and chromosomal regions have been implicated as common causes of a primary tic disorder, in Gilles de la Tourette syndrome, no gene or common variants of major effect have been discovered. Several large-scale collaborative genetic studies have started, and several recent studies are producing promising leads. It is suspected that many of the candidate genes will fall in the dopaminergic or serotonergic pathways, given the understanding of the pathophysiology of the disorder. Initial genome scans for copy number variants (defined as variation in the number of copies of one or more sections of DNA) and genome-wide association studies on Tourette syndrome have been published, which should increase the rapidly of gene discovery in this disorder. The genetic etiology of secondary tics, associated with medication use, autistic spectrum disorders, pervasive developmental delay, or other causes have not been determined.

Chorea

The genetics of HD have been reviewed in the chorea chapter (Chapter 6), see the "Tips and Tricks: Gene testing in HD." Other genetics causes of chorea have been summarized in Table 6.1, but will be mentioned in some detail here. Most of the autosomal dominant gene mutations causing chorea are due to a trinucleotide repeat expansion in the gene, similar to that seen in HD. There are two autosomal dominant genes that cause HD-like (HDL) phenotypes. HDL1 is caused by an insertion in *PRNP* and is associated with seizures and onset between 20–40 years of age. HDL2 is due to an expansion in junctophilin-3 (*JPH*), with patients having dystonia, parkinsonism, and hyperreflexia in addition to chorea. Several of the autosomal dominant SCAs have chorea as a feature and are detailed in Table 6.2: SCA1, SCA2, SCA3, SCA17. DRPLA is also an autosomal dominant cause of ataxia, with varying phenotypes in adult compared to pediatric presentations and is secondary to a mutation in *DRPLA* that codes for atrophin-1. Neuroferritinopathy, which results from an adenine insertion in the ferritin light chain (FTL) gene, has a variety of phenotypes in addition to chorea. Non-progressive chorea is seen in benign hereditary chorea, which is caused by a mutation in the thyroid transcription factor 1 (*TITF-1*) gene. Paroxysmal kinesigenic dyskinesia, which result in other phenotypes such as paroxysmal dystonia, is caused by a deletion or missense mutation in the glucose transporter 1 (*SLC2a1*) gene.

One of the common autosomal recessive causes of chorea is chorea-acanthocytosis, secondary to a mutation in *VPS13*, which codes for chorein. These patients have orofacial dyskinesia, self-mutilation, and dystonia (typically affecting the oromandibular region, often with prominent tongue-protrusion dystonia). Panthothenate kinase-associated neurodegeneration patients, from a mutation in the *PANK2* gene, typically present in childhood and often have acanthocytosis, in addition to characteristic imaging abnormalities. Aceruloplasminemia is due to a mutation in ceruloplasmin (*CP*), resulting in the absence of ceruloplasmin and high ferritin in adult patients with retinal degeneration, chorea, ataxia, and dystonia. Wilson disease, also associated with low ceruloplasmin, may present with many movement disorders or psychiatric disease, and is caused by a mutation in copper-transporting *ATPase 1* (ATP7B). Several autosomal recessive disorders that have prominent ataxia, in addition to chorea, include ataxia telangiectasia (AT), ataxia with oculomotor apraxia (AOA) 1 and 2, and Friedreich ataxia (FA) and are located in Table 6.1 and Table 6.3. Metabolic disorders that have associated chorea include the following: nonketotic hyperglycinemia and pyruvate dehydrogenase deficiency (also X-linked), which are caused by several different gene mutations; recessive hereditary methemoglobinemia type 2 from an abnormality in the NADPH-cytochrome b5 reductase (*DIA1*); and beta-ketothiolase deficiency from an abnormality in mitochondrial acetoacetyl-coA thiolase (*ACT1/T2*).

McLeod syndrome is X-linked and also causes acanthocytosis and is secondary to a mutation in *XK*. These patients may be older than the patients with chorea-acanthocytosis from mutations in *VPS13*. Lesch–Nyhan, also X-linked recessive, results from mutations in hypoxanthine phosphoribosyltransferase (*HPRT*), presents in infancy with hyperuricemia and associated chorea, dystonia, spasticity, and self-mutilation. Two mitochondrial diseases include Leigh syndrome and infantile bilateral striatal necrosis (from genes *NUP62* and *MT-ATP6*) and have the classic elevation in lactate/pyruvate ratio.

Dystonia

The terminology for genetic dystonia was established with the symbol "*DYT*" followed by a number after the discovery of the first gene in 1994. Eleven genes have now been confirmed as monogenic forms of dystonia (see Chapter 7 on dystonia) with an additional eleven loci that are unconfirmed.

Ataxia

Ataxia can be seen with almost every pattern of inheritance: autosomal dominant, autosomal recessive, X-linked, and mitochondrial. The genetics of ataxia are detailed in both the text and in Tables 8.3 and 8.4 of the ataxia chapter.

Hemifacial spasm

The majority of hemifacial spasm cases are sporadic, but families with multiple affected members are reported in the literature. The inheritance pattern appears to be autosomal dominant with low penetrance, but no genes have been identified to date.

Restless legs syndrome, periodic limb movements of sleep, and REM sleep behavior disorder

Patients with RLS frequently report a family history and there is a high concordance rate (83%) between identical twins with the disorder. However, no individual genes have been identified that are causal in primary familial RLS. Genome-wide association studies have identified several susceptibility loci that increase risk by 50%. This includes single nucleotide polymorphisms RLS3—protein-tyrosine phosphatase receptor-type delta (*PTPRD*); RLS6—BTB/POZ domain-containing protein 9 (*BTBD9*); mitogen-activated kinase 5 (*MAP2K5/SOCR1*), RLS7 (*MEIS1*); and four other sites. Linkage studies have identified the seven genetic loci, RLS 1–8, based on an inheritance pattern of autosomal dominant with variable expressivity or autosomal recessive.

A genetic variant was found to be associated with periodic limb movements of sleep in an Icelandic population. This common variant is located in an intron of *BTBD9* and was replicated in a second Icelandic sample and has an attributable risk of RLS with PLMS of 50%, but was not associated with RLS alone in the Icelanders. The variant was also associated with decreased serum ferritin levels. Although individuals with idiopathic REM behavior disorder have a higher likelihood of having a family history of RBD (OR = 6.1, 95%CI 2.1–18.1), no genes have been identified to increase risk.

Stereotypy

Stereotypies, which can be seen in normally developing individuals, are highly associated with many genetic disorders that cause intellectual disability. Some of these, like the Rett syndrome, are described in the stereotypy chapter (Chapter 12). Fragile X syndrome, caused by a CGG expansion in the fragile X mental retardation 1 (*FMR1*) gene and resultant silencing of the gene, is associated with stereotypies, especially in boys with lower intelligent quotients. Self-injurious behavior can be seen in neurodevelopmental disorders such as neuroacanthocytosis (described above) or inborn errors of metabolism. Lesch–Nyhan is caused by a mutation in the hypoxanthine guanine phosphoribosyltransference 1 (*HPRT1*) gene and manifests in self-destructive biting of fingers and lips. Cornelia de Lange syndrome is a multisystem malformation with facial dysmorphism, limb anomalies, and self-injurious behaviors. The majority of cases are secondary to mutations in the nipped-B-like (*NIPBL*) gene. The complex genetics of autism are not yet well defined, but as research progresses in this area, genes that are associated with stereotypy in autism are likely to be discovered.

Paroxysmal disorders

The genetics of the paroxysmal dyskinesias and episodic ataxias are described in the paroxysmal movement disorders chapter (Chapter 13).

Conclusions

Although the role of genetics in movement disorders is variable, it is likely that over time, most movement disorders will have an identified genetic cause or contributor. Understanding the basics concepts of inheritance and being up to date with clinical testing for these gene mutations is critically important for families who are interested in family planning, research, or gene-specific therapies in the future. Geneticists and genetic counselors have a key role to play for families experiencing rare disorders with unidentified genes, variants of unknown significance, or diseases with complicated molecular genetics. If the clinical provider does not have access to these specialized services, some of the aforementioned online resources can be used to effectively inform patients of their risks, testing options, and ultimately, genetic diagnosis.

Further Readings

Dauvilliers Y, Winkelmann J. Restless legs syndrome: update on pathogenesis. *Curr Opin Pulmonary Med* 2013; **19**(6): 594–600.

Hallett M. Myoclonus: phenomenology, etiology, physiology, and treatment. In Principles and Practice of Movement Disorders, 519–540. Fahn S and Jankovic J, eds. Oxford: Elsevier, 2007.

Kuhlenbaumer G, Hopfner F, Deuschl G. Genetics of essential tremor: meta-analysis and review. *Neurology* 2014; **82**(11): 1000–1007.

Merner ND, Girard SL, Catoire H, et al. Exome sequencing identifies FUS mutations as a cause of essential tremor. *Am J Human Genetics* 2012; **91**(2): 313–319.

Paschou P. The genetic basis of Gilles de la Tourette syndrome. *Neurosci Biobehav Rev* 2013; **37**(6): 1026–1039.

Walker RH. Chorea. *Continuum* 2013; **19**(5 Movement Disorders): 1242–1263.

20

Neuroimaging Finding in Movement Disorders

Kathleen L. Poston, MD, MS

Department of Neurology and Neurological Sciences, Stanford University, Stanford, California, USA

Introduction

Non-parkinsonian movement disorders are common conditions. For instance, essential tremor (ET) is present in up to 14% of people over the age of 60, and dystonia is diagnosed in almost 2% of people over the age of 50. Magnetic resonance imaging (MRI), computed tomography (CT), positron emission tomography (PET), and single-photon emission computed tomography (SPECT) have a considerable role in aiding the clinician in the diagnosis of a patient with movement disorders. In this chapter, we review the use of these readily available imaging modalities in the workup of a non-parkinsonian movement disorder patient. Transcranial ultrasound (TCU) is a growing technology currently being applied to the diagnosis of movement disorders patients, but the clinical diagnostic value in individual patients has not yet been established. Thus TCU is primarily a research tool at this time and will not be covered in this chapter.

Imaging findings in movement disorders by phenomenology

Non-parkinsonian movement disorders are collectively classified as hyperkinetic movement disorders. However, these movements can vary widely in frequency, speed, amplitude, and quality. In this review, we approach the use of imaging to aid in the diagnosis of non-parkinsonian movement disorders by individual phenomenological classification.

> ⭑ **TIPS AND TRICKS**
>
> In a hyperkinetic patient, the clinician must be certain to take time determining the phenomenology of the movement before deciding what imaging technique to use as part of the workup. The clinician must remember that patients can exhibit more than one type of movement disorder. For instance, a patient with fragile X tremor/ataxia syndrome could present primarily with ataxia or could have a predominant action tremor. These patients can also be parkinsonian. The key is to determine the prominent movement type and then determine if that movement is isolated or presents in addition to other movements or neurological findings. Once the syndrome is defined clinically, then the proper imaging technique can be determined.

Tremor

Tremor, which is defined as a rhythmic, oscillatory, involuntary movement, is a common movement disorder that can be associated with other neurological

Dr. Poston has received support from the NIH/NINDS (K23NS075097, R01NS065070, P50NS071675), the Michael J Fox Foundation for Parkinson's Disease Research, Neurologic Inc., and Ceregene Inc.

or medical conditions or can exist in isolation. Tremor must be clinically distinguished from dystonia (or "dystonic tremor") and myoclonus, both of which are non-rhythmic. Clinically, tremor is unlikely to be confused with ataxia or chorea, but like most movement disorders, tremor can coexist with either disorder. Standard magnetic resonance imaging (MRI) or computed tomography (CT) is helpful to clinicians in order to rule out secondary causes of tremor, such as tremor associated with multiple sclerosis or Wilson disease. However, standard structural imaging is unhelpful in the diagnosis of a primary tremor syndrome. In this section we focus on the use of neuroimaging to aid in the diagnosis of primary tremor syndromes.

The two most common primary tremor syndromes are ET and Parkinson disease (PD). The hallmark feature of ET is bilateral, high-frequency, postural, and kinetic tremor of the arms, head, and voice. By contrast, a parkinsonian tremor is best defined as an asymmetric, 4–6 Hz tremor that occurs when the limbs are fully rested. However, the clinical overlap can be significant, and some studies suggest that over 30% of patients diagnosed with ET have other tremor syndromes such as PD or dystonic tremor, which can lead to critical errors in medication selection, patient counseling, and disease prognosis.

diagnosis. Van Laere and colleagues examined the cost effectiveness of DAT SPECT and found that when the diagnosis was changed after DAT SPECT, patients gained an average of 1.2 potentially beneficial years of adequate treatment.

In addition, a number of patients with ET can develop concomitant PD, adding to the diagnostic challenge. Other diagnostic considerations in a patient presenting primarily with tremor include dystonic tremor, drug-induced tremor, orthostatic tremor, and psychogenic tremor.

Unfortunately, the standard structural 1.5 Tesla or 3.0 Tesla MRI is essentially normal in patients with ET, PD, and other common forms of tremor. However, MRI abnormalities are seen in a small number of rare, but important tremor disorders. Therefore MRI should be considered in the diagnostic workup of tremor to rule out these less prevalent etiologies. The most important disorder to rule out in a younger patient with tremor is Wilson disease, which is classically associated with basal ganglia T2 hyperintensities on MRI. While not diagnostic, these MRI findings strongly suggest Wilson disease, which can then be confirmed with a 24-hour urine excretion and serum ceruloplasmin.

EVIDENCE AT A GLANCE

ET is one of the most common neurological disorders, yet recent evidence suggests that up to one-third of patients diagnosed by physicians as having ET have a different disorder. In a study by Jain and colleagues, 37% of patients first diagnosed with ET had an actual diagnosis of PD (15%), dystonia (8%), PD and ET (7%), or another disorder (6%). Factors associated with a misdiagnosis included unilateral arm tremor, dystonic posturing of the hands, isolated thumb tremor, isolated leg tremor, and non-rhythmic tremor. Therefore careful clinical examination is the most effective method for improving the diagnostic accuracy of ET. However, in certain clinical situations where the expert examiner is unable to distinguish the tremor of ET from PD, the addition of a DAT SPECT can aid in the

⚘ SCIENCE REVISITED

Fragile X-associated tremor/ataxia syndrome (FXTAS) is a neurodegenerative disorder that can affect carriers of a premutation in the fragile X mental retardation 1 (FMR1) gene. This gene normally contains fewer than 40 CGG triplet repeats. The full mutation (repeat number >200) is responsible for fragile X syndrome. Repeat lengths between 55 and 200 constitute a premutation, which has been found to manifest as progressive ataxia, tremor, and cognitive decline in carriers over the age of 55.

In older patients with tremor, fragile X-associated tremor/ataxia syndrome (FXTAS) should be considered. This disorder is predominately found in men over the age of 50, but has been reported in a several dozen women as well. Symptoms usually begin in

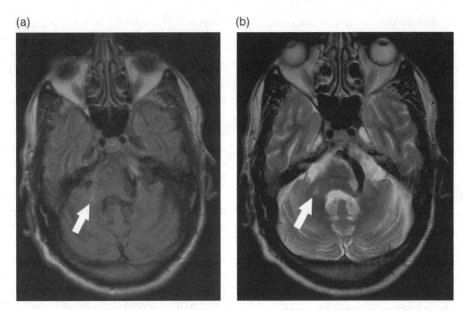

Figure 20.1 A patient with fragile X tremor/ataxia syndrome. (a) Axial fluid attenuated inversion recovery (FLAIR) and (b) axial T2-weighted MRI illustrating middle cerebellar peduncle hyperintensity (arrows).

the seventh decade and consist of action tremor, cerebellar ataxia, and parkinsonism, along with cognitive decline, neuropathy, and autonomic dysfunction. Many patients are found to have increased T2 signal in the middle cerebellar peduncles on MRI imaging (the MCP sign) but can also have cerebellar atrophy, cerebral cortical atrophy, and T2 signal hyperintensities in the deep white matter of the cerebellum (Figure 20.1). These MRI findings are suggestive of FXTAS, but they are not fully specific or diagnostic, and should be confirmed with commercially available genetic testing.

Finally, stroke is an uncommon cause of tremor, but it can be easily evaluated with an MRI scan. Hemorrhagic or ischemic lesions of the thalamus, midbrain tegmentum, superior cerebellar peduncle, and pons have all been associated with Holmes tremor, which is a combined rest, postural, and intention tremor associated with lesions of the dopaminergic nigrostriatal and cerebello-thalamic pathways. MRI is preferable to CT imaging for tremor because the midbrain, pons, and cerebellum are more difficult to visualize on CT.

While MRI and CT imaging are typically normal in patients with common causes of tremor, recent developments in nuclear medicine imaging can now aid in clarifying the underlying diagnosis in

some patients with primary tremor. This technique makes use of the unique underlying pathophysiology of PD to differentiate parkinsonian tremor from other tremors. Specifically, the core clinical symptoms of PD (i.e., bradykinesia, rest tremor, and rigidity) occur when at least 40–50% of dopaminergic cells are lost. Post-mortem examination in PD patients shows that the loss of dopaminergic cell bodies in the substantia nigra is associated with a depletion of dopamine transporter (DAT) density on the cell axon terminals in striatum. PD is the only etiology of primary tremor due to degeneration of these nigrostriatal dopaminergic neurons. Other neurodegenerative parkinsonian syndromes associated with nigrostriatal dopamine cell loss (e.g., multiple system atrophy (MSA) and progressive supranuclear palsy) are much less associated with tremor, and when tremor is present, it is not the primary symptom and does not typically exist in isolation. By contrast; ET, dystonic tremor, drug-induced tremor, and psychogenic tremor are not caused by nigrostriatal degeneration. Therefore direct imaging of the nigrostriatal dopaminergic pathway can help distinguish PD from these other primary tremor syndromes. PET and SPECT DAT tracers do just this—directly image the density of dopaminergic synaptic terminals in the caudate and putamen. Thus, for PD, we expect to see a reduction in DAT uptake, which is often asymmetric and more prominent in the posterior putamen (Figure 20.2). For ET, DAT uptake is indistinguishable from control subjects. While fewer studies have directly compared patients with PD to those with dystonic tremor, drug-induced tremor, and psychogenic tremor, DAT imaging is also thought to distinguish PD from these tremor syndromes.

> ✋ **CAUTION**
>
> When ordering DAT SPECT, it is important to know that certain medications can interfere with the imaging finding, and should therefore be discontinued before the scan. These medications include most antidepressants, antipsychotics, stimulants (e.g., methylphenidate or dextroamphetamine/amphetamine), antianxiety medications (e.g., buspirone), smoking cessation medications, and appetite suppressants. The amount of time each medication needs to be stopped before the scan varies for each individual drug; therefore you should check with the radiologist or radiology technician before ordering the test. In addition, one hour before the isotope is injected, patients should be given an iodine blocker, which typically needs to be ordered and obtained before the scan day.

Myoclonus

Myoclonus is defined as sudden, brief, shock-like movements caused by muscle contractions or inhibitions. There are several different classification systems for myoclonus. The physiological classification, which is based on the source and neurophysiology of the myoclonus, is most useful when considering a neuroimaging approach to diagnosis. For example, drug-induced, post-hypoxic, hepatic and uremic encephalopathies, and other secondary causes of myoclonus are frequent causes of cortical myoclonus. Neurodegenerative causes, such as Alzheimer disease, should also be considered. In most of these secondary and neurodegenerative causes, the brain MRI is often normal or shows nonspecific abnormalities, but the MRI should be included as part of the clinical evaluation if conditions such as Creutzfeldt–Jakob or Huntington disease are considered (Table 20.1).

Subcortical non-segmental myoclonus is thought to arise from a subcortical locus, resulting in widespread distribution of movements. While brain imaging is typically normal for most subcortical non-segmental etiologies such as essential myoclonus, a patient presenting with opsoclonus-myoclonus syndrome should undergo a CT of the chest and abdomen to evaluate for neuroblastoma in a child or paraneoplastic syndrome in an adult.

In addition to cortical and subcortical etiologies, the spine and peripheral nerves can be implicated in a patient with myoclonus. In such patients, specific imaging modalities should be part of the standard workup to investigate potentially treatable causes. For instance, propriospinal myoclonus is characterized by involuntary movements arising in the muscles activated via the propriospinal pathway. The thoracic spine is commonly implicated, and while spinal MRI can be normal in such cases, thoracic disc herniation has been a reported reversible etiology. Segmental myoclonus arises from segmental generators in the brainstem or spinal cord; thus the muscles affected correspond to segments that are closest to the level of the segmental generator. The common segmental myoclonus is palatal myoclonus arising from the olivo-dentate region of the brainstem. Other regions reported include spinal segmental myoclonus, abdominal myoclonus, and respiratory myoclonus. MRI imaging is recommended at the brainstem or spinal level (which is associated with the clinic findings) to investigate possible structural etiologies.

Finally, hemifacial spasm consists of unilateral, involuntary, irregular clonic or tonic movement of muscles innervated by the facial nerve (cranial nerve VII), and it is the common form of peripheral myoclonus. Over 60% of the cases are idiopathic, presumably due to vascular loop compression at the facial nerve root exit zone. However, other secondary etiologies, such as demyelination, mass lesions (e.g., meningioma or schwannoma), and bony lesions, and vascular insults, such as brainstem lacunar infarct, should be considered. The presence of persistent, sustained, tonic facial spasms can specifically indicate underlying brainstem pathology, such as tumors in the cerebellopontine angle or pontine gliomas, and should be evaluated by MRI. While an enlarged ectatic artery and vascular compression of

(a)

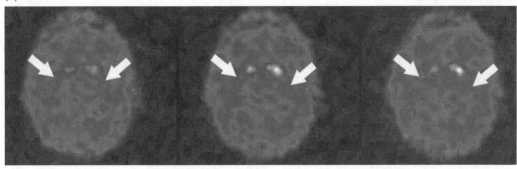

(b)

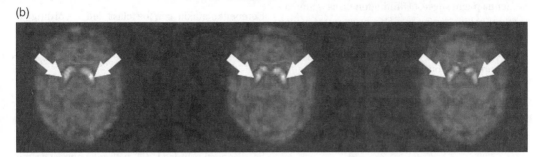

Figure 20.2 Two patients with tremor. (a) A patient with Parkinson disease where DAT SPECT shows asymmetric, posterior more than the anterior reduced uptake in the putamen (arrows). (b) A patient with essential tremor who has normal DAT uptake in the caudate and putamen (arrows) bilaterally. (*See insert for color representation of the figure.*)

Table 20.1 Clinical syndromes in a patient with myoclonus where the MRI can be helpful in determining the diagnosis

	MRI typically normal or nonspecific	MRI disease specific

Cortical myoclonus	Dementia with Lewy body disease
	Alzheimer disease
	Frontotemporal dementia linked to
	  chromosome 17 (FTDP 17)
	Corticobasal degeneration
	Parkinsonism-dementia
	  complex of Guam
	Drug-induced and toxic conditions
		Creutzfeldt–Jakob disease
		Huntington disease
		Dentatorubral pallidoluysian
		  atrophy (DRPLA)
		Storage diseases
		Posthypoxic myoclonus

Subcortical-non-
  segmental myoclonus
	Essential myoclonus (includes
	  myoclonus-dystonia)
		Opsoclonus-myoclonus
		  syndrome
		Propriospinal myoclonus

Segmental myoclonus		Palatal myoclonus Spinal segmental myoclonus
Peripheral myoclonus		Hemifacial spasm

the facial nerve root can be found on MRI with magnetic resonance angiography (MRA), it is important to note that this may not be specific for hemifacial spasm and can be found in otherwise normal individuals. The treatment of hemifacial spasm with surgical decompression remains controversial, the pros and cons of which are beyond the scope of this discussion.

Chorea and Ballism

Choreic movements are irregular, purposeless, involuntary movements that "flow" into one another in a random fashion. Ballistic movements are more proximal and larger amplitude than choreic and are often seen as "flinging" of a limb. By contrast to a patient with myoclonus, where the distribution of symptoms dictates the imaging workup, the differential diagnosis of chorea and ballism is largely based on the other neurological signs and symptoms found on the patient history and exam. For instance, chorea with psychiatric symptoms and dementia might suggest Huntington disease, dentatorubral pallidoluysian atrophy, or spinocerebellar ataxia 17, particularly in a patient with a family history of similar symptoms. By contrast, parkinsonism and chorea in a younger patient is concerning for Wilson disease. When evaluating a patient with acute onset chorea, a brain MRI is important to rule out vascular, structural, and inflammatory causes. Hemichorea or hemiballism, in particular, is suggestive of a vascular or structural lesion and should be emergently evaluated on MRI. Stroke and non-ketotic hyperglycemia are the two most common causes of hemiballism Non-ketotic hyperglycemia can be the initial presentation of diabetes mellitus, and in these cases, MRI T1-weighted images show hyperintensity in the putamen, caudate nucleus, and globus pallidus. These lesions are thought to result from ischemic injury due to hyperviscosity and regional metabolic failure. In general, resolution of MRI signal change correlates with clinical improvement in chorea.

Dystonia

Dystonic involuntary movements involve sustained muscle contractions that produce twisting and are often accompanied by abnormal posture. Adult onset focal or segmental dystonia and childhood onset generalized dystonia are not typically associated with abnormal imaging findings. However, structural lesions, such as posterior fossa tumors and cervical cord tumors, can present with acute neck dystonia in children. In addition, acute neck dystonia can follow a number of infections, including pharyngitis, tonsillitis, mastoiditis, or other infections involving the head or neck. In these cases, dystonia results from atlantoaxial rotatory subluxation secondary to infection involving the soft tissue surrounding the cervical spine, which typically causes a painful, fixed torticollis. This is a medical emergency and prompt recognition and treatment decreases the rate of subsequent neurologic complications, which can occur in 15% of cases. Therefore evaluation of a child with acute neck dystonia should include treatment of infection and cervical immobilization, followed by imaging of the head and neck with MRI or CT to look for an underlying space-occupying lesion or orthopedic abnormality.

Ataxia

Cerebellar ataxia can be classified according to several paradigms; for the purpose of illustrating the imaging characteristics of this class of disorders, we first discuss rapid onset or acute ataxias. Then, among the progressive onset group, we discuss general imaging findings, and last, more specific and potentially diagnostic imaging findings.

Acute onset ataxia is most suggestive of a stroke, which is a cause of ataxia in which CT scan can be diagnostic. Indeed, CT without contrast is the imaging modality of choice to diagnose cerebellar hemorrhage due to hypertension or secondary to bleeding within a neoplasm or a vascular malformation. However, a negative CT scan in the acute condition should always be followed by an MRI, as cerebellar ischemia is frequently undetectable on CT scan due to X-ray beam artifacts in the posterior fossa. Even small cerebellar hemorrhages or ischemic lesions are medical emergencies due to potential swelling in an enclosed space; therefore rapid diagnosis and assessment with brain imaging is critical for urgent decision-making and treatment.

In subacute or chronic ataxia, the workup should still begin with a brain MRI because a structural lesion such as a tumor or abscess needs to be excluded in all cases. In addition, there are several specific MRI abnormalities that can be identified to aid in the diagnosis of ataxia. Cerebellar atrophy is the common, nonspecific finding on MRI. This usually indicates a degenerative disease, but can also be seen in genetic ataxias and paraneoplastic cerebellar degeneration (see Schöls et al.). Three main atrophy patterns characteristic of degenerative ataxias can be visualized on MRI, and are best demonstrated by T1-weighted images in which the high signal intensity of CNS structures stands out on the background of the very low signal cerebrospinal

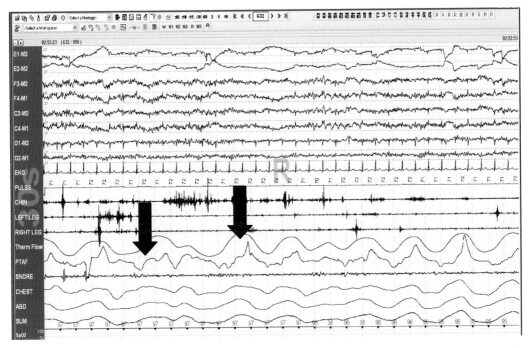

Figure 11.1 Excessive electromyographic activity in the chin and limbs during REM sleep in a patient with RBD (red arrows illustrate two episodes of movement).

Non-Parkinsonian Movement Disorders, First Edition. Edited by Deborah A. Hall and Brandon R. Barton.
© 2017 John Wiley & Sons, Ltd. Published 2017 by John Wiley & Sons, Ltd.
Companion website: www.wiley.com/go/hall/non-parkinsonian_movement_disorders

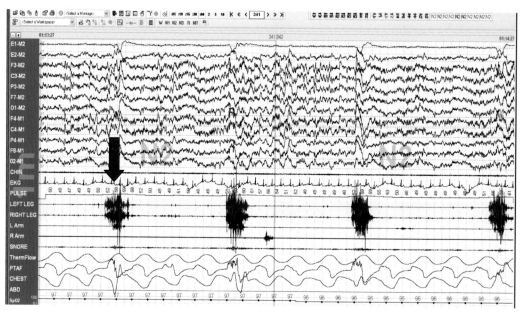

Figure 11.2 Sequence of four periodic limb movements of sleep from a polysomnography recording (red arrow illustrates the first limb movement).

(a)

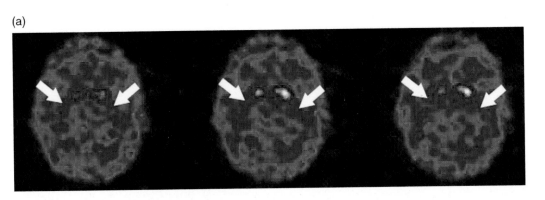

(b)

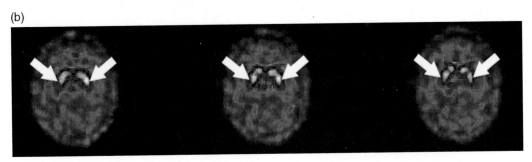

Figure 20.2 Two patients with tremor. (a) A patient with Parkinson disease where DAT SPECT shows asymmetric, posterior more than the anterior reduced uptake in the putamen (arrows). (b) A patient with essential tremor who has normal DAT uptake in the caudate and putamen (arrows) bilaterally.

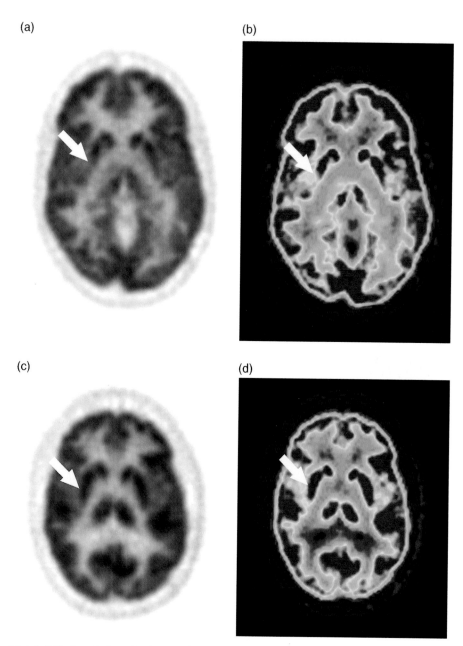

Figure 20.4 (a) Black and white display and (b) rainbow display on an FDG PET scan in a patient with pathologically confirmed MSA-C. Hypometablism in the putamen (arrow) is a suggestive feature of MSA in a patient with ataxia. (c) Black and white windowing and (d) rainbow windowing on an FDG PET scan with normal putamen (arrow) metabolism.

Table 20.2 Clinical ataxia syndromes and pathology associated with different patterns of brain atrophy of MRI

Atrophy pattern on MRI	Associated pathology	Associated etiology
Olivopontocerebellar atrophy (OPCA)	Damage of the pontine gray nuclei	SCA1, SCA2, SCA3, SCA7, SCA13, DRPLA, EOCA, MSA-C
Corticocerebellar atrophy (CCA)	Damage to the Purkinje cells	SCA4, SCA5, SCA6, SCA8, SCA10, SCA11, SCA12, SCA14, SCA15, SCA16, SCA17, SCA18, SCA19, SCA21, SCA22, SCA25, EOCA, AT, Gluten ataxia, ILOCA
Spinal atrophy (SA)	Damage of neurons of the sensory ganglion of the spinal nerves and of Clarke's column in the spinal gray matter	FRDA

Modified from Schöls et al. (2004).

AT = ataxia–telangiectasia; DRPLA = dentatorubral pallidoluysian atrophy ; EOCA = early onset cerebellar ataxia with retained tendon reflexes; FRDA = Friedreich ataxia; ILOCA = idiopathic late-onset cerebellar ataxia (pure); MSA-C = multisystem atrophy – cerebellar type; SCA = spinocerebellar ataxia.

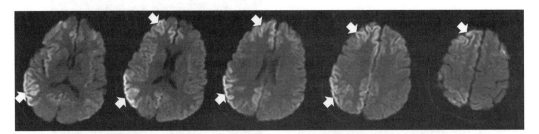

Figure 20.3 A patient with Creutzfeldt–Jakob disease. Axial diffusion weighted imaging showing "cortical ribboning" with decreased diffusion in the cerebral cortex (arrows).

fluid (CSF). Olivopontocerebellar atrophy characteristically includes atrophy of the lower and middle cerebellar peduncles, the cerebellar hemispheres, and vermis, often with widening of the fourth ventricle. Corticocerebellar atrophy usually includes atrophy of the cerebellum with widening of the cerebellar sulci and fourth ventricle with normal brainstem and spinal cord volume. Spinal atrophy typically includes atrophy of the spinal cord with widening of the fourth ventricle, but without significant atrophy of the cerebellum or cerebral hemispheres. The clinical syndromes most often associated with these three patterns are discussed in Table 20.2.

There are also several "classic" abnormal findings on MRI that are associated with specific ataxic syndromes, and these should be meticulously considered when reviewing a patient's imaging. This section reviews the "do not miss" and the common MRI findings associated with specific syndromes.

Sporadic Creutzfeldt–Jakob disease (CJD) is a rapidly progressive disorder that often includes the clinical syndrome of dementia and ataxia. While other neurological signs such as myoclonus and parkinsonism eventually develop, the ataxia can be the presenting feature and therefore proper workup can lead to earlier diagnosis. On diffusion weighted imaging (DWI), decreased diffusion in the cerebral cortex (called cortical ribboning), along with associated decreased diffusion in the basal ganglia, is a highly sensitive (91%) and specific (95%) diagnostic marker of CJD (Figure 20.3). Variant CJD more often presents with psychiatric symptoms before ataxia and other neurological findings, and is associated with a high signal in the pulvinar and dorsomedial thalamus (together giving the "hockey stick" sign) on T2.

(a)

(b)

(c)

(d)

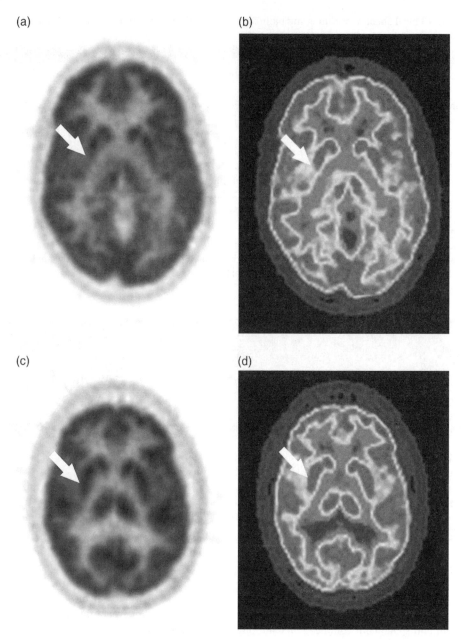

Figure 20.4 (a) Black and white display and (b) rainbow display on an FDG PET scan in a patient with pathologically confirmed MSA-C. Hypometablism in the putamen (arrow) is a suggestive feature of MSA in a patient with ataxia. (c) Black and white windowing and (d) rainbow windowing on an FDG PET scan with normal putamen (arrow) metabolism. (*See insert for color representation of the figure.*)

As previously discussed, the MRI in patients with FXTAS is associated with the MCP sign (Figure 20.1). Patients often present with gait ataxia and complain of frequent unexplained falls, noted on exam as difficulty with tandem gait. While, in general, the MCP sign appears to be relatively specific for FXTAS in an ataxic patient, it has also been reported to be present in patients with MSA, genetic recessive ataxia, and acquired hepatocerebral degeneration.

Patients with MSA can present with either a primary ataxic or parkinsonian motor syndrome. Both clinical presentations, however, have been associated with a cruciform hyperintensity in the pons observed on the T2-weighted MRI, referred to as the "hot cross bun" sign. A less specific finding is known as the "putaminal rim" sign, which is a high signal line extending laterally from a slightly darkened putamen. While these MRI findings are highly suggestive of MSA, and in one series found to be highly specific for MSA, when present, they are often a late finding in the disease course and therefore not a sensitive diagnostic tool. In addition, one study found the "hot cross bun" sign in 8.7% of patients with genetic spinocerebellar ataxia (SCA; see Jain, Lo, and Louis), so even when present, a genetic ataxic syndrome should be considered. Functional nuclear medicine imaging has also been found to be helpful when considering a diagnosis of MSA in an ataxic patient without parkinsonian features, and specific imaging findings were recently added as additional features of possible MSA in the second consensus statement on diagnosis. For instance, demonstration of striatal or brainstem hypometabolism by [18 F]fluorodeoxyglucose PET can suggest a diagnosis of MSA (Figure 20.4).

> **⚠ CAUTION**
>
> When ordering an FDG PET scan, it is important to remember that certain medications need to be stopped prior to the scan. In general, all short-acting dopaminergic medications should be stopped at least 12 hours before the scan, and all long-acting dopaminergic medications should be stopped at least 72 hours before the scan. In addition, benzodiazepines should not be taken the day of the scan and should be stopped at least 8 hours before the scan.

In addition, evidence of nigrostriatal dopaminergic denervation on DAT SPECT or PET in a non-parkinsonian, ataxic patient may point to the diagnosis of MSA. Taken together, these MRI and PET/SPECT features can aid the clinician in order to make an earlier, more accurate diagnosis. But it is important to remember than none have been found to be pathognomonic of MSA, and further longitudinal studies, ideally with pathology confirmation, are needed to determine the true sensitivity and specificity for each modality.

In summary, non-parkinsonian movement disorders are common, and multiple imaging modalities exist to evaluate patients both emergently and non-urgently. When coupled with the correct phenomenological diagnosis, neuroimaging is a powerful tool for diagnosis and investigation of many kinds of clinical situations.

Further Readings

Berry-Kravis E, Abrams L, Coffey SM, et al. Fragile X-associated tremor/ataxia syndrome: clinical features, genetics, and testing guidelines. *Mov Disord* 2007; **22**: 2018–2030.

Caviness JN, Truong DD. Myoclonus. In: William JW, Eduardo T, eds. *Handbook of Clinical Neurology*, 399–420. Amsterdam: Elsevier, 2011.

Gilman S, Wenning GK, Low PA, et al. Second consensus statement on the diagnosis of multiple system atrophy. *Neurology* 2008; **71**: 670–676.

Jain S, Lo SE, Louis ED. Common misdiagnosis of a common neurological disorder: how are we misdiagnosing essential tremor? *Arch Neurol* 2006; **63**: 1100–1104.

Lee YC, Liu CS, Wu HM, Wang PS, Chang MH, Soong BW. The "hot cross bun" sign in the patients with spinocerebellar ataxia. *Eur J Neurol* 2009; **16**: 513–516.

Leehey MA, Hagerman PJ. Fragile X-associated tremor/ataxia syndrome. In: Sankara HS, Alexandra D, eds. *Handbook of Clinical Neurology*, 373–386. Amsterdam: Elsevier, 2012.

Massey LA, Micallef C, Paviour DC, et al. Conventional magnetic resonance imaging in confirmed progressive supranuclear palsy and multiple system atrophy. *Mov Disord* 2012; **27**: 1754–1762.

Schöls L, Bauer P, Schmidt T, Schulte T, Riess O. Autosomal dominant cerebellar ataxias: clinical features, genetics, and pathogenesis. *Lancet Neurol* 2004; **3**: 291–304.

Van Laere K, Everaert L, Annemans L, Gonce M, Vandenberghe W, Vander Borght T. The cost effectiveness of 123I-FP-CIT SPECT imaging in patients with an uncertain clinical diagnosis of parkinsonism. *Eur J Nucl Med Mol Imaging* 2008; **35**: 1367–1376.

Yaltho TC, Jankovic J. The many faces of hemifacial spasm: differential differential diagnosis of unilateral facial spasms. *Mov Disord* 2011; **26**: 1582–1592.

Young GS, Geschwind MD, Fischbein NJ, et al. Diffusion-weighted and fluid-attenuated inversion recovery imaging in Creutzfeldt-Jakob disease: high sensitivity and specificity for diagnosis. *Am J Neuroradiol* 2005; **26**: 1551–1562.

Zeidler M, Sellar RJ, Collie DA, et al. The pulvinar sign on magnetic resonance imaging in variant Creutzfeldt-Jakob disease. *Lancet* 2000; **355**: 1412–1418.

21

Clinical Rating Scales in Movement Disorders

Padmaja Vittal, MD, MS[1,2] and Brandon R. Barton, MD, MS[1,3]

[1]Department of Neurological Sciences, Section of Movement Disorders, Rush University Medical Center, Chicago, Illinois, USA
[2]Northwestern Medicine Regional Medical Group, Winfield, Illinois, USA
[3]Department of Neurological Sciences, Rush University Medical Center; Jesse Brown VA Medical Center, Chicago, Illinois, USA

Introduction

Clinical scales for movement disorders can be routinely used in clinical practice. They afford the clinician the ability to assure patients of disease stability (or, conversely, deliver news of advancing disease), measure efficacy of between-visit interventions, and properly document key portions of the patient examination in relation to their movement disorder. While the scales may add to the burden of time for evaluation, when a clinician is familiar with the scales, they can be done fairly rapidly. Clinicians should thus familiarize themselves with rating scales for the disorders they see most often and consider adding the best scales for routine use in their practices. In many cases, the scales can be adapted for easy use and recording in an electronic medical record, along with the neurological examination and other measures of general health. In this chapter, rating scales for dyskinesia, tremor, dystonia, Huntington disease, Gilles de la Tourette syndrome, and functional movement disorders are discussed.

Rating scales in movement disorders focus on two primary concepts of dysfunction: impairment and disability. Whereas impairment relates to objective deficits, disability refers to the impact of disease on patient function. As such, items usually rated by the investigator and based on the neurological examination assess impairment, whereas interviews that involve the patients, caregivers, and investigator's assessments of activities of daily living or quality of life rate disability. Some scales are uniquely impairment ratings, others are uniquely disability assessments, and many combine the two in separate sections, allowing a total score to estimate a global level of disease severity. Global scales that combine the two also exist.

Objective measurement of movement disorders poses a number of implicit challenges, which must be accounted for by rating scales. First, even within a single diagnosis, there are a variety of movements and multiple variables that need to be measured, such as frequency of movements, number of different types of movements, intensity, complexity, body distribution, suppressibility, and interference. Second, symptoms may vary spontaneously under certain environmental conditions, such as stress or excitement. Third, patients with some movement disorders are able to suppress some of their symptoms voluntarily for minutes to hours. Studies even suggest that disease severity improves in the clinic. Fourth, there are often both motor and non-motor features that can contribute to poor quality of life, so scales must capture the broad range of possible symptoms. Finally, rater and subject biases are important limiting factors in rating scales. Personal expectations, mood disorders, and educational level can strongly impact the ratings, and the clinician raters may be influenced by their own expectations of change or stability.

Non-Parkinsonian Movement Disorders, First Edition. Edited by Deborah A. Hall and Brandon R. Barton.
© 2017 John Wiley & Sons, Ltd. Published 2017 by John Wiley & Sons, Ltd.
Companion website: www.wiley.com/go/hall/non-parkinsonian_movement_disorders

Dyskinetic/abnormal involuntary movements

The modified version of the *Abnormal Involuntary Movement Scale (AIMS)* is an objective scale that rates dyskinesia across body parts by severity. The AIMS is not disease specific: it was originally developed for the evaluation of tardive dyskinesia but has been widely used in Parkinson disease (PD) as well. This scale rates seven body areas at rest with a 0–4 severity rating. It also has three global assessments: overall severity, incapacitation for the patient, and patient awareness of dyskinesia. It is a simple and quick scale to complete, but it does not distinguish between choreic and dystonic dyskinesia. It does not include activation maneuvers that often increase dyskinesia nor provide information on severity that is likely more relevant to activities of daily living. It offers a quick, general way to rank the severity of global hyperkinetic movements with a numerical score.

Dystonia

Dystonia may be categorized by body distribution into focal (involving a single body area), segmental (involvement of two or more contiguous body areas), and generalized (involving at least one leg, the trunk, and some other body area). Dystonia rating scales, likewise, have been developed specifically to assess these categories of dystonia, with separate scales for generalized dystonia and for each body region affected.

The variable presentations of dystonia have made the development of reliable rating scales problematic and have necessitated the development of standardized examination protocols that include dystonia-activating maneuvers, such as writing, chewing, and speaking. The state-dependent (i.e., action vs. rest, presence vs. absence of compensatory maneuvers) character of dystonia has resulted in the addition of items that are intended to capture the effects of sensory inputs or to measure the duration of time that dystonia is present during the examination. Most rating scales additionally provide a uniform examination protocol to ensure consistent and complete assessments of patients.

- *Fahn–Marsden Dystonia Rating Scale (F-M)*: This is a standard instrument used to assess the severity of generalized dystonia. The F-M has two parts: a movement scale based on the motor features of dystonia and a disability scale based on a patient's subjective impairment in activities of daily living. The movement scale has two separate factors and assesses nine body regions: eyes, mouth, speech/swallowing, neck, bilateral arms, bilateral legs, and trunk. The factors include a severity factor.

- *Unified Dystonia Rating Scale (UDRS)*: This scale was developed in 1997 at a consensus conference of dystonia experts and was intended to address the potential limitations of the F-M scale by subdividing body regions and separately assessing a duration factor measuring the time dystonia was present during the examination. This scale rates 14 body regions for dystonia severity and duration, with each scored from 0 to 4.

The instruments used to assess the severity of cervical dystonia are numerous and include objective and subjective rating scales and quantitative measures. Several clinical rating scales have been developed, including the *Columbia torticollis scale*, the *Tsui scale*, and the *Toronto Western Spasmodic Torticollis Scale (TWSTRS)*. The TWSTRS is currently the most widely used. The TWSTRS consists of three subscales: motor severity, activities of daily living, and pain. The motor severity scale is a 10-item rater assessment that evaluates the severity of head posture in several axes of movement (turning, tilting, anterocollis, retrocollis, shoulder elevation), the effect of sensory tricks, range of motion, and the duration of dystonia during the examination. It can be done relatively quickly during a clinical visit to measure the outcome of interventions.

Another common form of focal dystonia is blepharospasm. A task force commissioned by the Movement Disorder Society recommends the *Blepharospasm Disability Index* as a scale for rating blepharospasm although others exist, including the *Craniocervical Dystonia Questionnaire* which rates both blepharospasm and cervical dystonia.

Chorea

The Unified Huntington Disease Rating Scale (UHDRS) was developed by the Huntington Study Group to describe clinical performance and functional capacity in patients with Huntington disease. It assesses 4 main domains of impairment in Huntington disease: motor performance, cognitive performance, behavioral abnormalities, and functional capacity. The scale assesses relevant clinical features of Huntington disease to allow comparison of clinical signs, disease progression, and effects of therapy. Given the progressive nature of this rare and severe disease, periodic measurements of disease features is prudent. The UHDRS is a useful clinical tool to follow disease progression and may be useful in assessing clinical changes in the setting of experimental interventions.

The motor section of the UHDRS assesses motor features of Huntington disease with standardized ratings of oculomotor function, dysarthria, chorea, dystonia, gait, and postural stability. The cognitive section of the UHDRS uses the verbal-fluency Symbol Digit Modalities Test and the Stroop Interference Test. The behavioral section measures the frequency and severity of symptoms related to affect, thought content, and copying styles. The Huntington Disease Functional Capacity Scale part of the UHDRS is reported as the total functional capacity score, and its items include ability to maintain occupation, ability to manage one's finances, ability to perform domestic chores, degree of independence with activities of daily living, and level of care required.

Tremor

Measuring tremor clinically is difficult because tremors behave in different and often complex ways. Tremor is influenced by a variety of factors, including natural fluctuations; the patient's physical, emotional, and mental state; and various environmental triggers. Therefore it is difficult to develop a tool that would allow measurements of a movement disorder that is rarely stable.

- *Clinical Rating Scale for Tremor*: Designed specifically for essential tremor, this scale assigned different point values of tremor to different body parts. A score for functional impairment was added to the sum of these products.
- *Fahn–Tolosa–Marin Tremor Rating Scale*: This scale assesses rest, postural, and action tremor. This scale also evaluates voice tremor,

handwriting and other tasks, as well as functional disability and tremor impact.

- Bain et al. *Severity of Tremor Scale*: This scale was devised to assess the severity of tremor in different body parts for different tremor components. For each body part, tremor is assessed during rest, action, and movement and during writing and spiral drawing.
- *Washington Heights–Inwood Genetic Study of Essential Tremor (WHIGET) Rating Scale*: A 26-item, 10-minute tremor examination designed to elicit tremor during two different postures, five different tasks, and two different positions at rest. Tasks included pouring water between two cups, drinking water from a cup, using a spoon to drink water, finger-to-nose movement, and drawing spirals. Each task is first performed with the dominant arm and then with the non-dominant arm.
- *Quality of Life in Essential Tremor Scale*: A 30-item questionnaire that assesses effect of tremor on physical, communication, psychosocial, leisure and hobbies, and work or finance.

Gilles de la Tourette syndrome

Although many clinical manifestations of Gilles de la Tourette syndrome (GTS) are visible or audible, there is considerable difficulty in objectively quantifying them. One factor contributing to this difficulty is the significant variety of tics that can affect an individual at any given time. To assess severity, one must consider multiple variables, such as frequency, number of tic types, intensity, complexity, body distribution, suppressibility, and interference. Second, symptoms vary spontaneously. Third, patients are able to suppress voluntarily their symptoms for minutes to hours. Situational stimuli also can change tic expression. For example, tics can increase when the examiner leaves the room. Hence information from multiple informants may be required to assess the multitude of clinical manifestations of tic disorders. As a result of the multidimensionality of GTS, it has been difficult to develop a single scale that can quantify the disease in a simple, accurate, and comprehensive way. The approaches to creating a GTS scale include the use of historical information, direct observation, or both. The clinician can choose one of the following scales based on time limitations and the necessary level of detailed involvement in managing TS patients:

- *Shapiro Tourette Syndrome Severity Scale (STSSS)*: A composite clinician rating of severity comprising five factors: the degree to which tics are noticeable to others, whether they elicit comments of curiosity, whether other individuals consider the patient odd or bizarre, whether tics interfere with functioning, and whether the patient is incapacitated, homebound, or hospitalized.
- *Tourette Syndrome Global Scale (TSGS)*: A multidimensional scale of GTS symptoms and social functioning comprising eight individually rated dimensions.
- *Yale Global Tic Severity Scale (YGTSS)*: Developed in response to criticism of TSGS and is designed for use by an experienced clinician following a semi-structured interview with multiple informants. YGTSS includes separate rating of severity for motor and phonic tics along five dimensions: number, frequency, intensity, complexity, and interference. It also includes a checklist for specific types of motor and vocal tics. An independent rating of impairment is added to the total tic score to obtain a final score.
- *Hopkins Motor and Vocal Tic Scale (HMVTS)*: A series of visual analogue scales (10 cm) on which both parent and physician separately rank each tic (motor and vocal), taking into consideration the frequency, intensity, interference, and impairment.

Myoclonus

The *Unified Myoclonus Rating Scale (UMRS)* is a quantitative 73-item scale developed by the Myoclonus Study Group and is a revised version of the scale introduced initially by Truong and Fahn. The UMRS contains a patient questionnaire, handwriting and spiral drawing samples, rating instructions, a score sheet, and a videotape protocol (approximately eight minutes). The scale consists of eight sections: patient questionnaire (11 items); myoclonus at rest (frequency and amplitude, 16 items); stimulus sensitivity of myoclonus (17 items); severity of myoclonus with action (frequency and amplitude, 20 items); performance on functional tests (5 items); physician rating of patient's global disability (one item); presence of negative myoclonus (one item); severity of negative myoclonus (one item).

Ataxia

Uncoordinated or "ataxic" movement can involve abnormalities of speech, eye movements, limb movement, and gait. The existing scales measure various combinations of these items.

- *International Cooperative Ataxia Rating Scale (ICARS)*: This scale was published in 1997. It has four subscales, including posture and gait, kinetic functions, speech disorders, and oculomotor disorders.
- *Scale for the Assessment and Rating of Ataxia (SARA)*: This scale was developed to assess only ataxia-related symptoms, including gait, stance, speech, sitting, nose-finger test, finger chase, heel-shin test, and rapid alternating movements. Mean time to perform the test is about 14 minutes.
- *Friedreich Ataxia Rating Scale* This scale combines ataxia and functional measures to evaluate progress and severity of this disease.

Further Readings

Albanese A, Sorbo FD, Comella C, et al. Dystonia rating scales: critique and recommendations. *Mov Disord*. 2013; **28**(7): 874–883.

Bain PG, Findley LJ, Atchison P, et al. Assessing tremor severity. *J Neurol Neurosurg Psychiatry* 1993; **56**: 868–873.

Burke RE, Fahn S, Marsden CD, et al. Validity and reliability of a rating scale for the primary torsion dystonias. *Neurology* 1985; **35**: 73–77.

Consky ES, Lang AE. Clinical assessments of patients with cervical dystonia. In: Jankovic J, Hallett M, eds. *Therapy with Botulinum Toxin*, 211–237. New York: Marcel Dekker, 1994.

Fahn S, Tolosa E, Marin C. Clinical rating scale for tremor. In: Jankovic J, Tolosa E, eds. *Parkinson's Disease and Movement Disorders*, 2nd ed., 271–280. Baltimore: Williams and Wilkins, 1993.

Frucht SJ, Leurgans SE, Hallett M, et al. The Unified Myoclonus Rating Scale. *Adv Neurol* 2002; **89**: 361–376.

Goetz CG, Nutt JG, Stebbins GT. The Unified Dyskinesias Rating Scale: presentation and clinimetric profile. *Mov Disord* 2008; **23**: 2398–2403.

Harcherik DF, Leckman JF, Detlor J, et al. A new instrument for clinical studies of Tourette's syndrome. *J Am Acad Child Psychiatry* 1984; **23**: 153–160.

Huntington Study Group. Unified Huntington's Disease Rating Scale: reliability and consistency. *Mov Disord* 1996; **11**: 136–142.

Leckman JF, Riddle MA, Hardin MT, et al. The Yale Global Tic Severity Scale: initial testing of a clinician-rated scale of tic severity. *J Am Acad Child Adolesc Psychiatry* 1989; **28**: 566–573.

Louis ED, Wendt KJ, Albert SM, et al. Validity of a performance-based test of function in essential tremor. *Arch Neurol* 1999; **56**: 841–846.

Schmitz-Hübsch T, du Montcel ST, Balikol, Berciano J, Boesch S, Depondt C, et al. Scale for the assessment and rating of ataxia: development of a new clinical scale. *Neurology* 2006; **66**: 1717–1720.

Trouillas P, Takayanagi T, Hallett M, et al. International Cooperative Ataxia Rating Scale for pharmacological assessment of the cerebellar syndrome. *J Neurol Sci* 1997; **145**: 205–211.

22

Videotaping Suggestions for Movement Disorders

Gian Pal, MD, MS and Deborah A. Hall, MD, PhD

Department of Neurological Sciences, Section of Movement Disorders, Rush University Medical Center, Chicago, Illinois, USA

Introduction

Videotaping of movement disorders patients is frequently done for several reasons. The videotape documents the patient's examination beyond what the written clinic report can demonstrate. It allows for independent consultation for unusual cases by other experts. Serial videos can demonstrate progression of both common and unusual diseases. Clips from videos can be used for teaching and publication of movement disorders cases. However, videotaping is a technical skill that is best performed with properly instructed staff, appropriate environment, equipment, and props, and with disease-specific protocols that capture the key aspects of the patient's movement disorder.

Environment

A designated room for videotaping is necessary to produce standardized videos reliably. The room should be near a quiet part of the office where there is not a large amount of traffic that could produce background noise and interfere with the quality of the video. The room should be well lit from many angles, and avoid casting shadows on the face or limbs. The color of the walls should provide a good contrast for taping; a light blue color is standardly recommended for this purpose. The dimensions of the room are important because patients must have ample room to ambulate and the room must be wheelchair accessible. The dimensions of the room should be at least 6 by 21 feet. A chair should be positioned at the rear of the room with the videographer filming directly across from the patient. Following these guidelines will prevent some of the common mistakes observed on poor quality videotapes (Table 22.1).

Equipment

Depending on the particular type of movement disorder being evaluated, different pieces of equipment may be necessary. The following are some recommendations.

Technical equipment

Microphone: Although many cameras capture sound, we have found a separate microphone is more reliable given the distance of the patient from the videographer and decreased volume of speech of many patients. Detachable Bluetooth microphones are particularly easy to handle, compatible with modern cameras, and produce good sound quality. The microphone should be hands-free (i.e., clipped to the shirt of the patient) so that it does not obscure any particular body region.

Camera: A high-quality camera that produces high-definition (HD) quality videos should be acquired. Given rapid advances in technology, excellent models of adequate quality are found in an affordable price range, and expensive professional-style recorders are not needed. A 16:9 widescreen ratio is recommended for

Non-Parkinsonian Movement Disorders, First Edition. Edited by Deborah A. Hall and Brandon R. Barton.
© 2017 John Wiley & Sons, Ltd. Published 2017 by John Wiley & Sons, Ltd.
Companion website: www.wiley.com/go/hall/non-parkinsonian_movement_disorders

Table 22.1 Common mistakes when videotaping patients

Video too brief to ascertain overall pattern of movements over time
Inadequate lighting with shadows cast over sections of the patient
Only one angle used to view the patient
Not observing the limbs in multiple positions for an adequate amount of time
Focusing on one small element of the exam
Omitting gait or attempts at gait
Shaky camera technique (lacking tripod or image stabilization, too much zoom)
Neglecting to collect important identifier data (e.g., date/medical record number) for future reference

playback on modern television sets. The camera should be affixed to a tripod for a stable video frame and should be centered on the patient. It is important to select a camera that is user-friendly and produces video files that can be edited easily.

Video processing software: In general, playback in multiple formats are supported by video player programs (e.g., Windows Media Player, QuickTime), although one should carefully test that the files play back correctly on the desired computers and presentation software. Videos can be saved or converted into many formats. Often during taping, the video must be paused, and some cameras will produce a new clip each time this occurs. Thus the taping of a single patient may result in 10–15 individual clips that then need to be combined and edited. Editing can be accomplished using editing programs that are purchased separately, provided with the computer´s operating system (e.g., Windows Movie Maker), or provided by the video camera manufacturer. Many types of video editing software are available at a broad range of costs, and the individual choice should depend on the types of files, type of computer, and commonly used files. Before purchasing a particular camera and video processing software, check with a technical expert to make sure both are compatible with your computer system and will allow for proper processing of the output files.

Storage device: A high-capacity storage device for the video files that has a network connectivity is important. Different storage models exist with varying capacities and costs. The system should have automatic backup in place and be able to hold up to 16 terrabytes. On- or off-site backup is critical to avoid losing files. Some hospital systems may provide IT support to store and backup videos. The ideal format in which the digital output is stored is a complex issue that depends on the user and the capabilities of available software and storage. Current common video file output formats include MEPG2 (.mpg), MPEG4 (.mp4), Windows media Video (.wmv), Quicktime (.mov), and Flash video (.flv).

Video room equipment

Chair: A comfortable chair for the patient to sit in that provides good support and an upright posture is needed. Armrests will allow the patient to push up from the chair if needed as well as to dangle their hands from the end of the armrests.

Coffee mug: The mug is used for patients with tremor when trying to capture a kinetic tremor, particularly since tremor can specifically affect drinking ability.

Two paper cups: For patients with tremor, one cup is filled with water and the other cup is left empty. The patient is instructed to pour water from one cup into the other.

Paper and pens: The patient's handwriting may need to be assessed as part of a dystonia or tremor protocol, so these should be available if needed. Since patients are asked to write with one hand, scotch tape should be available to affix the paper to a smooth surface for stability.

Rainbow passage: This passage should be printed in a large font and laminated for reuse. The passage is readily available online and is commonly used to assess speech (e.g., see Fairbanks, 1960).

Archimedes spiral: The Archimedes spiral should be printed in a large font and laminated for reuse. It is used to assess patients with tremor (Figure 22.1).

Blocks: Patients with myoclonus may not demonstrate symptoms unless a particular action occurs. Small blocks should be available for the children to play with in order to elicit action myoclonus.

Reflex hammer: Stimulus sensitive myoclonus should be assessed with a reflex hammer. Some people also use the light touch of a pin for this

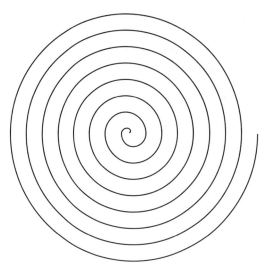

Figure 22.1 Archimedes spiral.

DOE, JOHN
DATE OF BIRTH – DATE OF VIDEO
[SEX] [RACE] ATT* [PROTOCOL]
MRN – TAPE: [TAPE #]

Figure 22.2 Cue card template. *Att = attending physician initials, MRN = medical record number.

purpose, but this should be done cautiously as not to puncture the patients skin should the sensation cause a limb to jerk.

Penlight or flashlight: If slight movements are difficult to visualize, a penlight or flashlight may help illuminate them. This is particularly important with intra-oral movements such as tongue dystonia and palatal tremor.

Cue card: The patient's name, date of birth, medical record number, date of video, and tape number should be recorded on a cue card. At the start of the video, the cue card should be shown to label the video clip visually. This cue card is typically deleted during editing prior to use for educational purposes (Figure 22.2).

Instructions for the Videographer

The videographer has a critical role. This individual helps pick the appropriate videotaping protocol, maximize accuracy and completeness of video exams, and interact with clinical staff to provide further clinical information about the patient. At our institution, anywhere from 2 to 12 videotaping sessions occur during the day, and one designated non-medical staff member performs all of the videos in a given day, with each video session lasting 15–20 minutes. However, in many institutions there may not be adequate staffing to accomplish this degree of detailed video documentation; in this case, the videographer (typically a physician or medical trainee) may only be able to highlight the main features of the examination. If taping is occurring for publication purposes, the videographer should try to capture an entire protocol in order to have all of the salient features, in the event additional video is requested from a reviewer at a later point.

In cases where a patient has poor mobility and has limited physical independence, a second person should be available if the videographer needs assistance. In many instances, the patient can be examined and videotaped without the presence of family members. However, in certain instances, a family member may have insight into how a particular movement is elicited. Some patients may need the support of the family member during taping, particularly in patients with dementia who may benefit from the presence of a familiar face. However, no more than one family member should be present during the taping, as it may impact the quality of the final video.

Videotaping goals relevant to the patient's movement disorder should be anticipated in advance, although some elements will be common to all patients (Table 22.2). The videographer should have access to the patient's chart to obtain the reason for referral in order to select the appropriate protocol. If it is not clear from the referral source or the chart as to the patient's possible diagnosis, the patient should be asked what their movement concerns are before the videotaping is started. Also the patient should be asked the setting in which the movement is most prominent. For instance, in a patient with dystonia that is present only when typing, a keyboard would be an important piece of equipment during the video process. Patients with musician's dystonia will generally only display their abnormalities when being filmed while playing their musical instruments. The goal of the video should be explained to the patient. Typically, the

Table 22.2 Key elements for any video protocol

Position	Phenomenology to observe
Seated at rest	Parkinsonian rest tremor, hyperkinetic disorders (chorea, ataxia, dystonia)
Standing	Parkinsonian posture, ataxic stance, dystonic posturing
Rapid movements of the limbs (finger tapping, hand opening, foot stomping)	Action dystonia, tremors, bradykinesia, ataxia, myoclonus
Speech	Dysarthria, hypophonia, tremor, dysphonia
Eye movements	Supranuclear ophthalmoplegia, square wave jerks, saccadic pursuit, ataxic saccades
Limbs sustained against gravity	Tremor, myoclonus
Gait: forward, backward, tandem	Parkinsonism, dystonia, ataxia, gait disorders
Coordination: Finger-to-nose, heel-to-shin	Ataxia, tremor

videographer will explain that the videotape is a part of the "visual medical record," and some of the tasks being performed will be repeated by the physician during an assessment following the video, if they are seeing the patient after the video. It should be explained that the videos are for educational purposes, as well as for review of the diagnosis. Consent for the taping should be obtained at this time, and ideally patients are informed ahead of their visit that this may be discussed, as this makes it more likely for them to give consent to be videotaped. Prior to taping, the videographer should ensure that the patient does not have anything in their mouth that would interfere with the videotaping. For example, gum chewing could be mistaken for tardive dyskinesia.

The protocol for each movement disorder should be followed as closely as possible. Prior to recording, the videographer must assess the proper visual frame in the camera for the particular movement being taped and should avoid excessive zooming in or out during the actual taping. While specific sections of the protocol are being taped, the videographer must also be aware of movements that may be occurring elsewhere. He or she must be flexible and adjust the frame of view to capture the most salient features of the patient's condition. Ultimately, time and experience are needed to make a smooth transition between videography and the clinical appointment and to maintain the flow of the workday.

Some patients will need to be video-recorded under suboptimal conditions, such as in the emergency room, intensive care unit, or while having an acute event in an examination room. In such cases, the videographer should attempt to videotape the parts of the body involved as best possible while positioning the patient safely. Sometimes the disorder can be so intermittent that it cannot be captured in the office and the patient will need to be instructed to take a video of the episodes at home. In this situation, mobile phone or smartphone cameras (now fairly ubiquitous in public use) can be used to film the episodes at home. The episodes can then be reviewed at future visits or, more ideally, mailed securely to the physician for review and storage.

Further Readings

Barboi AC, Goetz CG, Musetoiu R. The origins of scientific cinematography and early medical applications. *Neurology* 2004; **62**: 2082–2086.

Comella CL, Stebbins GT, Goetz CG, Chmura TA, Bressman SB, Lang AE. Teaching tape for the motor section of the toronto western spasmodic torticollis scale. *Mov Disord* 1997; **12**: 570–575.

de Leon D, Moskowitz CB, Stewart C. Proposed guidelines for videotaping individuals with movement disorders. *J Neurosci Nurs* 1991; **23**: 191–193.

Duker AP. Video recording in movement disorders: practical issues. *Continuum* (Minneapolis, MN) 2013; **19**: 1401–1405.

Fairbanks, G. *Voice and Articulation Drillbook*, 2nd ed., 124–139. New York: Harper Row, 1960.

Goetz CG, Nutt JG, Stebbins GT, Chmura TA. Teaching program for the unified dyskinesia rating scale. *Mov Disord* 2009; **24**: 1296–1298.

Goetz CG, Pappert EJ, Louis ED, Raman R, Leurgans S. Advantages of a modified scoring method for the rush video-based tic rating scale. *Mov Disord* 1999; **14**: 502–506.

Goetz CG, Stebbins GT, Chmura TA, Fahn S, Poewe W, Tanner CM. Teaching program for the movement disorder society-sponsored revision of the unified Parkinson's disease rating scale: (mds-updrs). *Mov Disord* 2010; **25**: 1190–1194.

Hornyak M, Rovit RL, Simon AS, Couldwell WT: Irving S. Cooper and the early surgical management of movement disorders: video history. *Neurosurg Focus* 2001; **11**: E6.

Jog MS, Grantier L. Methods for digital video recording, storage, and communication of movement disorders. *Mov Disord* 2001; **16**: 1196–1200.

Kompoliti K, Goetz CG, Gajdusek DC, Cubo E. Movement disorders in kuru. *Mov Disord* 1999; **14**: 800–804.

Rao AS, Dawant BM, Bodenheimer RE, Li R, Fang J, Phibbs F, Hedera P, Davis T. Validating an objective video-based dyskinesia severity score in Parkinson's disease patients. *Parkinsonism Relat Disord* 2013; **19**: 232–237.

Taylor K, Counsell CE, Gordon JC, Harris CE. Maximizing patient consent for video recording. *Mov Disord* 2004; **19**(9): 1116–1117.

Taylor K, Mayell A, Vandenberg S, Blanchard N, Parshuram CS. Prevalence and indications for video recording in the health care setting in North American and British paediatric hospitals. *Paediatr Child Health* 2011; **16**: e57–60.

Index

Indexer: Dr Laurence Errington
Note: Vs indicates the differential diagnosis of two or more conditions.

Non-Parkinsonian Movement Disorders, First Edition. Edited by Deborah A. Hall and Brandon R. Barton.
© 2017 John Wiley & Sons, Ltd. Published 2017 by John Wiley & Sons, Ltd.
Companion website: www.wiley.com/go/hall/non-parkinsonian_movement_disorders